RIGHT HEMISPHERE DAMAGE

Disorders of Communication and Cognition

RIGHT HEMISPHERE DAMAGE

Disorders of Communication and Cognition

PENELOPE S. MYERS, Ph.D.

Division of Speech Pathology
Department of Neurology
Mayo Clinic
Rochester, Minnesota

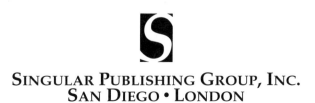

SINGULAR PUBLISHING GROUP, INC.
SAN DIEGO • LONDON

Singular Publishing Group, Inc.
401 West A Street, Suite 325
San Diego, California 92101-7904

Singular Publishing Ltd.
19 Compton Terrace
London N1 2UN, UK

Singular Publishing Group, Inc., publishes textbooks, clinical manuals, clinical reference books, journals, videos, and multimedia materials on speech-language pathology, audiology, otorhinolaryngology, special education, early childhood, aging, occupational therapy, physical therapy, rehabilitation, counseling, mental health, and voice. For your convenience, our entire catalog can be accessed on our website at *http: //www.singpub.com.* Our mission to provide you with materials to meet the daily challenges of the ever-changing health care/educational environment will remain on course if we are in touch with you. In that spirit, we welcome your feedback on our products. Please telephone (**1-800-521-8545**), fax (**1-800-774-8398**), or e-mail (*singpub@mail.cerfnet.com*) your comments and requests to us.

© 1999, by Singular Publishing Group, Inc.

Typeset in 10/12 Palatino by Thompson Type
Printed in the United States of America by Bang Printing

Library of Congress Cataloging-in-Publication Data
Myers, Penelope S.
  Right hemisphere damage : disorders of communication and cognition
  / by Penelope S. Myers.
      p.   cm.
    Includes bibliographical references and index.
    ISBN 1-56593-224-2 (pbk.)
    1. Communication disorders.   2. Cognition disorders.   3. Brain
  damage.   4. Cerebral hemispheres.   I. Title.
    [DNLM: 1. Brain Damage, Chronic—complications.   2. Laterality.
  3. Communication Disorders—complications.   4. Cognition Disorders—
  complications.   WL 354 M996r 1998]
  RC423.M83   1998
  616.85'5—dc21
  DNLM/DLC
  for Library of Congress   98-22184
                                                                        CIP

Contents

Preface

As we approach the end of the 20th century, the mysteries of what was once thought to be the minor hemisphere are beginning to be unraveled. It has become clear that the two cerebral hemispheres play cooperative roles in cognition and communication, and that the right hemisphere (RH) is dominant for certain attentional, perceptual, cognitive, and communicative functions. It also has become clear that damage to the RH can have devastating consequences for the quality of life of patients.

Increased understanding of the functions of the RH and the effects of right hemisphere damage (RHD) has been motivated by academic interest in how the intact brain works and by clinical interest in what happens when it does not. Although complementary, these two sources of inspiration often fail to intersect. Researchers who investigate brain-behavior relationships often study patients with focal RH damage to understand more about normal brain function. By its very nature, their experimental work isolates individual deficits for in-depth scrutiny. As a result, the complex web of intersecting deficits that define the clinical reality of the patients under study may not be appreciated. At the same time, clinicians and others involved in the care and rehabilitation of RHD patients may not

appreciate the value of this body of research for their clinical practice—not because they are too busy or lack scholarly interests, but because it comes from widely scattered sources that are often outside of their clinical and professional focus. For example, the study of left-neglect, one of the most common consequences of RHD, has inspired research by scientists interested in the computations necessary for spatial and visual cognition, in attentional mechanisms in the intact brain, and in its impact on motivation and insight, as well as by speech-language pathologists interested in its relationship to communication disorders, and by other rehabilitation professionals interested in its impact on recovering independence in daily activities. Similarly, the study of communicative deficits subsequent to RHD has come from speech-language pathologists, neurologists, neuropsychologists, psychiatrists, and linguists who are variously interested in the reduced discourse skills, impaired prosodic performance, changes in affective behavior, and altered cognitive status that can accompany RHD. The impact of RHD casts a wide net. My main motivation for writing this book has been to synthesize information available from clinical experience and from experimental and clinical research into a more complete picture of the impact of RHD on cognitive and communicative abilities.

RHD can alter cognitive and communicative experience in both subtle and dramatic ways that pose difficult challenges for clinicians concerned with the management of individuals with RHD. Particularly challenging are the communication disorders that can accompany RHD. They have been described, but have yet to be explained in a way that provides the basis for theory-driven versus symptom-driven assessment and treatment strategies. The signs and symptoms of RHD often are treated as a collection of independent disorders that bear little relationship to one another when, in fact, many of them may share common themes. In lieu of absolutes about their underlying cause, an understanding of some of the common threads running through the patchwork quilt of these disorders is a first step in the process of providing effective treatment. Where possible, this book highlights those connections in the hope that it will inspire new treatment models and approaches and promote research that is sensitive to the clinical realities of the disorders.

This book is intended primarily for clinicians, researchers, and graduate students in the discipline of speech-language pathology and for other professionals involved in the rehabilitation of patients with RHD. Physicians involved in the care of patients with RHD should find the discussion of deficits and their management helpful in their medical practice. Finally, scientists in a variety of disciplines investigating brain-behavior relationships in the intact brain may gain a deeper understanding of the constellation of symptoms that can affect this patient population.

The population of patients for whom this book is relevant includes those with focal damage from stroke or tumor. It also is relevant for patients who have diffuse or multifocal damage in which the area of damage includes the RH. Examples of such disorders include traumatic brain injury, dementing illnesses, asymmetric cortical

degeneration syndromes, and patients with a history of multiple strokes.

This book contains 10 chapters. Chapter 1 serves as an introduction and reviews some of the history of research and interest in the RH. It also paints a broad overview of patients with RHD deficits and lists some of the caveats to keep in mind when reviewing the current state of our knowledge about RHD.

Chapter 2 addresses neglect. It emphasizes its attentional mechanisms and suggests that it has far reaching consequences not only for visual and spatial perception, but also for cognitive and communicative performance. The various frames of reference, modalities, and input and output channels in which neglect can occur are explored as are some of the behavioral anomalies such as anosagnosia that may accompany it.

Chapter 3 addresses deficits in attention. It expands the discussion of attentional deficits by exploring deficits in various attentional operations that can occur subsequent to RHD. Together, Chapters 2 and 3 provide the attentional background considered crucial to understanding the various cognitive and communicative impairments that can affect patients with RHD.

Chapter 4 discusses deficits in prosodic production and comprehension that may occur with RHD. Emotional and linguistic prosodic disorders are reviewed with an emphasis on the perceptual basis of some of these impairments.

Chapter 5 addresses the linguistic disorders that can occur with RHD. Specific linguistic deficits and theories about specialized RH contributions to semantic processing are reviewed.

Chapter 6 continues the discussion of communication impairments by reviewing deficits in discourse and the pragmatic aspects of communication. These disorders are explored in light of their cognitive, semantic processing, and attentional bases.

Alterations in affective behaviors are reviewed in Chapter 7. Connections between impairments in emotional communication and the pragmatic and cognitive disorders discussed in Chapter 6 are highlighted. The impact of attentional disturbances and neglect on alterations in emotional and cognitive status are explored. This chapter also reviews theories about the mechanisms underlying specific delusions that are sometimes a consequence of RHD.

Chapters 8 and 9 are devoted to evaluation and management of patients with RHD. Chapter 8 reviews assessment techniques for attentional and communicative deficits as well as for neglect under the assumption that neglect influences cognitive and communicative performance. Chapter 9 discusses treatment approaches and includes strategies that promote compensation for deficits and as well as some that may promote recovery of function.

Finally, Chapter 10 offers some concluding observations and suggestions for future research on the theory, assessment, and management of the cognitive and communicative impairments associated with RHD.

Because the focus of this book is on disorders of cognitive processing and communication, visuoperceptual disturbances are covered only as they relate to these problems. Many of the visuospatial problems associated with RHD stem from problems in visual integration, neglect, and visual attention. Visual integration deficits are discussed in light of their connections to other deficits in information integration. The impact of neglect and impaired attention on visual perception is extensively reviewed in Chapter 2.

It is hoped that this book will provide clinically relevant ways of conceptualizing the deficits associated with RHD, useful suggestions about their management, and inspiration for developing new treatment interventions that will improve the lives of those afflicted with damage on the right side of the brain. Finally, it is hoped that this book may add to our understanding of brain function and will inspire research that continues to unlock the mysteries of the once silent right hemisphere.

Acknowledgments

No achievement is realized in isolation. This book represents the contributions of many people to my work in this area. My mentors include Terry Wertz, Jay Rosenbek, and Chick LaPointe who took my interest in the possibility of communication disorders in RHD patients seriously back in 1975, who gave me the confidence to pursue that interest, and who became lifelong friends. I also would like to thank all those who contributed to my work at The George Washington University from 1974 to 1987, former students, patients, and staff. I would especially like to thank my friend and colleague, Craig Linebaugh, whose creativity, enthusiasm, and excellent research skills sparked all of my early work and made collaboration all that it should be. My thanks, as well, to Louise Mackisack, dear friend and fellow traveler in RH territory, whose clinical insights and originality are scattered throughout this book. My good friend, Bob Brookshire, deserves special recognition and thanks for his mentorship and collaboration during my years at the University of Minnesota and beyond.

There are a number of people directly connected to the writing of this book who deserve special mention. Hiram Brownell, Joe Duffy, and Craig Linebaugh edited drafts of the entire book. I greatly appreciate the expertise they brought to the task and their insightful comments and sug-

gestions. Thanks also to my sister, Patty Starratt, who contributed editorial advice mixed with humor and support. I am grateful for the good working relationship I have had with Sadanand Singh and the staff at Singular Publishing Group, particularly Marie Linvill, who supported this effort since its inception with good cheer, helpful suggestions, and patience.

There are many whose gift of friendship has sustained my efforts, including especially Eleanor Challen. My friends from the Clinical Aphasiology Conference, too numerous to mention by name, have my gratitude for their humor and wisdom, their genuine interest in the "other" hemisphere, and the excellent contributions many of them have made to our understanding of RHD deficits.

I am deeply grateful to my family—my parents, Anne and Alfred Starratt, my sisters, Polly and Patty, and the entire Duffy Clan—for their inestimable gift of love which translated into a haven of support. My heartfelt thanks to my family here at home who never once let me feel guilty for the time and energy this book has taken. Thanks to my ever-enthusiastic stepson, Matt, for his infusions of levity and consistent interest in my progress. Thanks to my daughter, Melanie, the special light of my days, who has been there since the beginning with her generous heart, her cheerful countenance, and her never-ending encouragement and faith in me. Finally, thanks to my husband, Joe Duffy, whose camaraderie, intellectual support, patience, humor, honesty, and consistent willingness to edit throughout the process have helped see this work to fruition. He is my companion on the high road, my anchor in troubled seas, and the best friend anyone could hope for. I cannot believe my good fortune.

DEDICATION

To

My mother, Anne,

who inspired a desire to help others

My father, Alfred,

who fostered a love of learning

and to

My husband, Joe,

My daughter, Melanie,

and my stepson, Matt

who strengthen and uplift me with their love

Introduction to the Right Hemisphere

HISTORICAL OVERVIEW OF THE ROLE OF THE RIGHT HEMISPHERE

The cognitive and communicative deficits associated with right hemisphere damage (RHD) have been given serious consideration only in the last quarter century. Prior to that time, communication impairments associated with left hemisphere damage (LHD) dominated the research and rehabilitation efforts of professionals involved with the cognitive consequences of brain-damage in adults. In the late 1860s, neurologists Paul Broca and Karl Wernicke had identified aphasia as a distinct language disorder that was associated with left hemisphere lesions. For the next 100 years, neurologists, speech-language pathologists, psychologists, and linguists studied aphasia and, later, apraxia of speech, for clues about how humans process language, the nature of language breakdown, and the best means of remediating these breakdowns. Language *was* communication, and the left hemisphere (LH) was where it all happened. The LH appeared to house that which distinguishes us in a fundamental way from other living creatures; we could communicate using speech, and they could not. So powerful was this notion that the LH became known as the "dominant" hemisphere. Little regard was given to the right hemisphere (RH), which was rather ignominiously dubbed the *silent* or *minor* hemisphere.

That is not to say that the RH went unnoticed. As early as 1865, Hughlings Jackson had suggested the possibility that the RH played a role in perception (Taylor, 1958). In the late 1940s, data from studies of people with brain damage from a variety of causes, including missile wounds sustained during World War II, appeared to confirm Jackson's suggestion (Springer & Deutsch, 1981; Weisenburg & McBride, 1935). It was found that the RH played an important role in visual perception, although the nature of that role was not well understood. For many years, the story of the two hemispheres remained the same. The LH, dominant for language, was cast as the active participant in processing information. The RH, with some special contributions to visuospatial processing, was cast in a more passive role and remained a rather shadowy presence in neurologic models of cognitive function.

Things began to change in the early 1960s, about 100 years after the identification of the LH as dominant for language. A new surgical technique allowed access to the independent functions of the two hemispheres. The operation, called a *commissurotomy,* had been developed in the late 1940s by William Van Wagenen to control the seizure activity of patients with severe epilepsy. It involved separating the hemispheres by severing parts of the corpus callosum, the fiber group that connects the two cerebral hemispheres. In this way, it was hoped that seizures would be limited by preventing their activity from spreading from one hemisphere to the other. The initial results were disappointing. However, in the early 1960s, two other neurosurgeons, Philip Vogel and Joseph Bogen, achieved greater success with commissurotomies in which the corpus callosum was more completely severed. In addition, be-

cause the hemispheres had been more completely disconnected, the surgery provided an opportunity to investigate the independent operations of the two hemispheres. Patients undergoing the procedure became known as *split-brain* patients, and the subsequent research as *split-brain research.* Much of the original split-brain research was conducted by Roger Sperry, Michael Gazzaniga, and Steven Hillyard, with later contributions by Jerre Levy, Robert Nebes, Harold Gordon, and Eran Zaidel. Detailed information about the results of their research is available elsewhere (Gazzaniga, 1970, 1983a, 1983b; Gazzaniga, Bogen, & Sperry, 1962; Nebes, 1972; Sperry, 1974; Zaidel, 1983, 1985). In general, it confirmed the view that the RH played a prominent role in visual perception and added to information about its capacity to decode simple linguistic forms.

In the 1970s, two other techniques, *dichotic listening* and *hemifield tachistoscopy,* allowed researchers to examine the functions of each hemispheres in non-brain-damaged people. Soon, this type of investigation, called *laterality research,* played a prominent role in scientific inquiry into the operations of the brain and the mind-brain connection. In the heyday of laterality research, it was difficult to pick up a scientific journal on the brain without finding at least one article about hemispheric specialization. The search was on to identify more completely the disparate functions of the two hemispheres.

Differences between the two hemispheres began to be analyzed not in terms of function alone, but also in terms of "cognitive style" and "cognitive strategies" for processing information. In these conceptualizations, the RH was considered important not only in visuospatial processing, but in holistic, nonlinear, or parallel processing. It was considered important to information synthesis, apprehending the "gestalt" or whole picture, and dealing with novel input for which there are no rules. The LH was seen not only as dominant for language, but also as important to analytic, linear processing of the type that is bound by rules like those that govern linguistic processing. The idea that the hemispheres processed information differently led to increasing interest in the operations of the intact RH and the effects of damage to that hemisphere. It was noted that RHD could affect body image, visual memory, visual imagery, visual perception, spatial orientation, and awareness of illness.

In the popular press, the RH became the seat of artistic capacity and creativity, less bound by rules, more fluid and flexible, and more adept at managing novel input than the LH. Allusions to the two sides of the brain appeared in all sorts of social contexts. People talked about whether they were more "right-brained" or "left-brained." A popular automobile ad detailed the car's features in printed text on the left page, and pictured it speeding up a twisting mountain road on the right page with the words, "A car for the left side of your brain, and a car for the right side of your brain" written across the two-page layout.

At the same time that scientific inquiry and the popularization of the RH were altering traditional notions of what did and did not constitute dominance, traditional concepts of communication were expanding. Communication came to be thought of as more than speech and language. There was a new emphasis on communicative style, on the importance of body language and other nonverbal aspects of communication. In research of both language development and of aphasia, the importance of language *use*, or pragmatics, was recognized. The focus shifted from semantics and syntax to discourse as a whole, from what was *said* to what was *meant* from what was said. The expanded role of the RH in the intact brain, combined with the more inclusive concept of communication, began to erode the concept of dominant and nondominant hemispheric control over cognitive functions.

Laterality research had much to tell us about how the brain operated, but it began to fall into decline as problems of reliability became apparent. Laterality effects were found to vary with task familiarity and instructions, type of stimulus material, response mode, sensory modality, and a number of other factors (Zaidel, 1985). By the mid-1980s many of the narrow, overly precise, and somewhat oversimplified assumptions about hemispheric specialization and localization of function had given way to newer models of neurobehavior. *Connectionist* or *neural network*, and most recently *interhemispheric inhibition*, models of how the brain processes information emphasize cooperation among areas in the brain, including the two hemispheres. The significance of nonverbal processing in cognition in general, and in communication in particular, and the contribution of the RH to intellectual function had been recognized. The RH would never again be considered a minor participant in cognitive processing.

The particular role of the RH in communication was originally thought to occur at the level of language. Results of split-brain and laterality research had revealed that, although speech is in the purview of the LH, the intact RH was capable of some simple language comprehension, especially at the single word level. This finding, however, did little to explain the impaired communicative abilities subsequent to RHD.

In addition, by the mid-1970s, various researchers and clinicians noted that RHD patients did not perform normally in certain communicative situations. Gardner and his colleagues at the Aphasia Research Center in Boston observed certain abnormal behaviors in the RHD patients they were using as control subjects in their aphasia research. Their observations led to a series of investigations of RHD communication problems (Gardner & Denes, 1973; Gardner, King, Flamm, & Silverman, 1975; Wapner, Hamby, & Gardner, 1981; Winner & Gardner, 1977). At the same time, some clinicians working with stroke patients to remediate dysarthria noted that quite a few RHD patients, although free of aphasia, did not seem to communicate adequately (Collins, 1975; Myers, 1978, 1979). These early studies were among the first to investigate the effects of RHD on communicative abilities in a controlled and systematic way. Impaired prosody was added to the list of potential RHD communication deficits by Ross and Mesulam in a 1979 article entitled, "Dominant functions of the right hemisphere?" The title attests to the shifting landscape in which the RH began to assume a more powerful role in communicative and cognitive operations.

Research on communication deficits associated with RHD has been largely descriptive, and rightly so. Researchers and clinicians interested in RHD communication deficits needed first to identify the signs and symptoms of communicative impairment through systematic observation. Investigations of cause and mechanism had to wait for symptom description.

It was quite clear from the outset that the communication problems faced by RHD patients were not language-based. Despite apparently adequate linguistic processing, RHD patients had problems in the broader context of communication. Early descriptions characterized the RHD patient as a kind of "language machine," someone for whom the subtleties and nuances of communication were lost and whose use of language seemed restricted to a rather literal decoding of information (Gardner et al., 1975; Myers, 1978). Problems noted in the 1970s included impaired prosody, impaired sense of humor, problems with emotional language, and deficits in the use and comprehension of figurative language.

Initial efforts at describing RHD communication deficits focused on a litany of difficulties without entertaining the idea that they were connected. Subsequent investigations have added many more deficits to the list, provided an increasingly complex picture of deficit areas, and suggested connections among them. As a result, a new wave of research has begun to address the underlying mechanisms that result in the complex symptomatology as-

sociated with RHD. Work by Brownell and his colleagues, for example, has suggested possible explanations for the communicative disconnection experienced by many RHD patients. Work by Tompkins and others has begun to specify the ways in which RHD may affect the processing of complex inferences and alternate meanings in discourse. Work by Van Lancker has suggested new hypotheses about the underlying nature of some affective impairments associated with RHD. Using new techniques to study neglect, Heilman and his colleagues and Halligan, Marshall, Posner, Robertson, and a host of others have provided a better understanding of this complex phenomenon. And finally, as the pages of this book reflect, attentional deficits specific to RHD have assumed more of an explanatory role in our understanding of RHD communication disorders.

PORTRAIT OF THE PERSON WITH RHD

Patients with damage limited to the RH can have a variety of deficits, some of which affect communication and cognition directly and some of which exert indirect effects on the ability to participate in communicative events and to interact successfully with the environment. Table 1–1 lists the range of deficits associated with RHD. It is important to remember that these are *possible* but *not absolute* consequences of RHD. Just as not all adults with damage in the LH are aphasic, not all RHD adults have problems in perception, cognition, and/or communication. At this point, however, it might be useful to give a general description of RHD patients who do have communication problems.

The type of RHD patients described by experienced clinicians as having "typical" RHD signs almost always communicate adequately in superficial conversation. There may be a flatness in the voice and affect and a general sense of reduced arousal, but as long as conversation is brief

TABLE 1-1. Deficits associated with right hemisphere damage.

Attentional Deficits
- Arousal
- Orienting
- Vigilance
- Sustained attention
- Selective Attention

Neglect
- Reduced attention to left-sided input
- Reduced use of left limbs
- Reduced awareness of and recognition of left-sided body parts
- Reduced awareness of illness

Visuoperceptual Deficits
- Visual attention
- Visual integration
- Visual memory
- Spatial orientation
- Topographical orientation

Cognitive and Communicative Deficits
- Reduced discourse comprehension and production
- Reduced communicative efficiency and specificity
- Reduced capacity to process complex inferences
- Reduced capacity to process alternate and ambiguous meanings
- Reduced sensitivity to contextual information
- Reduced sensitivity to emotional tone
- Reduced use of prosodic information
- Reduced appreciation of shared knowledge
- Reduced reflection (shallow responses)

Affective and Emotional Deficits
- Reduced use of facial expression to convey emotion
- Reduced sensitivity to facial expressions of others
- Reduced use of prosody to convey emotion
- Reduced comprehension of emotional prosody
- Misidentification syndromes (rare)
- Agitated confusion, delirium, psychosis (rare)

and covers familiar territory, one might not detect any communication deficits. Problems begin to emerge in more extended and complex conversation. Patients may seem disinterested and somewhat insensitive as communicative partners. They may begin and end conversations abruptly, fail to follow social conventions, and even appear rude. They may interrupt and fail to make eye contact. If they are no longer interested in what someone is saying, or can no longer sustain attention, they may turn without apology to something else, apparently unaware of the disruption they have caused to the conversational flow. They may be perfunctory, making the least effortful response to questions, regardless of the consequences of their answers.

Alternately, they may be verbose and rambling. They may have trouble getting to the point. Their discourse may seem to be made up of an assembly of facts without the glue that holds them together in an overriding structure. They may be led by internal associations to related but tangential issues, as if they are thinking out loud, rather than having a conversation.

As listeners they may focus on bits of information in a piecemeal way without integrating them into the larger picture. They may fail to respond to situational variables that specify the nature of the communicative event—lighthearted banter, serious discussion, superficial social exchange. They may have problems recognizing when people are kidding, sarcastic, or ironic.

Patients with RHD may appear distant, remote, and bound up in themselves. They may have trouble adopting other people's point of view, or recognizing what their listeners know and what they do not know. They may show little appreciation for shared knowledge and may not take contextual variables into consideration. Vague references to unfamiliar people, places and events may force the listener to make the connections that have been omitted.

Their capacity to attend may be reduced or fade in and out so that they miss crucial information. They may have trouble interpreting others' intended meanings, and have difficulty conveying their own. They may fail to follow the gist of conversation, written narratives, television news, and so on when information is presented too quickly or when core concepts are subtle and require high levels of inference. When overwhelmed by the speed of complexity of information, they may look down into their laps, feign sleep, or simply tune out while appearing to attend. Rarely, however, will they ask someone to repeat or re-explain information. Failure to admit to confusion and uncertainty can accompany reduced insight into both physical and cognitive problems. Called *denial of deficit* or *denial of illness*, this symptom may give the impression that RHD patients are unconcerned about their current status and about their future adjustments. They may report their plans to return to work, for example, with an almost cavalier disregard for their physical, let alone their cognitive, deficits.

Failure to respond appropriately to their deficits is characteristic of patients who have left-neglect. These patients may not notice their left arm dragging in their wheel chair spokes. They may not attend to people, events, or even sounds to their left. They may be less attentive to visual input at any location, not just the left. Many patients with neglect seem "hypoaroused," bringing less energy and less interest to physical tasks and conversational speech.

Unlike some patients with diffuse damage, patients with focal RH damage are neither incoherent nor generally confused. They usually are oriented to time, person, and place. In rare cases, however, unilateral RHD may cause affective disturbances that can include agitated confusion and certain types of delusions. Sometimes, patients who are not otherwise confused will confabulate elaborate justifications to cover for cognitive uncertainty. This may occur specifically in response to lack of insight about their physical disabilities in a disorder called *anosognosia* (e.g.,"someone took my arm and left me this one"). It also can occur as they negotiate information that is conflicting, ambiguous, makes no sense to them, makes no sense to others, or is in some way at odds with known phenomena. Rather than questioning, reflecting, analyzing, or dismissing it, they construct elaborate explanations to justify it, as if all must be right with the world or something may be wrong with them.

Patients may appear unresponsive to the emotional tone of the exchange and have problems conveying their own emotions through prosody, facial expression, gesture, and body language. Their speech may sound flat and uninflected. The problem may be subtle but evident enough to give the listener pause. Their words may be embedded in a sort of stereotypic prosodic pattern that does not differentiate well among sentence types or emotional content, making listening difficult.

Some patients, because of the size and/ or site of their lesions or because of the way their particular brains are wired, may be almost free of these signs. Among those who do have cognitive and communicative deficits, there is a range of impairments. Aside from prosodic deficits, communicative, cognitive, and attentional impairments typically co-occur. Communication disorders in this population may be obvious or subtle. But even when the problems are not severe, people interacting with RHD patients can come away feeling a little tense, a little uncomfortable, a little worn out. The sense is of someone using language, but not as effectively as expected; of someone communicating, but not quite connecting.

UNDERSTANDING AND CATEGORIZING RHD COMMUNICATION IMPAIRMENTS

Table 1–1 highlighted the variety of deficits that can affect RHD patients. As stated earlier, the body of work on the cognitive/communicative deficits associated with RHD is only beginning to address underlying cause. Effective treatment, of course, is as dependent on understanding the *why* of behavior as it is on understanding the *what*. Because deficits have been identified, but not explained, therapy generally has focused on the symptoms, but not the cause. As a result, there has been little generalization from one task to another. Adopting a theory of the nature of RHD deficits is crucial to therapy that attempts remediation by addressing underlying disordered processes.

The search for mechanism and explanation necessarily begins with a search for possible themes that tie deficits together. Until recently, RHD cognitive deficits have been conceptualized as disparate entities. This book emphasizes the connections among RHD impairments so that the constellation of deficits emerges in a clinically useful and relevant way.

To illustrate, impaired appreciation of figurative language subsequent to RHD was originally seen as an independent problem. Tests of RHD deficits typically included figurative language tasks that asked patients to use or interpret idioms or metaphors. The assumption was that, if a figurative language impairment was present, it should be treated. Naturally, one might question the expenditure of time, effort, and rehabilitation dollars toward the remediation of such a problem. Does it really matter very much in the real world whether a patient can use, explain, or interpret the phrase, "He had a heavy heart"? It might be valuable in some circumstances, certainly. For example, it might help understanding that when the late President Johnson said to the nation, "I come to you tonight with a heavy heart," he was referring to his spirit, not to his physical condition. But in the main, problems with figurative language probably would assume a low priority in the larger rehabilitation picture.

Later, problems with figurative language were seen as part of a larger tendency among RHD patients to restrict themselves to the concrete or denotative rather than the connotative aspects of language use. Under such an umbrella, remediation of figurative language assumes more importance. Still later, such deficits were conceptualized as part of an even more fundamental problem in generating alternative meanings, a problem that has a wide-ranging impact on the ability to adopt alternative viewpoints, manage new information, revise original expectations and interpretations, and assess the plausibility of facts, all of which may be impaired by RHD. This reinterpretation of figurative language impairment is not merely a different way of categorizing the problem. It is a way of giving it stronger clinical meaning. Remediation of the more fundamental disorder should have an impact on a variety of discourse interpretation deficits as well as on figurative language itself.

Improving rehabilitative efficiency is not the only reason why understanding the relationship among deficits is important. It also improves the level of inquiry into underlying mechanisms. For example, having identified deficits in alternate meanings as a core problem with multiple implications, various hypotheses have been generated to explain it. The results of testing these hypotheses will enhance our ability to address underlying cause in patient management.

The above example helps us recognize that there are relationships among identified RHD disorders. Other overriding themes have emerged as well. This book gives serious consideration to attentional deficits as a possible mechanism for many of the cognitive and communicative impairments in this population. Neglect is presented as a symptom of a more profound attentional problem in arousal and orienting, as a deficit which crosses spatial borders, one that goes beyond visuospatial processing and has an impact on cognitive function. Other attentional disorders such as deficits in vigilance, maintenance, and selective attention are considered as fundamental impediments to cognitive and communicative performance. Also addressed are specific cognitive, semantic, and affective impairments that impact on discourse performance and may be somewhat independent of deficits in attention (to the degree that any process can be independent of attention).

CAUTIONARY NOTES

There is much we know and much we do not know about the cognitive and communicative impairments associated with RHD. Several things are important to keep in mind when reading this book, when reading the literature, and when interacting with patients. First, there is no label for the collection of communication disorders associated with RHD. Second, we know little about their course of recovery or response to treatment. Third, we are only beginning to address localization issues and, as a result, we know little about which patients are at risk for communication im-

pairments based on lesion site. These issues are reviewed below.

Labeling RHD Cognitive/ Communicative Deficits

We do not have a label for the communication disorders that can accompany RHD. What we have instead is a location. This single fact has led to confusion in promoting an understanding of these deficits among professionals and the public. The term "RHD" on its own or as a symptom descriptor (e.g., "RHD communication disorders") conveys nothing about the nature of the impairments associated with it. In addition, as a lesion locator, the term "RHD patient" is used interchangeably to describe patients *with* and those *without* cognitive and communicative impairments.

Compare this to the term "aphasia," which refers to a specific disorder of acquired speech and language. It is understood that not all LHD patients are aphasic. As the name of a disorder, "aphasia" calls up a constellation of symptoms, regardless of the location of the damage. Aphasia can occur in patients with RHD as in cases of *crossed aphasia*. If one found RHD deficits in the LH would they be called "crossed right hemisphere damage?" If so, what would that mean?

Although it is true that labels can oversimplify, mislead, and confuse, it is better to have a term or terms that refer to deficits in cognitive and communicative function than one that refers to location. Lack of a label makes it difficult to discuss the problems with patients and their families. It is problematic enough to explain that disorders of communication can exist in the face of intact speech and language. It is even more difficult to do so without a label. For example, one cannot expect to communicate much by walking into a patient's room and saying, "Mr. Jones, you have RHD communication deficits," or "You have a problem in generating alternate meanings," or "problems with the pragmatic aspects of language." One might avoid jargon and discuss "problems in complex levels of communication," but the patient, his family, and even the physician may point out that he does not have trouble talking. It may not be until he leaves the hospital and resumes his former life that Mr. Jones and his family will note that he "talks, but it isn't the same." Had they had a name for the symptoms, the symptoms themselves might have seemed more legitimate, and patients and families more able to deal with them. More than once, after explaining and demonstrating a particular deficit to a given patient, the author has found he or she responds with relief, saying they were afraid they were going crazy because everyone else thought things were fine. That which is nameless can generate fear and confusion.

The dearth of public education on the cognitive and communicative impairments is in part the result of the lack of a label for these disorders. Although there are support organizations and foundations for those with aphasia, there are none that specifically address problems associated with RHD. The public has a hard enough time understanding the term "aphasia," but when they see it in a friend or family member, the term assumes reality because it is a description of a disorder. Confronted with the term "RHD deficits," they hear what they already know—the stroke, lesion, tumor, or disease process is on the right side of the brain.

The location-as-disorder problem has affected the research literature as well. Studies of aphasia usually are conducted on aphasic patients whose aphasia is well documented and whose performance may be compared across aphasia type or with non-aphasic subjects. In RHD research, on the other hand, damage restricted to the RH is often the criteria used for inclusion in the experimental group, regardless of whether subjects in the study have the deficits under investigation. This is fine for studies of incidence, but not for studies investigating the nature of a given deficit. Until this state of affairs changes, one should be careful to note the individual performance of subjects in group studies. When our understanding of the cause of cognitive and communicative deficits associated with RHD improves, we should be able to arrive at a general agreement about the core definition of RHD communication deficits and find appropriate labels for the problem or problems we have identified.

Predictors of Recovery

We do not know much about predictors of recovery because the thrust of research has been deficit description and identification. One cannot follow the course of an impairment until one knows what one is following. Recovery data are more available for deficits such as neglect than for cognitive/communicative impairments, but even there, new methods of identification and testing suggest that neglect may exist subclinically with potential impact on cognitive processing, even when functional recovery appears to have occurred.

Localization

There also is little information connecting lesion location to deficit type. It was enough for early studies to restrict lesion site to the RH because, at the time, it was so extraordinary to consider that RHD might have an impact on communication. In addition, most studies then and now did not have enough subjects to break them into groups according to intrahemispheric lesion location, and intrahemispheric lesion location has not been the thrust of many studies of the nature of the deficits. Many of the subjects in the literature on RHD communication deficits have had large lesions in the territory of the middle cerebral artery with damage to the frontal, parietal, and temporal lobes. Other studies have had subjects with more circumscribed lesions, and the differences between small and more extensive lesions are not clear. For example, we do not know whether small and selective lesions can be as disruptive to communication as larger lesions. There may be certain functional/anatomic systems that can be disrupted by selective damage and with wide-ranging consequences for a variety of communicative functions.

As it has become more accepted that RHD can affect communication, researchers have become more aware of the need to group patients according to intrahemispheric site of lesion. It is important to do so, not only to understand the nature of functional systems within the brain, but also to understand the consequences of pathology. For example, some of the discourse-level disorders associated with RHD such as verbose production, tangentiality, inference deficits, and failure to integrate discourse have also been found to occur in bilateral dorsolateral prefrontal lesions (see McDonald, 1993 for a review). As pointed out by McDonald, differing theories have been posited to explain these deficits by researchers studying the effects of RHD and by those looking at the effects of pre-frontal damage. Sorting out the explanations depends in part on isolating differences between the behavioral effects of anterior versus posterior RHD.

Another factor that impacts on the relationship of deficit and lesion site is the nature of anatomical/functional organization in the RH. The RH is purported to be more diffusely organized and the distribution of functions within it less focal, and hence, localization of function may be less precise in the RH than it is in the LH (Goldberg & Costa, 1981; Gur et al., 1980; Semmes, 1968). Semmes (1968), for example, found that although specific sensorimotor deficits occur with discrete lesions in the LH, the same type of deficits are less dependent on locus of lesion in the RH. In addition, Gur et al. (1980) found that the distribution of white matter (axons) to gray matter (cell bodies) differed across the two hemispheres. The ratio of white to gray matter was found to be higher in the RH than in the LH. The authors speculated that the RH is characterized by a neural organization in which there is more connectivity *among* regions whereas the LH is characterized by greater connectivity *within* a given region. These anatomical/functional findings are in concert with the fact that lesions in a given area of the RH may produce very different deficits, and various lesion sites may result in the same deficit (Tompkins, 1995). For example, many of the attentional operations that have been mapped out appear to depend on anatomical/functional networks that require various cortical and subcortical structures to be fully operational. Both frontal and parietal areas contribute to a wide variety of attentional functions and are themselves extensively interconnected. Damage in one part of the system may have distant effects on other parts of the system. Nonetheless, as deficits are more systematically and universally defined, it is likely that more investigators will take specific lesion site into account and that we will learn more about the functional organization within the RH.

SUMMARY

1. *The recognition of cognitive and commuicative disorders associated with RHD has occurred only in the past 25 years.* Until the late 1960s and early 1970s, the RII was associated with visuospatial processing and was relegated to the role of the "minor hemisphere" in other areas of cognition.

2. New surgical and research techniques from the 1970s and 1980s suggested that the two hemispheres differed not only in function, but also in cognitive strategies for processing information. *The RH was considered important in nonlinear, parallel processing and information synthesis. RHD was thought to affect body image,*

awareness of illness, and visuospatial orientation, imagery, and memory.

3. Newer models of how the brain processes information were developed in the mid-1980s and emphasized cooperation between different areas of the brain, including the two cerebral hemispheres. These new models include *Neural Network* or *Connectionist* models and models of *Interhemispheric Inhibition.*

4. *Communication deficits associated with RHD were first noted in the late 1970s as understanding of RHD increased and the definition of communication expanded to include more than linguistic function.* Early work described the deficits and, more recently, researchers have begun to look at underlying mechanisms that may explain them. *Impaired attention and specific cognitive disorders have been proposed to account for many of the communication impairments associated with RHD.*

5. *RHD may affect overall communicative skills without disrupting language. RHD patients with communication deficits may appear disconnected, abrupt, verbose, less*

sensitive to situational and affective cues, less insightful, less animated, less efficient, and/or less informative than they once were.

6. *Just as not all LHD patients have aphasia, not all RHD patients have cognitive and communicative impairments.* For those who do have communicative impairments, there is no single label to describe their deficits other than one connected with their location (e.g., "Right Hemisphere Communication Deficits" or "Right Hemisphere Syndrome"). *Lack of a label has inhibited understanding of the problems among professionals and the public.*

7. *Deficits typically associated with RHD include problems in attentional functions, left-sided neglect, visuoperceptual deficits, cognitive impairments, communicative disorders, and affective and emotional deficits* (see Table 1–1).

8. *There is little information on predictors of recovery or lesion localization. Only recently have investigators begun to identify lesion sites within the RH with specific RHD cognitive and communicative deficits.*

CHAPTER

2

Neglect

Chapter Outline

DEFINITION

Who, What, Where

Simply stated, patients with neglect *fail to respond to information presented on the side opposite to their brain lesion.* That is, they fail to respond to "contralateral" or "contralesional" input which, in the case of RHD, is input from the left. Neglect, or "left-sided neglect," as it is sometimes called, is often considered a hallmark of RHD. Although it can occur in LHD patients, it is *more frequent, more severe,* and *longer lasting* with RH lesions (Brain, 1941; Chedru, Leblanc, & Lhermitte, 1973; Columbo, De Renzi, & Faglioni, 1976; Hecaen, 1962; Levine & Kinsbourne, 1986; Mesulam, 1981, 1985; Schenkenberg, Bradford, & Ajax, 1980; Weintraub & Mesulam, 1988). Neglect is one of the most familiar, but least understood, of the disorders that can accompany RHD. Typically thought of as a deficit in spatial attention, it appears to be related to other attentional impairments. Very often, patients with neglect appear less responsive and less aroused than do RHD patients without neglect. Clinical experience suggests that the presence of neglect may be a good indictor of impaired cognitive and communicative processing.

The simple definition of neglect as failure to report or respond to contralesional input is a good descriptor of neglect behavior, but does not tell us about the *who, what,* and *where* of neglect. It does not tell us, for example, where the side opposite a brain lesion begins or ends. Does "side" refer to the left side of the body, to the left half of space relative to the body, or to the left side of objects located anywhere in space? Is there an absolute demarcation between sides of space or does neglect occur on a graded scale? Is there a chunk of space simply missing from the patient's awareness or does awareness vary relative to the significance of the stimuli and the conditions of the environment?

As to the "what," there are several major theories that address the nature of neglect, not one of which can account for all of the phenomena associated with it. Theories attempting to explain neglect have tied it to a perceptual disorder, to a deficit in the representation of space, to a directional impairment, to a bias in orienting attention, and to a more general attentional disorder. These theories are not mutually exclusive, and they may be valid explanations of various *types* of neglect. Theories that tie neglect to an attentional disorder account for more neglect behaviors than do other hypotheses.

As for the "who," not all RHD adults have neglect. It has been said, however, that "with appropriate measures, neglect can be identified in a majority of patients with damage or disease of the right hemisphere," and that "neglect may be as common in right-hemisphere damaged patients as language disorders are in left-hemisphere-damaged patients" (Schenkenberg et al., 1980, p. 517). This may seem surprising. It seems less surprising when one understands that certain subtypes of neglect may not be detected by traditional tests nor readily observed in patient behavior.

Estimates of the incidence of neglect range from 31% to 66% in RHD patients and from 2% to 15% in LHD patients (Ogden, 1987; Schenkenberg et al., 1980). Estimates depend on several variables including the type of patients tested and the type and number of tasks used to identify neglect. Some investigators have suggested that the higher incidence of neglect among RHD patients compared to LHD patients may be due to a sampling bias that excludes aphasic patients (Albert, 1973; Battersby, Bender, Pollack, & Kahn, 1956). However, as Ogden (1987) points out, a higher incidence of neglect is found in RHD even when this possible sampling bias has been reduced by using tests that aphasic patients can comprehend. For example, Faglione, Scotti, and Spinnler (1971) found neglect on a simple paper and pencil task in 45% of their RHD and only 9% of their LHD subjects. Only 10% of their sam-

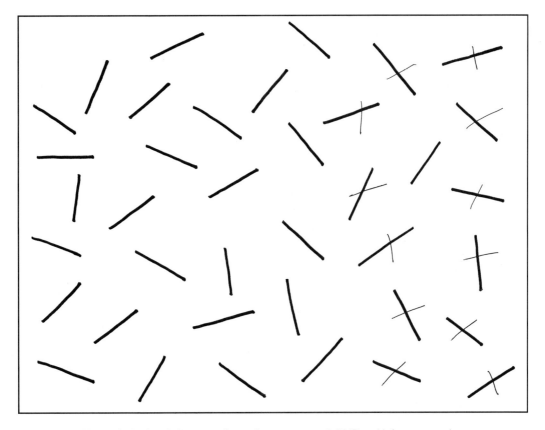

Figure 2–1. Simple line cancellation by a patient with RHD and left severe neglect.

ple were unable to participate, and that 10% included an equal number of RHD and LHD subjects.

Estimates of incidence also depend on the type of tasks used to measure neglect and on the interpretation of the results. Albert (1973), for example, found no difference between in the occurrence of neglect between RHD and LHD subjects on a line cancellation task in which subjects must make a mark through every target to demonstrate that they have seen it (see Figure 2–1). However, in that study neglect was defined as failure to cancel *any line,* and location was not considered. In fact, the number of lines missed was much higher for the RHD group and their omissions occurred primarily on the left. LHD subjects' omissions occurred more frequently in the center and also on the left (i.e., their *ipsi-*

lesional side), a sign of visual inattention, but not neglect.

Early reports of incidence often used a single test. More recently, recognition of subtypes of neglect has suggested that a single test may not be sufficient because neglect may be task dependent (Columbo et al., 1976; Horner, Massey, Woodruff, Chase, & Dawson 1989; Schenkenberg et al., 1980). For example, Schenkenberg et al. identified neglect in 90% of their RHD subjects on a drawing task, but in only 30% on a line-bisection task. Horner et al. (1989) identified it in 83% of their subjects in a drawing task, but in only 61% on a writing task.

Finally, the type of patients sampled can affect estimates of incidence. Studies finding a higher frequency of neglect in RHD typically are based on a sample of subjects with unilateral lesions of either hemisphere. A study by Ogden (1987) found neglect in 50% of the LHD and in 44% of the RHD subjects in her sample. However, the sample included both children and adults, and subjects with tumor, hemorrhage, abscesses, and arteriovenous malformations, as well as infarcts. Tumor was the etiology in 66% of the LHD and in 67% of the RHD subjects whereas only two of the 56 LHD and only 6 of the 45 RHD subjects had cerebrovascular infarcts. Use of patients with tumors in lesion localization studies is generally considered risky because edema, compression, and infiltration can affect areas that are distant from the tumor site.

Clinical reality supports the literature. Neglect is much more frequently observed among RHD than LHD patients. It is doubtful that aphasia masks neglect in LHD patients, as has sometimes been suggested. Rather, neglect may be so mild in LHD patients that it barely affects their behavior, whereas in RHD patients, the symptoms have a much greater impact on attention, motivation, and cognitive processing.

Manifestations of Neglect

RHD patients with severe neglect typically ignore all manner of input from the left, be it the food on their plates, their left limbs, the telephone ringing, or people standing to their left (Table 2–1). Their left arms may drift unnoticed into the spokes of their wheelchairs. They have trouble navigating without bumping into walls and doorways on the "neglected" side. They may ignore the left half of compound words, the left half of sentences, the left half of a paragraph, or the entire left page of a book. Their writing may be characterized by excessive left-hand margins and extraneous and perseverative strokes on the right. They may not be able to read the newspaper, follow a TV show, read important personal documents, manage a checkbook, or pay their bills. They may not notice traffic on the left when crossing a street. They may be a risk to themselves and others.

Despite the physical capacity to master the tasks of daily living such as cooking and cleaning, they may ignore the burners on one side of the stove or the ingredients on one side of the cupboard. They may have difficulty dressing, grooming, and bathing because they ignore one side of their body. In fact, hemiplegic patients may not even recognize their impaired left limbs as their own. They may not use their left limbs to their full capacity, in some cases giving the impression that they are hemiplegic when they actually are not.

In addition to these obvious contralesional deficits, many patients with neglect pose problems in the rehabilitation process because they seem singularly disinterested in it. They may seem less alert, aroused, responsive, and motivated. They may deny or minimize their problems and respond with a sort of passive resistance, give a blank stare, shrug, or confabulate an explanation when deficits are pointed out to them. Reading problems may be dismissed with statements like, "Oh, I guess I need new glasses," "There must be something wrong with that book," or "I never did like to read." The vast majority of patients with neglect do not complain of it and will deny the disorder. Others acknowledge it verbally, but fail to compensate for it behaviorally. Still others recognize it in some circumstances, but not in others. Neglect does not always manifest itself as dramatically or as explicitly as the above picture suggests. It may take sensitive testing to tease it out, but even so, it can exert an influence on the patient's experiential processing.

Although there is much we do not understand about neglect, there are a few certainties in our knowledge. Once the subject of intense debate, we know now that neglect is not caused by a primary sensory deficit (e.g., visual field cuts, hemisensory loss), nor by a primary motor impairment (e.g., hemiplegia). It often accompanies sensorimotor impairments, but can occur in their absence. Patients with neglect are not *unable* to shift their eyes or their attention toward contralesional stimuli. They

TABLE 2–1. Commonly observed left neglect behaviors in RHD patients with moderate to severe neglect.

Problems:
- Responding to people and objects to the left of their body midline
- Attending to the left while conducting self-care activities (grooming, bathing, eating, dressing)
- Moving, attending to, and recognizing their left limbs
- Navigating through halls and doorways without bumping into left-sided walls
- Reading the left half of printed materials
- Appropriate use of margins and spacing when writing
- Following presentations in films, videos, or on TV
- Localizing sounds emanating from the left
- Insight into and awareness of deficits including hemiplegia and neglect
- Actively participating in the rehabilitation process

are not *unable* to move their arm toward the contralesional side. Rather, they appear reluctant or unmotivated to do so. Sensory awareness as demonstrated by physiologic measures may be intact, but the patient's response to incoming stimuli is not. Motor capacity may be intact, but use of the contralesional limbs is not. The contralesional side of space is not "missing," any more than are the contralesional limbs. They are there, but not responded to. The nature of that lack of response is important to our understanding of the patient's cognitive experience.

Ramifications of Neglect

At first glance, and as manifest in casual observation, neglect appears to be a spatial problem, affecting only the patient's perception of space and response to left-sided information. In fact, neglect *has meaning for patients' motivations, expectations, attention to and experience of the physical and abstract world around them, and a potentially significant impact on their communication of that experience.* To understand how this is so is to understand neglect as an *attentional* disorder, related to a variety of other attentional deficits that extend beyond spatial cognition to other cognitive processes.

Damage to the neural network supporting spatial attention is rarely discrete, and thus affects other aspects of attention. For example, neglect may narrow attentional focus, not only toward right-sided information, but also in the realm of ideas. Deficits in selective attention may interact with neglect such that each disorder has an influence on the other. Selective attention deficits may make neglect worse, and neglect may impede selective attention. Understanding neglect is important to understanding many of the attentional, cognitive, and communicative impairments that can accompany RHD.

Certainly, neglect is a factor in, and has a negative impact on, functional outcome. *Patients with neglect are less successful in recovering independence in the activities of daily living (ADLs) than are patients without neglect* (Denes, Semenza, Stoppa, & Lis, 1982; Kinsella & Ford, 1980; Kinsella, Olver, Ng, Packer, & Stark, 1993; Marquardsen, 1969; Sundet, Finset, & Reinvang, 1988). Even when patients are matched at initial evaluation for independence of ADLs, sensory, motor, and intellectual function, those with neglect regain less independence in the long term (Denes et al., 1982). As Kinsella and Ford (1980) stated, "The implication is the intellectual deficit of neglect adds another debilitating factor to the known handicap of hemiplegia and impaired mobility" (p. 665).

Duration and Severity

The duration of neglect is variable. It has been reported to last from 6 months

(Campbell & Oxbury, 1976; Denes et al., 1982) up to 12 years and more (Zarit & Kahn, 1974). Zoccolotti et al. (1989) found that, depending on the measure used to assess it, neglect was present 2 months post-onset in anywhere from 26% to 52% of the 104 patients they tested. Traditional screening tasks are not designed to measure *degree* of deficit. In the future, severity might be determined not only by test performance, but by the number of types of neglect a patient has. When severity has been addressed, some studies have found it follows a bi-modal distribution. That is, neglect tends to be either very mild or very severe, rather than moderate (Plourde, Joanette, Fontaine, LaPlante, & Renaseau-Leclerc, 1993). Severity has been linked to the extent, rather than to the location, of brain damage (Hier, Mondlock, & Caplan, 1983). Studies of recovery tend to focus on complete remission of symptoms, rather than on improvement, in part because so few tests of neglect addressed severity of deficit.

In the past 15 years the study of neglect has changed considerably, altering traditional notions of the symptoms, and moving beyond behavioral description and localization toward explanation. Recently, it has captured the interest of researchers in a variety of disciplines. Our understanding of neglect has benefited from experimental rigor in studies addressing normal spatial cognition, normal and disordered attention, normal and disordered visual representation, and the multiple dissociations that occur under the name "neglect." It is popular now to talk of the "fractionation" of neglect. It may occur in one or several modalities (olfaction, touch, audition, as well as vision). It may occur in motor behavior as well as in sensory awareness. It may occur in some sectors of space and not in others. It has been said that "it appears that the profusion and diversity of the signs of hemi-neglect are limited only by the imagination of the patient and the attentiveness of the examiner" (Friedland & Weinstein, 1977, p. 3).

Since the mid-1980s, findings of multiple dissociations of the syndrome of neglect have helped both to clarify and to muddy the picture of what was once thought to be a unified, if little understood, disorder. Understanding the types and subtypes of neglect is important to our understanding of its underlying mechanisms and its impact on other cognitive operations.

TRADITIONAL MEASURES OF NEGLECT

To understand the impact of neglect, one must start with the signs and symptoms of the disorder. Outside the laboratory, in a medical setting, the presence of neglect usually is determined by informal observation and testing. These tests and observations are used to determine the presence, but rarely the severity, of neglect. The tasks reviewed here are used to establish the presence of neglect. They provide a survey of the phenomena associated with neglect and introduce the reader to the terminology used to describe and explain it. These are the tasks most often used in an initial work-up and most commonly understood and referred to in the vernacular by rehabilitation professionals.

Tests of Extinction

Extinction refers to failure to respond to stimulation on one side of the body when both sides are stimulated simultaneously (Bellas, Novelly, Eskenazi, & Wasserstein, 1988a). Extinction is evoked by a test of *double simultaneous stimulation* (DSS) in which the patient is asked to respond to single and to competing stimuli. Stimuli are usually tactile or visual, but may be auditory as well. For example, while facing the patient, the examiner may tap the patient's left and right knees one at a time and then simultaneously in random order. The patient's task is to point to whichever knee was tapped and, in the case of DSS, to point to both knees. Patients with left-sided ex-

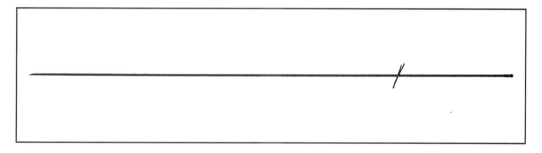

Figure 2–2. Line-bisection by a patient with RHD and severe left neglect.

tinction, for example, are successful in reporting sensation on the right or left in isolation, but fail to report left-sided stimulation when both knees are tapped. It is assumed that the failure is linked to the effect of competing stimuli, in which the right-most stimuli have a greater impact on the patient's awareness. On the other hand, patients with diffuse damage may fail to report or "extinguish" stimuli on either side of the body.

Often when testing RHD patients, the examiner will present the two stimuli together on the right or the left side of the patient's body. Patients with neglect may fail to report the most contralesional of two competing stimuli in either hemispace (i.e., when the left and right sides of the right knee are tapped simultaneously) (Feinberg, Haber, & Stacy, 1990).

Extinction often is considered a mild form of neglect, especially when it occurs in the absence of other signs of neglect. Although some researchers have suggested that neglect evolves into extinction as it resolves (Heilman & Watson, 1977), there are those who disagree because neglect can occur without accompanying extinction (De Renzi, Gentilini, & Barbieri, 1989a). Most typically, however, extinction and neglect occur together.

Tests of Visual Neglect

Visual neglect appears to be the most common form of neglect, but that may be because it is the most commonly tested and most frequently and easily observed type of neglect. In any case, most patients who have neglect in other modalities also have visual neglect. The following tasks are those typically used to screen for neglect and most frequently referred to in the literature.

Line Bisection

The goal of line bisection is to assess the patient's estimation of the center of space by asking them to bisect a horizontal line. The line is usually from 6 to 10 inches long, drawn on a sheet of paper placed at the patient's midline. The patient is asked to make a vertical mark through its center. Deviations to the right of the geometric midpoint are considered an indication that the patient's concept of center is skewed to the right and that he or she is neglecting a portion of the line to the left of true center (Figure 2–2). Recent research demonstrates considerable individual differences among normal subjects in line bisection (Manning, Halligan, & Marshall, 1990; Nichelli, Rinaldi, & Cubeli, 1989; Schenkenberg et al., 1980). Slight deviations to the right or left may be normal, but substantial deviations are indicative of neglect.

Cancellation

The goal in cancellation tasks is to determine if a patient can find specific targets in a visual array. The array is placed at the patient's midline and may consist of short

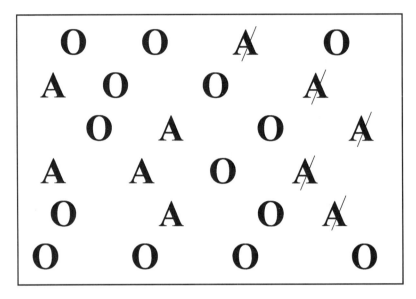

Figure 2–3. Target-foil cancellation task by a patient with RHD and neglect. Targets: the letter A; foils: the letter O.

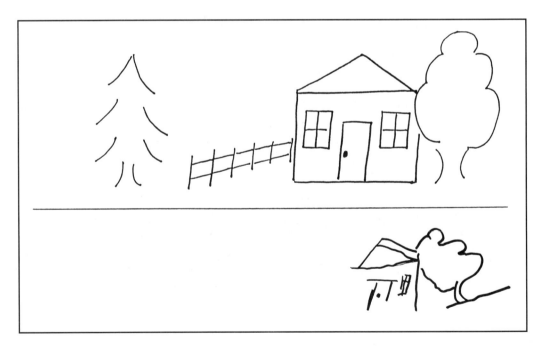

Figure 2–4. Copy-drawing by a patient with RHD and severe neglect. The scene above the line was in view as the patient copied it.

lines, letters, numbers, objects, or geometric forms. Patients are asked to put a mark through or "cancel" each occurrence of the target. Scoring typically is based on the ratio of targets cancelled to the right and left of center. Figure 2–1 showed the perfor-

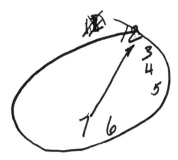

Figure 2–5. Free-hand clock set for 7:15 drawn by a patient with RHD and severe neglect.

mance of a patient with left neglect on a simple cancellation task originally designed by Albert (1973). An example of a more complex cancellation task consisting of targets embedded in foils is found in Figure 2–3.

Drawing

Drawing tasks require patients to copy or spontaneously draw simple symmetrical forms such as a daisy, clock, or man. The goal is to compare the amount of detail produced on the two sides of the figure. Left neglect is present when the left half of the figure is incomplete relative to the right half. Examples of the copied and spontaneous drawings of patients with left neglect are found in Figure 2–4 (which depicts a simple scene) and in Figure 2–5 (which depicts a clock set for 7:15).

Reading

Patients typically are asked to read aloud a series of compound words, sentences, and/or a paragraph presented at their midline. Patients with neglect may read the word "Whitehouse" as "house" or the sentence, "Joe and Ella came over last night" as "Ella came over last night." An example of a patient's rendition of the first several lines of the Grandfather Passage is found on page 36.

Writing

Patients are asked to write or copy a sentence. Patients with neglect tend to squeeze written samples over to the right, leaving a wide left margin. There may be extra strokes in some letters and omitted strokes in others as seen in Figure 2–6.

Together these tasks are considered the standard method of screening for neglect. Variants of these tasks have been used extensively in the experimental literature to investigate the underlying nature of neglect and to explore subtypes of the syndrome. As traditionally administered, most of them define left as the area to the left of the patient's midline. As we shall see in the following section, "left" can have more than one definition.

FRAMES OF REFERENCE

To understand the "left" in left neglect, one must recognize that neglect can occur in different *frames of reference.* Frames of reference are a means of conceiving of how space and spatial relations are coded in the brain, a concept that helps us understand the breakdowns in spatial cognition that may occur in neglect. The concept of left space in neglect is not static, but can vary with the nature of the stimulus, the task, and the type of neglect a patient has. We typically think of left neglect as occurring on the horizontal plane in left lateral space as defined by the midline of the body. However, the fact that patients may neglect the left sides of objects in both central and in right hemispace tells us that left is not defined by hemispatial coordinates alone. The picture is far more complex. Neglect is a dynamic deficit that occurs not in a single sector of space, but changes with the position of the viewer and with the conditions of the environment.

Two fundamentals are important to remember. First, *neglect is a subjective experience that occurs inside the mind of the neglector.* Areas of space do not actually dis-

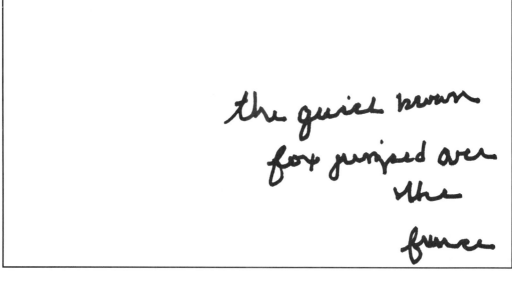

Figure 2–6. The sentence, "The quick brown fox jumped over the fence," written to dictation by a patient with RHD and neglect.

appear; they disappear or are diminished in the awareness of the patient. Second, *the concept of space is a mental or psychological construct.* It is based on the perception of the relationships among items in the environment. Spatial locations and relations are translated into representations that are internal to the observer and are used to manipulate and organize the external environment. *The spatial coordinates used to generate the representation of spatial location are called "frames of reference."* Understanding the frames of reference in which neglect can occur is a relatively new idea and one that is important to the conceptualization, identification, and remediation of neglect.

Essentially, there are three frames of reference within which spatial locations are specified: *viewer-centered, environment-centered,* and *object-centered* (Arguin & Bub, 1993; Farah, Brunn, Wong, Wallace, & Carpenter, 1990). Each of these frames of reference and their relevance to neglect are discussed below.

Viewer-Centered Neglect

In *viewer-centered frames of reference, the location of objects is defined relative to the viewer.* Within viewer-centered space are various body-centered coordinates that include the trunk, the eyes, and the head. For example, an umpire standing at home plate on a baseball diamond, facing the pitcher's mound, will see first base to his right and third base to his left. If he turns his head sharply to the right, he might determine that first base is now to his left. What he sees as right and left space has now been coded according to the position of his head and eyes, not his body. Yet, relative to his trunk, first base continues to be to his right and third base to his left (see Figure 2–7). Thus, viewer-centered frames of reference can change depending on the frame of reference on the body that the viewer adopts (head, eyes, or trunk).

As traditional tests of neglect demonstrate, neglect occurs to the left of the mid-

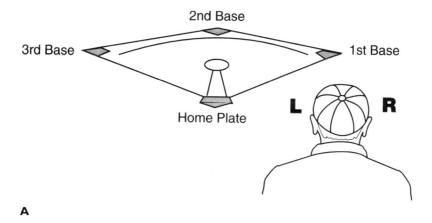

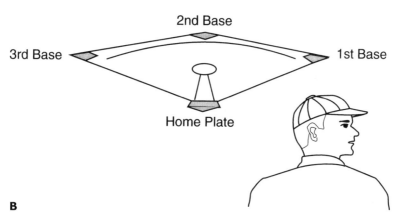

Figure 2–7. Examples of viewer-centered and environment-centered frames of reference on a baseball diamond. In the viewer-centered frame of reference, first and third base are to the right and left of the umpire as he faces the pitcher's mound (A). When he turns his head to his right (B), right and left shift relative to his head, but remain the same relative to his trunk. In the environment-centered frame of reference, home plate and second base are the invariant front and back of the diamond, and first and third base are always to the right and left, respectively, of the pitcher's mound.

line of the patient's body when head, eyes, and trunk are aligned. However, when their head or eyes are turned to the right, patients may ignore stimuli that are on the left in what would be considered right hemispace relative to their trunk. In other words, "left space" may shift according to the direction of gaze, regardless of the alignment with the trunk.

Other coordinates such as top and bottom are important in viewer-centered ne-

glect as well. The lower left quadrant appears particularly vulnerable to neglect (Halligan & Marshall, 1989a; Mark & Heilman, 1988), and some patients may have neglect for the entire bottom half of space (Rapcsak, Cimino, & Heilman, 1988). Mark and Heilman (1988) found lower left quadrant neglect even when patients were asked to begin a cancellation task by starting at the bottom left side of the page. Thus neglect occurs more intensely in the lower half of space according to viewer-centered coordinates.

Viewer-centered neglect informs us that the position of the patient's head, eyes, and trunk will define in part what he or she neglects. If the patient's head is turned 90 degrees to the right, for example, two areas of neglect may exist (see Figure 2–7). These dual areas of neglect may be demonstrated by the fact that the patient fails to search visually to the left of his head (i.e., in what appears to be right hemispace), and simultaneously fails to search manually to the left of his trunk in left hemispace. In addition, viewer-centered neglect tells us that the lower left relative to the body itself (leg versus arm) or to a visual array (bottom versus top) will be particularly problematic.

Environment-Centered Neglect

Environment-centered frames of reference specify the location of objects relative to one another and relative to fixed environmental boundaries (e.g., the edges of a page or the walls of a room). They are more stable than viewer-centered frames, which are subject to changes in the position of the viewer. This stability and invariance helps us navigate successfully through the world without our every step altering our concept of the spatial arrangement of objects in the environment. In the baseball field, because it has an invariant front and back, the perimeter can be used to specify the locations of the bases within that boundary. Thus, third base is considered to be on the left of the field and first base on the right, regardless of where the umpire is looking. If he drops to the ground and lays sideways, he will continue to conceive of the bases in those spatial relationships when using "environmentcentered" (versus viewer-centered) coordinates for coding spatial location. What was once top and bottom (sky and field) are now to his left and right in viewer-centered coordinates, but remain top and bottom in environment-centered coordinates.

It has been found that environment-centered and viewer-centered neglect can, and probably often do, occur together (Calvanio, Petrone, & Levine, 1987; Farah et al., 1990; Ladavas, 1987). For example, Calvanio et al. found that, when subjects are lying on their right sides, they report fewer items from both the top of a display (i.e., to their left) and from the left of the display itself. Fewest items were reported from the upper left quadrant which encompassed both subjects' left and the left of the display (see Figure 2–8). Thus, when the body is not aligned with environmental left and right, neglect can occur both to the left of the body and the left side of the environment simultaneously. *In the normal upright view, the most neglected area is usually the lower left quadrant.*

Environment-centered frames of reference also include the *position of objects relative to one another*. In a horizontal array of two objects, one is to the left of the other even if they are both in right hemispace relative to the viewer or relative to the boundaries of the environment. At the top of Figure 2–9, there are four squares, two in right and two in left hemispace. When the four squares are arrayed across the midline, patients with neglect will typically neglect the two to the left of the midline in accordance with viewer-centered neglect. In the second row, all four squares are arrayed in left hemispace. Rather than neglecting all four squares, most patients with neglect will neglect the two most leftward squares. That is, they will move their attention to the left because there is nothing in right hemispace to capture their attention, but they will stop moving their attention at around the midpoint of the squares. Their neglect is not a function of hemispatial coordinates alone, but of the stimulus environment.

In the lowest row, all the squares are arrayed in right hemispace where one would not expect to see neglect. Nonetheless, patients with severe neglect often will not attend to the two left-most squares in right hemispace because the ones farthest to the right attract their attention. Thus, the most

L   R

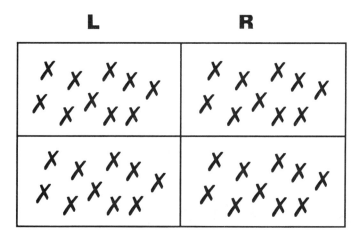

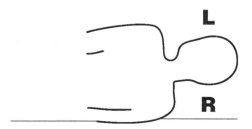

Figure 2–8. Example of the combined effects of viewer-centered and environment-centered neglect in a search task, described by Calvanio et. al. (1987). In an upright position, the person with viewer- and environment-centered left neglect would report fewest objects from the lower left quadrant of the display which is the most neglected area when viewer-centered and environment centered coordinates match. Lying on his right side, as depicted here, the person with viewer- and environment-centered left neglect viewer would report the fewest objects from the upper left quadrant, which is to the left in both viewer-centered and environment-centered coordinates.

leftward object in a row will be neglected, regardless of its hemispace location relative to the body midline. Clinically, this is called *ipsilesional neglect* because it occurs on the same side as the lesion.

Numerous studies have found ipsilesional and central neglect in RHD patients (Feinberg et al., 1990; Gainotti, D'Erme, Monteleone, & Silveri, 1986; Posner, Walker, Friedrich, & Rafal, 1987; Weintraub & Mesulam, 1987, 1988). Arguin and Bub (1993), for example, found that in non-

brain-damaged (NBD) subjects the speed of response to a target's appearance was not affected by where it occurred relative to the edge of a computer screen, the other stimuli displayed on the screen, or the subject's midline. However, the RHD subject was slower to respond the further to her left the target appeared (viewer-centered neglect), the further it was to the left of the array of foils (environment-centered neglect), and the further it was to the left of the display screen (environment-centered

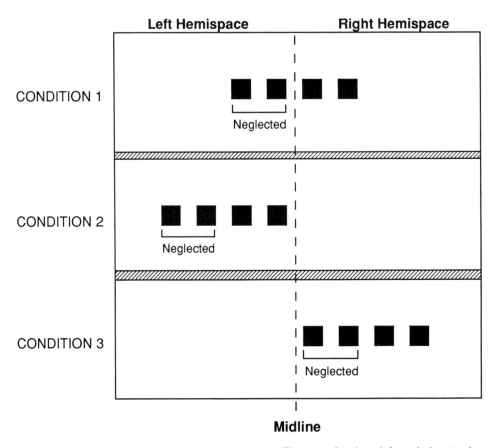

Figure 2–9. Example of the dynamic nature of neglect. The area of neglect shifts with the stimulus environment. As they count the number of squares in each row, RHD patients with neglect tend to ignore the two most leftward squares, regardless of whether they are centered at midline (condition 1), to the left of midline (condition 2), or to the right of midline (condition 3).

neglect) Numerous other reaction time studies measuring the time taken for patients with neglect to orient attention to targets in various spatial locations also have found that the relative rightward position of a target increases its saliency and the relative leftward position decreases its saliency, regardless of its absolute hemispace location (Butter, 1992; D'Erme, Robertson, Bartolomeo, Daniele, & Gainotti, 1992; De Renzi, Gentilini, Faglioni, & Barbieri, 1989b; Farah et al., 1990; Ladavas, 1987, 1990; Ladavas, Del Pesce, & Provinciali, 1989; Posner, Walker, et al., 1987). That is, in neglect relative left operates independently of visual field or hemispace presentation (Ladavas,

1987; Ladavas et al., 1989). Even when stimuli are displayed only in right hemispace, subjects with left neglect take progressively more time to respond to the most leftward stimuli (De Renzi et al., 1989). Deficits in orienting attention in neglect support the concept that the problem is a directional one in which the *relative*, rather than the *absolute*, location of stimuli matters. Neglect, then, is influenced by the position of targets relative to both the boundaries of a field, the stimuli in that field, and the position of the viewer. Hence, "left" in patients with left neglect is not restricted to their left, but may occur to their right and in the center of space as well.

Environment-centered neglect tells us that neglect can be defined by the boundaries of space and by what is present within those boundaries. Understanding it prepares us for the possibility of ipsilesional neglect and for relative degrees of neglect in left hemispace. It also reminds us that the higher the concentration of objects to the right of a target, the more difficult it may be to find the target, regardless of its hemispace location. That is why a blank right space so often improves patient awareness of objects on the left.

Object-Centered Neglect

Finally, there are object-centered frames of reference in which there is a left and right side of each object as well as a top and bottom. Object-centered coordinates help us recognize objects even when they are in unusual orientations. For example, the doors of a car are considered to be on the sides, and the wheels underneath, regardless of whether the viewer is inside, outside, on top of, or underneath the car or whether the car is upside down or right-side up. Although many objects have an invariant top and bottom, not many have an intrinsic left and right side. A teapot cover is always the top, but the left-right position of the handle and spout change with the viewer's position. One class of objects that does have an invariant left and right is printed English words and sentences. The beginning of a word is considered to be the first letter to the left in horizontal displays. In vertical displays, it is considered to be the first letter at the top. The beginning of the word remains invariant relative to the end of the word, regardless of its orientation. If a word is upside down, the beginning occurs on the right.

There is little if any evidence for object-centered neglect in RHD patients (Farah et al. 1990). The evidence suggests that RHD patients treat printed words in a viewer-centered and environment-centered frame of reference, but not in an object-centered frame. That is, RHD patients with neglect, ignore the beginnings of words in their upright position, and the ends of words when words are inverted (Ellis, Flude, & Young 1987; Riddoch, Humphreys, Cleton, & Fery, 1990).

Caramazza and Hillis (1990), however, reported a different result with an LHD patient who had right neglect. He had difficulty reading the ends (right side) of words, and continued to do so even when words were inverted and appeared in left hemispace, suggesting that, in this patient, the intrinsic right side of the word was neglected. The same results have not been demonstrated in RHD patients. Marr (1982) suggested that there are stages of object recognition, the earliest of which rely on viewer-centered representation, and the last of which relies on object-centered representation. Caramazza and Hillis refer to similar stages in their account of their patient's neglect. Given that RHD does not appear to engender object-centered neglect in reading, and LHD does, it is possible that LHD disrupts word representations at a later, *semantically based* stage of processing whereas RHD disrupts the *spatial configurations* of words at an earlier, more primitive, viewer-centered stage of processing.

Neglect in Other Frames of Reference

The literature on neglect sometimes includes two other frames of reference: *personal* and *extrapersonal* space. *Personal space refers to the body as divided by the midline,* and to specific areas within one or the other side of the body. Patients may neglect their left arms, legs, hands, shoulders, the left side of their faces, and so on. They may extinguish touch on the hand, for example, when the face is also touched on either the right or left side of the body (Feinberg et al., 1990). Personal neglect also can take the form of *anosognosia* in which patients deny, ignore, or reject their left limbs. This disorder is reviewed later in the chapter.

Extrapersonal space refers to areas within reach of the viewer. It is the area of space in which most traditional paper-and-pencil tests of neglect are conducted. Extrapersonal neglect often occurs in the absence of personal neglect, but the reverse is rarely the case. Most patients with personal neglect have extrapersonal neglect as well, although there have been reports of dissociations (Bisiach, Perani, Vallar, & Berti, 1986). Guariglia and Antonucci (1992), for example, reported a man with severe personal neglect, characterized by failure to groom himself on the left, inability to look at his left leg while walking, and underutilization of the residual motor functions of his left side. However, he had no evidence of extrapersonal neglect in tests like line cancellation or reading. There has also been an attempt to find dissociations in neglect between near and far extrapersonal space, but without success (Pizzamiglio et al., 1989).

NEGLECT ACROSS MODALITIES

Up to this point, our discussion has focused on visual neglect, the most commonly found type of neglect. Neglect can and does occur in other input channels, although almost always in conjunction with visual neglect. Studies of neglect in specific modalities have several goals. One, of course, is to establish whether neglect occurs in a given modality. Another is to distinguish the input from the output channels in which neglect may occur. That is, does the patient fail to cancel lines on a page because of reduced input (visual attention) or because of reduced output (motor production) that inhibits movement of the right arm into left hemispace? A third goal is to distinguish neglect from a primary sensory and/or motor loss in a given modality. Neglect has been found across modalities (i.e., auditory, tactile, visual, and even olfactory channels), and it can be distinguished from primary sensory and motor impairments.

Auditory Neglect

Patients with neglect may not answer the telephone or notice people talking to them on their left side. Because sound reaches both ears in free field, their failure may be attributed to a motor problem in that they simply fail to reach toward the left to get the telephone or fail to turn their heads to the left to talk to people. However, there appears to be a directional component in auditory neglect, which suggests patients may be less responsive to left-sided auditory input. Auditory neglect has been demonstrated in studies in which subjects are asked to localize sounds that are presented binaurally (De Renzi et al., 1989a) and dichotically (Bisiach, Cornacchia, Sterzi, & Vallar, 1984) and to localize a sound emitted from one of several loudspeakers arrayed in a seimicircle in front of them (Pinek, Duhamel, Cave, & Brouchon, 1989; Ruff, Hersh, & Pribram, 1981). RHD patients with posterior lesions may have trouble localizing sound, regardless of where it occurs (Ruff et al., 1981), suggesting that sound localization may be a problem independent of neglect. In some cases, subjects mistakenly localize sounds heard in left hemispace to the right hemispace in a disorder called *alloacusis* (Heilman & Valenstein, 1972a). Typically, patients with auditory neglect also have visual neglect, but not always. De Renzi et al. (1989) found that only 15 of 25 RHD subjects with auditory neglect demonstrated neglect on a visual cancellation task.

Because most sounds reach both ears, auditory neglect probably is not much of a functional problem unless one is driving or in a situation in which localizing sound is crucial. However, as a sign of neglect and perhaps of a more general attentional disorder, its presence is important, regardless of its more immediate functional significance.

Tactile Neglect

Tactile neglect may take several forms. Extinction to competing touch stimuli (Ito et al., 1989; Schwartz, Marchok, Kennick, &

Flynn, 1979) has been discussed earlier. Additionally, researchers have investigated the ability to search space manually (De Renzi, Faglioni, & Scotti, 1970; Gentilini, Barbieri, De Renzi, & Faglioni, 1989; Weintraub & Mesulam, 1987). Others have attempted to distinguish a primary sensory loss from neglect in the contralesional limbs (Vallar, Bottini, Sterzi, Passerini, & Rusconi, 1991; Vallar, Sandroni, Rusconi, & Barbieri, 1991).

Tactile extinction has been studied in several formats. In simple extinction tasks, subjects must verify the presence of touch on one or both sides of their bodies with their eyes shut. In complex extinction tasks, subjects must identify or differentiate among materials presented to each hand (e.g., plastic, sponge, sandpaper) (Schwartz et al., 1979). Sometimes, subjects extinguish contralesional stimuli only in these more complex tasks, but not in the simple tasks (Ito et al., 1989). Subjects who extinguished stimuli in both types of tasks reported feeling either nothing or something very faintly. Those who extinguished only in the complex task, reported feeling something, but they were not certain what it was. The results suggested to the authors that tactile neglect can occur at several levels—at the level of sensory awareness, perception, and/or at the level of sensory recognition.

Manual search tasks compare the number of targets found or the time taken to locate targets in the right and left side of space. Subjects typically are blindfolded. When they are not, visual input and feedback actually may impair performance (Gentilini et al., 1989). Tactile and visual neglect may interact because the presence of visual stimuli in right hemispace captures visual attention (i.e., environment-centered neglect) and may inhibit motivation to manually search to the left.

Naturally, tactile neglect of the hand may reduce patients' ability to explore the environment manually and may affect self-care activities as well. Patients may be less aware of somatosensory feedback on their left side even when sensation is intact. Reduced tactile awareness on the left can ex-

tend to eating and swallowing, a factor to consider in dysphagia. Patients with neglect may not be aware of food collecting on the left side of their mouths, for example, and may not swallow as often as they should while eating. Because tactile neglect typically co-occurs with visual neglect, it is worth keeping in mind when working on swallowing with patients who have documented visual neglect.

Olfactory Neglect

Extinction of olfactory sensation consists of reduced sensitivity to sensory input to one nostril when a competing stimulus is presented to the other nostril. Studies of olfactory neglect have been particularly important in establishing that neglect is not a primary sensory problem. Most sensory pathways are crossed so that the majority of visual, auditory, and tactile stimulation is projected to the contralateral hemisphere. It was argued that left neglect might be due to reduced capacity of the RH to process sensory information presented in the left visual, auditory, and/or tactile fields. Olfaction is largely ipsilaterally innervated. The left nostril projects mainly to the LH and the right nostril to the RH. If neglect were the result of a sensory loss, one would expect olfactory neglect in RHD patients to occur in right nostril stimulation because of its projections to the RH.

In fact, just the opposite has been found (Bellas et al., 1988a, 1988b; Mesulam, 1981). Patients with left neglect in other modalities neglect the left, but not right, nostril stimulation. Thus, neglect has been shown to be independent of sensation. Although of little functional significance, this finding provided clear evidence that neglect is a spatial, not a sensory, deficit.

NEGLECT AND SENSORIMOTOR DEFICITS

There tends to be a higher incidence of hemiplegia and hemisensory impairments in RHD compared to LHD patients (Sterzi et al., 1993). Although neglect is not a primary sensory deficit, it appears to be a factor in the sensory and motor loss in some patients. Sometimes neglect may masquerade as hemiplegia, hemisensory loss, and/or visual field cuts.

Visuosensory Deficits and Neglect

Differentiating neglect from primary visual sensory impairments, particularly visual field defects, has been the subject of numerous investigations. Because neglect is so often associated with posterior lesions, many patients with neglect also have visual field defects. A *visual field defect (or field cut) is a primary visuosensory impairment caused by interruption of the visual pathways (optic tract) projecting to visual cortex (occipital lobe), interfering with vision.* Visual field defects cause a blind area in corresponding visual fields of both eyes. The area of impairment in visual field cuts is thus *eye-centered and moves with the eyes.* People with RHD and a visual field cut cannot see in some area of the left visual field of each eye, regardless of whether they are looking ahead or to the right or left. The most common type of field cut is *hemianopia or loss of vision in the hemifield contralateral to the lesion* (Zihl, 1989). It occurs following posterior lesions.

Although neglect and hemianopia can both interfere with visual performance in left hemispace, there are fundamental differences between them that are outlined in Table 2–2. Hemianopia affects the visual fields, regardless of the hemispace location of gaze. Neglect, on the other hand, does

not occur in a visual field, but in various sectors of space. It is not eye-centered; it is space-centered. Patients fail to report stimuli in the neglected area, not because they cannot see them, but because they do not *notice* them. Mesulam (1985) put it well when he said that visual field cuts interfere with seeing whereas neglect interferes with looking and searching.

Patients may have field cuts without neglect, neglect without field cuts, or both neglect and a field cut simultaneously (Albert, 1973; Chedru et al., 1973; Girotti, Casazza, Musicco, & Avanzini, 1983; Halligan, Marshall, & Wade, 1990; Vallar & Perani, 1986). To determine the presence of a field cut, the examiner asks the patient to keep his or her eyes fixed forward and to report whether they see stimuli in their peripheral vision. A field cut is said to be present when the patient fails to report stimuli in the area subtended by the visual field. For example, patients with left hemianopia have a blind area in the sector encompassed by the left visual field. Without further testing, it may be difficult to determine if the patient also has left visual neglect.

Kooistra and Heilman (1989) suggested one way to distinguish neglect from hemianopia is to test the visual fields in right hemispace with the patient's head aligned with the body, facing forward. The patient is asked to direct his or her gaze toward left and then toward right hemispace. If the apparent field cut disappears when the gaze is directed toward right hemispace, the problem can be considered a left-hemispatial disorder (neglect). If the field cut remains when gaze is directed toward right hemispace, it can be considered a left hemifield or visual disorder that moves with the eyes.

Another way of differentiating neglect from a field cut is through physiologic measures of responsivity to visual input. That is, if sensation is intact, the stimulus will register at a physical level, even if it has not done so at a perceptual level. Vallar, Sandrioni, et al. (1991) used visual evoked

TABLE 2–2. Hemianopia versus neglect.

Hemianopia	Neglect
Retinotopic	Spatial
Affects seeing	Affects looking and searching
Awareness of deficit	Denial of deficit
Compensation	Lack of compensation

potentials to measure neural activity in response to a visual stimulus. They found that patients with neglect who failed to report visual stimuli in neglected space had normal evoked potentials to the input. Thus, although subjects did not consciously perceive it, the stimuli had undergone some form of early processing, arguing against the type of sensory loss seen in hemianopia or other forms of visual field defects as a factor in neglect.

Another difference between patients with neglect and those with hemianopia is awareness of their deficits. Patients with hemianopia complain of their visual disorder in reading and in locating objects. Those with neglect alone or with both neglect and hemianopia rarely do. Awareness often leads to compensation, and most clinicians find that hemianopic patients without neglect learn to compensate, usually unconsciously, by turning their heads or altering their eye movements. Patients with neglect, on the other hand, have difficulty learning to compensate even when they are taught how to do so.

Compensation in hemianopia occurs with changes in both eye movements and search patterns. Oculomotor performance in hemianopic patients differs from that of patients with neglect and from NBD adults (Girotti et al., 1983; Meinberg, Zangemeister, Rosenberg, Hoyt, & Stark, 1981). In pursuit of a visual target, NBD adults tend to make smooth *saccades*, the rapid eye movements from one point of fixation to another. They typically make a single saccade to reach a target in a known location. When searching for one whose location they are unsure of, they tend to start in the upper left quadrant of a display and to proceed in a circular pattern (clockwise or counter-clockwise) as they continue searching (Chedru et al., 1973; Meinberg et al., 1981).

Patients with hemianopia perform quite differently. Aware of their inability to see targets in their blind hemifield, they compensate by adjusting their eye movements and search patterns. They tend to begin their search by exploring the whole of the normal visual field in a circular pattern and then proceed to the opposite hemifield (Chedru et al., 1973). There they adjust their gaze until the target appears in an unimpaired region of the field (Nagel-Lieby, Buchtel, & Welch, 1990). Short jerky saccades replace the smooth pursuit of normal search. Meinberg et al. (1981) described these short stepwise saccades as a slow but safe strategy in which the blind hemifield (which moves with the eye) is "pulled back like a curtain" until the target is revealed (p. 540). In visual search tasks, hemianopic patients make every effort to find targets. When possible, they use previous knowledge and make fairly accurate saccades to anticipated locations even when targets are in the blind hemifield (Meinberg et al., 1981).

Patients with neglect may also use short stepwise saccades to find targets, but their search patterns are disorganized and their effort to search in left hemispace is impoverished and feeble (Chedru et al., 1973; Girotti et al., 1983; Hornak, 1992). Also, unlike hemianopic patients, they do not improve performance in conditions in which target location can be predicted (Girotti et al., 1983).

Surprisingly, hemianopia does not appear to exacerbate symptoms of neglect (Halligan, Marshall, & Wade, 1990; Ogden, 1987). Halligan et al., for example, measured severity of neglect on six paper-and-pencil tasks in patients with neglect and found no significant differences between patients with and those without field cuts. In addition, perfomance between hemianopic and neglect patients differs on some neglect tasks. For example, whereas patients with left neglect bisect lines to the right of center, those with hemianopia bisect lines to the left of center (Werth, 1993). Eye movement recordings during line bisection have demonstrated that neglect patients tend to limit line exploration to the right of the midpoint of the line (Ishiai, Furukawa, & Tsukagoshi, 1989; Ishiai, Sugishita, Mitani, & Ishizawa, 1992).

Hemisensory Deficits and Neglect

Depending on its location, damage in the RH can produce a hemisensory loss in which there is reduced sensation in the left arm, hand, leg, and/or foot. Sometimes in patients with neglect, these sensory deficits are exaggerated because of their neglect. Indeed, in some patients without true hemisensory deficits, neglect may even masquerade as a hemisensory loss. That is, RHD patients with neglect may not perceive tactile stimulation even though it registers in their nervous systems. Investigators have used both skin conductance response and somatosensory cortical evoked potentials to monitor physiologic responses to tactile stimulation (Vallar, Bottini, et al., 1991; Vallar, Sandroni, et al., 1991). For example, Vallar, Sandroni, et al. (1991) found that patients with neglect, left hemiparesis, and hemisensory loss had normal evoked potentials to stimulation of the contralateral (left) hand even when they had no conscious perception of it. In contrast, when the contralateral (right) hand of LHD subjects was stimulated, cortical evoked potentials were absent, indicating a primary sensory deficit. The findings in the RHD patients help explain the greater prevalence of hemisensory deficits in the RHD compared to LHD population. Of course, that is not to discount the existence of true hemisensory loss in RHD patients with such impairments, but it tells us that in some cases neglect can exacerbate hemianesthesia or even look like it. The effect may be the same. To feel but fail to perceive a stimulus is not much different from failing to feel it at all. The difference between the two lies in the approach taken toward their remediation.

Hemiplegia and Motor Neglect

Neglect has an impact on motor movement as well as on sensory awareness and perception. Two types of motor neglect have been identified. The first, referred to simply as *motor neglect*, involves *movement of the contralesional limbs anywhere in space*. The second, called *directional hypokinesia*, has a directional component and refers to *difficulty in moving the ipsilesional limbs into or toward contralateral space*.

Motor Neglect

Motor neglect is an underutilization of the contralesional extremities in the absence of a primary motor deficit (Bisiach, Geminiani, Berti, & Rusconi, 1990; Laplane & Degos, 1983; Vallar, 1993). Like other types of neglect, it is more common following RHD than LHD (Barbierie & DeRenzi, 1989). Patients with motor neglect may act as if they have hemiplegia when, in fact, they are capable of near-normal movement. In some cases, hemiplegia, like some cases of hemisensory loss, actually may be a manifestation of neglect.

Motor neglect can exist in the absence of, but often is accompanied by, other signs of neglect (Barbierie & DeRenzi, 1989; Laplane & Degos, 1983). It is not considered a form of anosognosia. Patients with anosognosia are likely to explain the lack of voluntary movement in their extremities by stating that their limbs, "do not belong me," or are "dead," "lazy," "unreliable," or "useless." Motor neglect, on the other hand, is a disturbance of spontaneous movement "involving one half of the body and having the appearance of hemiplegia, yet with normal strength and dexterity, which can be proven by prompting an extraordinary effort on the part of the patient" (Laplane & Degos, 1983, p. 152). Patients with motor neglect do not show a marked reduction of reflexes nor impaired sensation.

Based on their investigation, Laplane and Degos (1983) described numerous clincial characteristics of motor neglect. Table 2–3 contains a list of signs of motor neglect. *Inappropriate placement of the extremities* refers to the fact that, while sitting, patients may allow their left arms to hang down or leave their hands between their legs instead of placing them on the arm of the chair or on

TABLE 2–3. Clinical signs of motor neglect.

- Inappropriate placement of left extremities
- Dragging left arm or leg
- Feeble participation of left limbs in bilateral movements
- Failure to use left limbs for balance
- Failure to withdraw extremities from painful stimuli

their thighs. When shifting position, their left arms may be dragged passively along the bed or table. The arm might end up in an uncomfortable position, twisted, for example, or underneath the patient's body. The arm or leg might be left dangling off the bed or in the spokes of a wheelchair. The leg, too, might be left in an uncomfortable position. Laplane and Degos reported that, in their experience, patients rectify the inappropriate posture when asked to assume a more comfortable position.

A second characteristic is the *tendency to lose balance.* Faulty posture can lead to falling without attempts by the patient to regain balance or minimize the fall through postural readjustment (e.g., reaching out with the left hand to break the fall). For example, the patient might leave his leg on the bed as he attempts to get up and immediately fall onto the floor.

Third, patients *may not withdraw from painful stimuli,* just as they do not move out of uncomfortable positions. Laplane and Degos noted that, even as patients complain of painful stimuli, they make no attempt to move away from them. Some of the patients in their study actually used their unaffected right hands to pull the left hand away, even though they were capable of moving the left hand.

Lack of or *feeble participation of the contralateral limb in bimanual tasks* such as opening a jar, clapping, or gesturing is another characteristic. Patients also may be reluctant to let the affected arm swing and may allow their affected leg to drag when walking. In some cases the authors reported that there appeared to be a problem in appreciating

the energy needed for a given movement. For example, patients moved their heads down to their hands when asked to touch their nose with their left hand.

Often when a patient with motor neglect does move his or her left extremities, the movement is slower, less forceful, or decreased in amplitude compared to movement in the right limbs. Coslett and Heilman (1989) refered to problems in moving the contralesional extremities as "hemihypokinesia," a term that combines the notion of failure to move (akinesia) or failure to move fully (hypometria) with the hemispace location of the affected limb. They addressed the incidence of hemihypokinesia in RHD and LHD patients by comparing shoulder elevation in matched subject pairs. Shoulder movement often is influenced less by lesions of the motor cortex and pyramidal tracts than are movements of the arm and hand. As expected, all subjects were able to move their ipsilesional shoulders higher than their contralesional shoulders. However, although the two groups did not differ in arm and hand strength, there were marked differences between them in contralesional shoulder elevation. LHD subjects could elevate their contralesional shoulders to within 43% of the height to which they elevated their ipsilesional ones. RHD subjects were able to elevate their contralesional shoulders to only 4% of the height of their ipsilesional shoulders. There was a positive relationship between the level of elevation and arm and hand strength in LHD, but not in RHD subjects. Many of the RHD subjects did not elevate their contralesional shoulders at all. Only two of the RHD subjects had other signs of neglect, supporting the notion that motor neglect may exist independently of other neglect symptoms.

The nature of motor neglect remains elusive. There are those who question whether neglect can occur at the level of elementary motor organization without an explanatory or scanning component (Weintraub & Mesulam, 1987). It represents neither a primary motor deficit, as the patient is capable of movement, nor an apraxia, as movements are formed adequately when the underutilized limb actually moves.

Laplane and Degos (1983) referred to motor neglect as a deficit in movement "preprogramming and organization" (p. 155), suggesting a deficit at an earlier stage than motor programming. Spontaneous movement requires a reason or intention to act, and intention to act is considered by some to be connected to premotor aspects of movement. Lesions associated with motor neglect involve areas that affect motor preparation and planning, such as the parietal association areas, the premotor cortex, supplementary motor areas, and the thalamus (Coslett & Heilman, 1989; Weintraub & Mesulam, 1987). These are areas in which neuronal activity increases *before* movement is initiated. Intention has been described as the "physiologic readiness to respond" (Heilman, Valenstein, & Watson, 1984, p. 215). Thus, motor neglect might be the result of a deficit in the intention and preparation for movement which, once initiated, is executed normally. Intention is, of course, closely tied to attention, which is a factor in all forms of neglect. Motor neglect is important to patients' physical recovery and should be considered a factor in the greater incidence of contralesional motor impairments found among RHD patients.

Directional Hypokinesia

Directional hypokinesia also is considered a disorder of premotor movement or motor preparation that is relatively independent of primary motor deficits. It refers to a direction-specific disorder in initiating movements toward contralesional space (Heilman, Bowers, Coslett, Whelan, & Watson, 1985). That is, patients with the disorder have problems *moving either the contralesional or the ipsilesional limbs into, toward, or within, contralesional space* (Bisiach et al., 1990). First noted in primates (Watson, Miller, & Heilman, 1978), Heilman et al. (1985) demonstrated it in humans in a simple task

that showed that initiation of movement toward contralesional space was slower than the initiation of movement toward ipsilesional space. Because the task did not require attention to a visual stimulus in left hemispace, the authors attributed their findings to an independent deficit in directional hypokinesia.

Several investigators have tried to determine if directional hypokinesia may play a role in the impoverished manual exploration of left hemispace and in "visual" scan and search tasks such as line bisection and cancellation. There is some evidence for the contribution of directional hypokinesia to performance on these tasks by patients with neglect (Bisiach et al., 1990). Some researchers, however, have not found it to be a factor (Mijovic, 1991). Others have found it is a factor in some neglect patients but not in others (Coslett, Bowers, Fitzpatrick, Haws, & Heilman, 1990). Some have found it to be only one of several directional-component factors contributing to neglect (Reuter-Lornez & Posner, 1990).

Directional hypokinesia helps us understand that moving the limbs in a leftward direction in either left or right hemispace may be a factor in neglect. It may play a greater role in some tasks compared to others, depending on the manual demands of the task. Clinicians should consider its possible contribution to impaired cancellation and visual search tasks that call for a manual response. It also may be a factor in activities of daily living that involve bilateral limb movement, such as dressing, grooming, cooking and eating, and in any situation in which manual exploration of left space is called for. Finally, it may play a role in visual (nonmanual) search tasks that require leftward eye movements.

VISUAL LINGUISTIC NEGLECT: READING AND WRITING

Patients with left neglect may omit letters and strokes in writing and make inappropriate use of margins because of neglect.

This disorder is sometimes called *neglect dysgraphia* or *spatial agraphia*. Patients with left neglect also may ignore the left side of words, sentences, or the page of written text. This disorder is sometimes referred to as *neglect dyslexia*. Both forms of neglect are almost always accompanied by other signs of visual neglect, but in rare cases, neglect dyslexia has appeared in isolation (Halligan & Marshall, 1993). Typically, patients with neglect dyslexia also have neglect dysgraphia (Ardila & Rosselli, 1993). Some patients with neglect dyslexia ignore the left half of words that are positioned horizontally, but are able to read the same words when they are presented vertically and read from top to bottom. Other patients may have problems in both formats, suggesting that they not only have left neglect, but a lower quadrant neglect that interferes with attention to the bottom half of a display.

In the cognitive science literature, there is debate about the nature of neglect dyslexia and the stage of processing in which it occurs (Caramazza & Hillis, 1990; Ellis et al., 1987; Nichelli, Venneri, Pentore, & Cubelli, 1993). When words are presented in nonstandard formats (rotated or mirror-reversed), it has been found that some patients neglect the initial (left) half of words in all presentations (Ellis et al., 1987). That is, whatever part of a word occurs in left space, it is ignored whether the word is presented upright or upside down or mirror reversed, which argues for a spatial attention deficit. Other patients have been found to neglect the same half of words, regardless of their spatial orientation (upside down or mirror reversed) (Caramazza & Hillis, 1990). For example, the beginning of the word "sidewalk" might be neglected even when presented in a rotated display, suggesting a problem not with the spatial presentation of the stimulus so much as with its internal representation (i.e., neglect operating on the internal word-map rather than on external space). Exploration of these issues is helpful in developing models of the mechanisms and stages of normal

reading and in improving our understanding of various reading disorders, including neglect dyslexia. Clinically, most patients are tested for neglect in standard formats aimed at uncovering problems at the level of spatial attention. As our understanding of other levels of disruption improves, patients may be examined with more sophisticated measures. However, at this point, they typically are given single words and passages to read in standard format, which is reflected in the clinical descriptions presented below.

Single Word Reading

Reading single words that are not embedded in a text can result in the types of errors listed in Table 2–4, of which letter substitutions are the most common, and additions are the least common (Ellis, Young, & Flude, 1993). Substitutions often contain the same or nearly the same number of letters as the target word (e.g., "cable" for "sable" or "nibble" for "scribble"). Neglect often gets worse as the horizontal length of the word increases (i.e., longer words or wider letter spacing) (Behrmann, Moscovitch, Black, & Mozer, 1990; Ellis et al., 1993). RHD patients with neglect typically will ignore the *left* side (versus the beginning) of a word, regardless of whether the word is in an upright, inverted, or mirror-reversed position (Ellis et al., 1993; Riddoch et al., 1990). As stated earlier, however, they may have problems reading the bottom

TABLE 2–4. Single word reading errors in neglect.

- Omission of left-most letters ("order" for "disorder")
- Omission of the left half of compound words ("house" for "greenhouse")
- Initial letter substitutions ("fine" for "pine")
- Initial letter additions ("class" for "lass")
- Left-most letter substitutions and additions ("compute" for "refute")

half of words in a vertical array if the bottom letters are in the lower quadrant of the page.

Hemianopia and neglect result in different types of single word errors. Patients with neglect ignore the left sides of words even when the word is presented in the right visual field (Ellis et al., 1987; Kinsbourne & Warrington, 1962; Young, Newcombe, & Ellis, 1991). Patients with hemianopia, on the other hand, make errors only when portions of words fall in their left visual field. They read words in their unimpaired visual field normally. Finally, neglect results most often in letter substitutions while hemianopia results in letter omissions.

For patients with both neglect and hemianopia, the hemispatial location of a word may make a difference in the type of errors made. When words are in central space, these patients have a tendency to omit letters on the left, particularly if another word is embedded to the right (e.g., "bin" for "cabin"). When words are moved into the right visual field (which is also right hemispace if the patient's eyes and head are aligned forward), hemianopia is overcome and letter *substitutions* (characteristic of neglect) will occur because the neglect continues to disrupt reading, but allows for some level of unconscious processing (i.e., the first two letters of "cabin").

Substitutions of the same length support the idea that letters are seen, but not fully processed, in neglect. This type of processing is called *implicit processing*, and it occurs in various other forms of neglect. It may be a factor in performance variability when real words versus nonwords or letter strings are used. Most studies, for example, have found that neglect is worse when reading nonwords (Behrmann et al., 1990; Brunn & Farah, 1991; Sieroff, Pollatsek, & Posner, 1988). The ability to recognize the difference between a word and a letter string suggests that neglect patients have processed the letters on the left at some level and that top-down processing has contributed to the process. In this sense,

words may operate much like objects (Brunn & Farah, 1991; Farah, Wallace, & Vecera, 1993). Farah et al. (1993) suggested that patients with neglect are more likely to process patterns that represent objects as complete or whole patterns than those that represent nonobjects. Words can be considered objects even though their properties are more abstract than those of physical objects. Exactly how patients can determine that a string of letters is a word or object without recognizing the word itself is not clear and continues to be explored experimentally. Whatever the mechanism, it must be assumed that some processing has taken place, even if it is not available to the conscious mind of the patient.

Ellis et al. (1993) suggested that much depends on expectations. If patients expect a real word, they may more readily substitute a real word for the partial word they perceive (i.e., "sofa" when they perceive "ofa"). If they know in advance that the word is a nonsense word, they have no resources to draw on, and they may not make the effort to overcome the orientational bias that draws them to the right-most letters in the string. Even when reading real words, once they are satisfied that they have read an actual word, patients with neglect usually make no effort to determine if it is correct.

Cuing patients to the left typically improves performance whether the cues are verbal reminders to look to the left or some other means of enhancing the saliency of the left-sided letters such as boldface print (Ellis et al., 1993). The effectiveness of cues is transient, however. Nonetheless, it suggests that voluntary attention to the left can, if briefly, overcome neglect in reading.

Text Reading

Patients with neglect are usually much better at single word reading than text reading (Kartsounis & Warrington, 1989). This difference is demonstrated nicely by the following example of a patient who read four

---

GRANDFATHER *PASSAGE*

You wish to know all about *my grandfather. Well,*
he is nearly 93 years old, yet *he still thinks as swiftly as*
ever. He dresses himself in *an old black frock coat,*
usually with several buttons missing. *A long beard clings to*
his chin, giving those *who observe him a pronounced*
feeling of the utmost respect. *When he speaks, his*
voice is just a bit cracked and *quivers a bit. Twice each*
day he plays skillfully and *with zest upon a small organ.*
Except in the winter when the *snow or ice prevents, he*
slowly takes *a short walk in the open air each day. We*
have often urged him to *walk more and smoke less, but*
he always answers, "Banana oil!" *Grandfather likes to*
be modern in his *language.*

Figure 2–10. The "Grandfather Passage" as read out loud by a patient with severe neglect. The underlined words in italics are the only words the patient read.

out of six single words correctly, but had extreme difficulty reading a short passage. The passage is printed in Figure 2–10 as it was presented to the patient. He was asked to read it out loud, and the words he read aloud are underlined and italicized.

The patient's reading was halting and slow with a number of phrase repetitions, as if he were trying to make sense of what he was reading as he went along. Not surprisingly, when finished, he said, "I don't get it at all." As one can observe in the example, patients often stop at a point at which a part of a sentence makes sense on its own, even if it does not make sense within the context of the text as a whole. If the examiner points out that their reading of a passage makes no sense in the wider context, some patients confabulate to make the text make sense as they have read it, or find fault with the material or even with the examiner for giving them something nonsensical to read. Others, like the patient in the above example, act resigned, but

show no interest in understanding *why* the text is confusing.

Karnath and Huber (1992) recorded the eye movements of a left-neglect patient as he read a text and found that, unlike normal readers who make a sweeping leftward saccade once the right margin is reached, his leftward saccade ended approximately at midline. He then made several short leftward saccades that were indicative of silent backward reading. His eyes moved in a right-to-left direction with fixations on each word until an appropriate, if inaccurate, continuation of the text was found. Thus, the extent of leftward omissions varied, a finding commonly observed clinically. Another subject in their study, however, stopped at the same place of the initial return sweep every time and kept reading, regardless of how nonsensical the text became. When patients do this, it seems that each line is processed as a unit that bears no relationship to the text as a whole.

Writing

Neglect dysgraphia, as neglect in writing is sometimes called, usually co-occurs with neglect in reading. The most notable sign is underutilization of the left margin. Writing typically is squeezed onto the far right side of the page (Figure 2–6). What is written there often contains letter and stroke omissions and sometimes extra strokes. In addition, the lines of writing typically slant up toward the right. Sometimes there are random blank spaces between the letters, and sometimes words are split inappropriately, particularly when the right edge of the page is reached. The left margin established by the patient, regardless of how far over to the right it is, may not be maintained. For example the first line may have four words, the next may have two or three, and the rest trail down the page, one word to a line in a cascading pattern.

Omissions and extra strokes are error patterns similar to those of NBD subjects when writing with their eyes closed. This suggests that neglect patients may suffer from reduced visual and kinesthetic feedback when writing (Ellis et al., 1993). Omissions may be explained by the occurrence of neglect in right or ipsilesional hemispace. Extra strokes and letter repetitions could be attributed to a narrowed focus of attention in which a given letter is over attended to. Usually, there also is a failure to dot *i*'s and cross *t*'s. One explanation for these omissions is that these marks typically are produced after one is finished writing a word, requiring a leftward hand movement and leftward visual scan (back to the beginning of the word) (Ellis et al., 1993).

Ardila and Rosselli (1993) found that error type differs according to lesion site within the RH. They found that frontal damage resulted in feature and letter iterations, which they suggested might be associated with motor perseveration. Postrolandic damage resulted most often in spatial disruptions such as under-use of the left half of the page, line slanting, instability of the left margin established by the patient, and other spatially based errors.

BEHAVIORAL ANOMALIES ASSOCIATED WITH NEGLECT

Unconscious Perception

The frequency of letter substitutions, as opposed to omissions, in neglect dyslexia suggests that, at some level, the physical stimulus has been processed, albeit not consciously. Examples of implicit or unconscious perception, sometimes called blind sight, abound in neglect. One of the best examples of this phenomenon is in a study by Marshall and Halligan (1988) who asked a woman with left neglect to determine if two drawings of a house were the same or different and to state which house she would rather live in (see Figure 2–11 for a similar type of drawing). She consistently said that the houses were the same, but also quite consistently picked the intact house as the one she would like to live in. Later, when the flames appeared on the right side of one of the houses, she noticed them. When the flames again were on the left, she still claimed the houses were identical until the fifth trial when she suddenly exclaimed that one house was on fire. The authors speculated that the picture of the flames on the right side had primed her so that insight was finally achieved. Her consistent preference for the intact house in all trials, however, demonstrates that she had processed the fire at some level.

Bisiach and Rusconi (1990) used the same paradigm with a group of RHD patients who were presented with pairs of objects, one of which was intact and one of which was damaged on the left side (e.g., broken glass, torn banknote). Subjects' responses about which object they would prefer were inconsistent. Some chose the broken objects and confabulated reasons why. Others chose the intact objects, but did not refer directly to the damage in their explanation. For example, one subject said

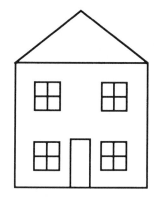

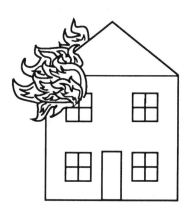

Figure 2–11. A rendition of the type of stimuli used by Marshall and Halligan (1988) to demonstrate unconscious perception on the part of a patient with RHD and neglect. Patients with neglect tend to claim the two houses are identical, but choose the one free of flames as the one they would like to live in.

he chose the intact glass because the other one had less capacity.

The objects in the above studies were arrayed vertically. When objects are presented horizontally, patients with neglect often are able to detect differences between them, but they may be unable to name the left-sided object (Volpe, Le Doux, & Gazzaniga, 1979). That is, they can detect enough to discriminate left-sided input, but not to name it accurately. As Farah, Monheit, and Wallace (1991) pointed out, discrimination can be based on low-level stimulus properties whereas naming depends on more complete visual information. According to Ladavas (1990), one must focus attention on and be consciously aware of a given stimulus before one can produce an arbitrary response, such as naming it. She suggested that left-sided input is not "aligned" with the focus of attention so, although it may influence unconscious processing, it has no impact on conscious awareness. That which does not stimulate a response automatically requires a "commitment of conscious attention" (Ladavas, 1990, p. 1537), which is often lacking in patients with neglect.

Anosognosia

Anosognosia, another behavioral anomaly associated with neglect, is quite the opposite of unconscious perception. A term first coined by Babinski (1914), *anosognosia means lack of knowledge or awareness of disease.* In particular, in patients with neglect, it refers to failure to recognize hemiplegia and/or hemianopia and hemisensory loss. It may extend to failure to recognize one's hemiplegic limbs as one's own. Patients may claim their arm or leg is missing, has been replaced by a useless or "dummy" arm, or even by someone else's arm. Alternately, they may claim that nothing whatever is wrong with their limbs, yet fail to move them, and state emphatically that they have done so, even when they have not. Occasionally, confusion between what they believe and reality will result in confabulatory explanations such as, "I would have moved my own arm, but somebody took it and left me with this one that doesn't work right."

Anosognosia, thus, can include three types of symptoms: (a) *failure to notice and/or use the contralesional limbs,* (b) *denial of hemiplegia or minimizing its impact,* and (c) *recognition of hemiplegia, but failure to claim ownership of contralesional limbs.* Any or all of these symptoms may lead the patient to overestimate his or her physical capacity and to adopt a cavalier attitude toward the need for physical rehabilitation. Typically, these deficits go along with denial of neglect itself and speak to the lack of awareness and insight that sometimes can be intractable to external explanation and demonstrations. Anosognosia is associated with RHD and rarely occurs with LHD (Bisiach, Vallar, Perani, Papagno, & Berti, 1986; Cutting, 1978; Green & Hamilton, 1976; see McGlynn & Schacter, 1989 for a review). It can occur in other disorders such as Anton's Syndrome in which there is unawareness of blindness. And it can occur without other signs of neglect, at least as measured on traditional tasks (Bisiach, Vallar, et al., 1986; McGlynn & Schacter, 1989). In general, however, anosognosia is accompanied by other signs of neglect (Heilman & Valenstein, 1972b; Hier et al., 1983; Willanger, Danielsen, & Ankerhus, 1981) and may be considered part of the syndrome when it occurs in neglect patients with unilateral RHD.

Interestingly, anosognosia usually is specific to a localized deficit, whereas other, more global deficits are acknowledged (Cutting, 1978). For example, patients often state that they have had a stroke or a heart attack or suffer from some other disease, while denying specific impairments such as hemiplegia. Thus, patients may admit to the stroke, but not to its consequences. Even when discussing the stroke, anosognosic patients are often indirect, saying things like, "They tell me I've had a stroke," rather than "I had a stroke."

Anosognosia is not considered a form of denial in the psychological sense of a defense mechansim motivated by unwillingness to confront physical or psychological problems (McGlynn & Schacter, 1989). Its greater incidence in RHD versus LHD, its consistent association with specific lesion sites (parietal and frontal), and its specificity relative to type of deficit denied argue against defensive denial.

Early investigators suggested that anosognosia was the result of a disturbed "body schema" due to failure to integrate perceptual information in the parietal lobes (Denny-Brown, Meyer, & Horenstein, 1952; Frederiks, 1969). However, damage to the frontal lobes also can produce anosognosia, and not all parietal patients with hemiplegia have anosognosia.

Most modern theories attribute anosognosia to a disturbance in an internal monitoring system that involves both the parietal and frontal lobes. The frontal lobes have been thought to monitor various cognitive functions (Stuss & Benson, 1986). The parietal lobes are considered an area of sensory association and integration. The parietal and frontal lobes are extensively interconnected (Mesulam, 1981; Heilman, Valenstein, et al., 1984), and there is evidence that there are areas in both parietal and frontal cortex where visual, somatosensory, and auditory pathways converge (McGlynn & Schacter, 1989).

Several models of cognitive monitoring have been proposed to explain anosognosia. Bisiach, Vallar, et al. (1986) suggested that cognitive monitoring may be modality-specific, resulting in denial of specific deficits. McGlynn and Schacter (1989) agreed that there may be modular representation in an overall system they called the "conscious awareness system" or CAS. In their model, input to the CAS comes from the output of perceptual, memory, and knowledge modules. The output of the CAS itself flows to an "executive system" in the frontal lobes, which is involved in the "initiation, organization, and monitoring of complex sequences of ideas and actions" (p. 190). The frontal lobes are known to be associated with integrative functions and with what are sometimes called "executive" functions such as planning and organizing. In their model, damage to the CAS would create a general awareness deficit. Damage to one of its input modules would create an anosognosia for a specific disorder. Both a general and a specific anosognosia could occur as a result of parietal damage. Damage to the "executive system" in the frontal lobes would result in unawareness of more complex and less physically obvious cognitive deficits such as problems in planning, problem solving, and the behavioral changes typically associated with head injury. As the authors pointed out, however, their model makes no attempt to explain the prevalence of anosognosia with RH versus LH lesions.

Yet, it is not surprising that anosognosia is so often associated with neglect and hence with RHD. The effects of damage in the RH on attentional processes in general and on directional scanning in particular suggest that impaired attention may be a factor in the laterality of anosognosia and in the specificity of the deficits that are denied. Hemiplegia, for example, occurs on the left of the body and the left side of space relative to midline. Without active attention to and monitoring of this part of the patient's universe, it slips from conscious awareness and presumably is more readily denied.

LOCALIZATION

Several factors should be taken into account in the following discussion of lesion location and neglect. First, different researchers use different types of tests to establish the presence of neglect (e.g., paper-and-pencil tasks, computerized reaction time tasks, behavioral observation). Some studies use only one task; others use several. Second, the criteria used to define neglect may vary. It may be defined very loosely (e.g., missing any target on a cancellation task) or have a very restricted definition (e.g., missing one third of the targets to the left of center in a cancellation task). Third, the time post onset and the etiology among subjects in localization studies is not consistent.

Numerous cortical and subcortical sites have been associated with neglect (see Table 2–5). The number of sites associated with neglect suggests that there may be different sites for different *types* of neglect. Finally, it suggests that the functions disrupted by neglect may be part of an attentional network that involves a variety of cortical and subcortical structures to be fully operational (Heilman & Watson, 1977; Heilman et al., 1987; Mesulam, 1985). Damage to one part of the system may have distant effects on other parts of the system. Metabolic studies suggest that the mechanism for the representation of space also involves neural networks with contributions from both cortical and subcortical structures (Vallar, 1993). For example, directional hypokinesia has been found in parietal and frontal lesions (Bisiach et al., 1990; Coslett et al., 1990; Heilman et al., 1985; Tegner & Levander, 1991). Motor neglect has been associated with frontal lesions (Laplane & Degos, 1983) and parietal lesions (Barbieri & De Renzi, 1989), as well as with subcortical lesions (Watson & Heilman, 1979; Vallar, 1993). Clinically, patients with large middle cerebral artery infarcts that result in fronto-parietal lesions often demonstrate neglect on traditional measures and in their activities of daily living. Severity and persistence of neglect have been associated with large lesions that encompass the parietal lobes as well as subcortical regions (Egelko et al., 1988; Hier et al., 1983). Hier et al. found that neglect following restricted lesions in cortical and subcortical areas often is transient and not very severe. Horner et al. (1989), on the other hand, found no significant correlation between size of lesion and severity of neglect on a variety of tests.

Cortical Lesions

Left neglect is associated most frequently with damage in the right parietal lobe, particularly its inferior and posterior portions (Vallar, 1993; Vallar & Perani, 1987). Types of neglect specifically associated with parietal lesions include: (a) *multimodal extinction* (Heilman & Valenstein, 1979), (b) *neglect of the left half of visual images* (Bisiach, Capitani, Luzzatti, & Perani, 1981), (c) *difficulty disengaging from right-sided stimuli* (Posner, Walker, et al., 1987); and (d) *directional hypokinesia* (Heilman et al., 1985).

TABLE 2–5. Association of types of neglect with lesion site.

Lesion Site	Type of Neglect
Cortical Sites	
Right Parietal Lobe	Multimodal extinction
	Viewer- and environment-centered visual neglect
	Perceptual aspects of visual scanning
	Difficulty disengaging right-sided focus of attention
	Directional hypokinesia
Right Frontal Lobe	Motor aspects of visual scanning
	Visual orientation
	Directional hypokinesia
Subcortical Sites	
Right Thalamus	Difficulty engaging attention toward contralateral stimuli
	Aspects of arousal and selective attention
Basal Ganglia	Extinction
	Visual scanning

Lesions restricted to the frontal lobe are less frequently associated with neglect, but are thought to affect motor aspects involved in visual scanning and orientation (Mesulam, 1981, 1985). For example, the frontal eye fields, which are just rostral to premotor cortex, are connected to various cortical and subcortical structures that play a role in visual scanning. Mesulam, among others, has suggested that frontal neglect produces a motor neglect whereas parietal neglect is more perceptual in nature. Indeed, Bisiach et al. (1990) found that directional hypokinesia was much more pronounced in patients with frontal damage than in patients with posterior damage.

Subcortical Lesions

Neglect can occur with subcortical lesions, although less often than with cortical lesions. Subcortical lesion sites associated with neglect include the thalamus, the basal ganglia, and the internal capsule. Thalamic neglect has been reported most often (Rafal & Posner, 1987; Vallar & Perani, 1986; Watson & Heilman, 1979; Wat-son, Valenstein, & Heilman, 1981), and appears to affect the ability for contralateral stimuli to engage (versus disengage or move) attention toward contralateral stimuli (Rafal & Posner, 1987). Posterior thalamic lesions are more likely than anterior damage to produce neglect (Vallar, 1993). Medial and posterior areas of the thalamus have been considered by some to be part of an attentional network that also includes association cortex and the reticular formation, which mediates aspects of arousal and selective attention (Watson et al., 1981; Mesulam, 1985).

Lesions of the basal ganglia and the internal capsule also have been linked to neglect (Damasio, Damasio, & Chang Chui, 1980; Fero, Kertesz, & Black, 1987; Fromm, Holland, Swindell, & Reinmuth, 1985; Vallar & Perani, 1986), although much less frequently than thalamic lesions. Vallar (1993) suggested that the posterior thalamus and the posterior limb of the internal capsule may be associated with neglect as part of a neural circuit that includes posterior and inferior parietal cortex and plays an important role in visual attention.

THEORIES OF NEGLECT

Theories about the nature of neglect are constantly evolving, but fall into two general categories, representational and attentional, each of which specifies different mechanisms for the observed symptoms. *Representational theories* attribute neglect to a *disruption of the internal representation of space. Attentional theories* attribute it to *impaired attentional mechanisms that disturb the ability to orient, select, and/or distribute attention across spatial boundaries.* Theories of neglect must account for several key phenomena, including: (a) *the greater frequency of neglect with RHD versus LHD,* (b) *the occurrence of neglect in ipsilesional as well as contralesional space,* and (c) *the occurrence of neglect in internal images, independent of external stimulation.* It is hoped that the following discussion will help the reader understand more about the manifestations, complexities, and impact of neglect on the daily life and cognitive function of patients with the disorder.

Representational Theories

As stated in the section on frames of reference, space exists outside of us, yet the concept of space is a mental or psychological construct. Most cognitive scientists agree on the existence of mental representations of external input, but there is considerable uncertainty and disagreement about their form and the mechanisms supporting them. A representation is an abstract code or mental construct that specifies the external world. We use this abstract form of space and spatial relations to perform operations such as navigating, reaching, and searching. We also construct internal images of space. When we close our eyes, we can access a mental image of a room through visual imagery without any direct visual input to support the image. That is, we can access visual memories that help us construct the spatial configuration of visual images.

There are two basic tenets in the representational theory. The first is that *the representation of space and spatial relations is mapped topologically across the two hemispheres.* That is, space is considered to be coded in an iconic fashion like a map with the left half of space (or left half of objects) represented in the RH, and the right half of space (or of an object) in the LH (Bisiach et al., 1981; Ogden, 1985a). The second tenet is that *the contralesional half of these mental representations is under-represented in patients with neglect.* Because the left half of space is under-represented in the RHD patient's mental construct, he or she has no expectation for events occurring there. Support for neglect as a disruption of the internal representation of space comes from studies in which neglect can be demonstrated in the absence of external sensory input.

For example, while sleeping, neglect patients may have a reduction of rapid eye movements (REMs) toward the contralesional side (Doricchi, Guariglia, Paolucci, & Pizzamiglio, 1990). Because patients with neglect are capable of making eye movements in a contralesional direction and REMs occur in the absence of sensory input, these results support the idea that, in neglect, the mental representation of space is impoverished. Hornak (1992) found the same pattern when subjects were asked to search a darkened room to determine if a light was present. Unlike control subjects, subjects with neglect confined their search in the dark almost exclusively to the right side of the room, suggesting that their internal image of the room was under-represented. When questioned, subjects with neglect said they were not aware that they had not fully searched contralateral space. Their responses contributed to the sense that the left side of space may be attenuated in their internal conceptualization of it.

The main support for representational theories comes from studies demonstrating that patients may neglect the left half or contralesional side of recalled or reconstructed images. In the classic experiment of this type, Bisiach and his colleagues asked several subjects to verbally recall a familiar city plaza in Milan from different vantage points (Bisiach & Luzzatti, 1978; Bisiach et al., 1981). In the first condition, subjects were asked to imagine themselves standing at one end of the square, facing the cathedral. In the second condition they were asked to imagine themselves at the opposite end of the square, with their backs to the cathedral. In both conditions the number of details they reported from the left was compared to the number they reported from the right of the imagined scene. Subjects reported fewer details from the left side of the scene in both conditions (i.e., regardless of the vantage point subjects were asked to adopt). In addition, details (shops, landmarks, etc.) from the left side often were transposed to the right in the subjects' descriptions. Subjects' failure to fully describe the left side could not be attributed to impaired memory because they were able to transpose their memories of the scene from one side to the other. It appeared instead that, regardless of the image they were trying to reconstruct, they omitted left-sided information. Using the baseball diamond example mentioned at the beginning of this chapter, if one imagined oneself at home plate, second and third base might be absent in the mental picture. If one shifted one's perspective to center field, facing home plate, first base would be absent in the mental image conjured up.

Another type of study dealing with imaginal space uses the reconstruction of images that are presented to subjects in segments as they pass behind a small slit-like aperture or opening (Bisiach, Luzzatti, & Perani, 1979; Ogden, 1985b). In these investigations, cloud-like shapes are passed horizontally in a right- or leftward direction behind a screen with a centrally located slit. Only a small portion of a given pattern or shape is visible to the subject through the opening as it passes from right to left or from left to right. Subjects must create or reconstruct a mental image of the shape based on successive presentations of only portions of it. They are then asked to make same-different judgments about pairs of shapes that they have mentally reconstructed as the cloud-like shapes pass behind the aperture. Findings suggest that subjects with neglect are less accurate when the crucial information about shape is located on the contralesional side. The implication is that subjects "neglected" the contralesional side of the internal image they generated to represent the pattern. Recall that the pattern was never displayed as a whole; subjects had to generate an image or representation of it, and it was this internal image that was flawed.

Evidence of impaired left-sided representations also comes from studies of olfactory neglect in which RHD subjects extinguished left-sided stimulation (Bellas et al., 1988a, 1988b; Mesulam, 1981). Because the olfactory system is predominantly ipsilaterally innervated, most of the sensation of smell from the left nostril goes to the intact left hemisphere. Thus, left-sided extinction of olfactory stimuli suggests that it is the representation of space, not sensation or perception, that has been disturbed. Finally, motor neglect and anosognosia have been cited in support of the representational theory. It is thought that such problems lie in an under-representation of the left side of the body so that in the patient's mind left-sided body parts are not there and thus cannot be moved.

The representational theory offers an explanation for why patients demonstrate neglect in constructing internal images of scenes, images, patterns, body parts, and dreams. However, dissociations between neglect of perceived input and neglect of imaginal space have been reported that contradict the explanation that neglect of visual or external space can be explained by distorted mental images (Bartolomeo, D'Erme, & Gainotti, 1994; Coslett, 1997; Guariglia, Padovani, Pantano, & Pizzamiglio, 1993). That is, there are some patients who neglect the left half of mental images, but perform well on tasks in which they must attend to the left half of external images (e.g., paper-and-pencil tests of neglect). There are other patients who demonstrate the opposite pattern. These dissociations suggest that neglect may operate on more than one mechanism for spatial construction. Coslett (1997) suggested that there may be one mechanism that controls external scanning and one that directs internal scanning of mental images and that these two systems can be disrupted independently of one another. Thus, disruptions in the representation of space do not necessarily explain neglect of external visual input, because some patients may show neglect in internal images, but not in visuospatial tasks. In addition, it has been proposed that impaired production of mental images may be accounted for by failure to direct attention toward the left-half of fully formed mental images, rather than by a weak representation of the image itself (Meador, Loring, Bowers, & Heilman, 1987).

There are several things the representational theory cannot explain. First, it cannot explain why neglect is more frequent and severe in RHD compared to LHD. Why would not the right side of space be just as vulnerable to damage in the LH as the left side of space is to damage in the RH? Second, it cannot explain neglect of ipsilesional stimuli. If spatial representations were mapped across the hemispheres in topological fashion, one would not expect neglect of contralesional information in ipsilesional space. Third, it cannot explain the apparent hyperattraction of rightward stimuli seen in many cases of left neglect. And finally, it cannot explain the ameliorative effect of cueing attention to the left. Attention theories are better able to explain these phenomena.

Attention Theories

Attention theories of neglect propose that *neglect is the result of abnormalities in the dis-*

tribution of attention. Theories differ in the emphasis placed on various attentional operations proposed to account for impaired attentional distribution, but they are united in their proposition that both reduced perception of external input and deficient internal images are the result of deficits in attention. Attentional theories are supported by an undisputed fact: *When attention is cued to the contralesional side, neglect is almost always reduced, regardless of the task.* Patients cued to look to the left, for example, typically discover information previously ignored. The facilitatory effect of cueing suggests that voluntary attention can be used to overcome deficits in more automatic aspects of attention. In addition, attention theories can explain the phenomena cited to support representational theories. Riddoch and Humphries (1987), for example, suggested that representational neglect may be explained just as easily by failure to direct attention toward and/or covertly scan the contralesional side of mental images as it can be by invoking a distorted representation as the primary deficit or cause. According to them, attention theories help explain why the recall of left-sided detail was improved by cueing in the scene-recall task of Bisiach et al. (1979). Cueing can be considered a manipulation of attention, and it would not have been facilitatory had the image itself been under-represented on one side. One cannot attend to what is not there.

It is understood that no one type of attentional deficit can explain all aspects of neglect. Attentional operations potentially impaired by RHD include *arousal, orienting, vigilance, selection, and intention,* all of which may impact on spatial attention. Different types of neglect, may, in fact, represent deficits in separate components of the attentional system. Attentional theories include *orienting bias theories* that suggest neglect is an impairment in orienting attention, and *directed attention theories* that relate it to a more general attentional impairment. According to attentional theories, the left side of space or objects is not under-represented in the brain. It simply is not attended to and, hence, has no impact on awareness.

Impaired Attentional Orienting

Attention theories help to explain why neglect is so much more prevalent and more devastating in RHD than in LHD patients. It is accepted that each cerebral hemisphere directs attention toward the opposite side of space. That is, the LH directs attention rightward and the RH directs attention leftward. The two hemispheres act as opponent processors that mutually inhibit one another to achieve balance in orienting to the right and left. When damage occurs to one hemisphere, the other takes over or is disinhibited, directing attention in a contralesional direction. Thus, the unopposed LH directs attention rightward when RHD occurs, and the unopposed RH directs attention leftward when LHD occurs. Damage to the RH appears to upset this balance in orienting more than damage to the LH because, unlike the LH, the *RH is considered to have the capacity to distribute attention across hemispatial boundaries* (Heilman, Valenstein, et al., 1984; Heilman et al., 1987; Heilman & Van Den Abell, 1980; Ladavas et al., 1989; Mesulam, 1981). That is, the RH, like the LH is strongly oriented toward contralateral space, but it also appears to have some capacity to attend to ipsilateral space (Figure 2–12). Thus, when damage occurs in the LH, attention toward the right is diminished, but the RH is able to compensate somewhat by attending to the right, reducing the impact of neglect. When damage to the RH occurs, however, the LH is unable to compensate and the ensuing left neglect is more severe. A more detailed review of the dominance of the RH in this and other forms of attention is covered in the chapter on attention. For now it is necessary only to understand that an attentional account of neglect helps us understand the reasons why left neglect subsequent to RHD is so much more devastating than the right neglect that can occur subsequent to LHD.

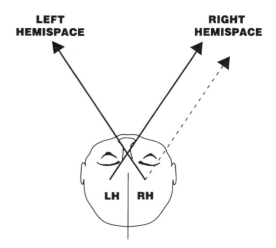

Figure 2–12. Right hemisphere dominance for attention. The two hemispheres direct attention toward the opposite hemispace (solid lines), but it is thought that the RH has some capacity to attend to right as well as to left hemispace (dotted line). When damage occurs in the LH, the RH can compensate somewhat by attending to right hemispace. When damage occurs in the RH, neglect is more severe because the LH lacks the capacity to compensate.

The strongest support for attention theories of neglect comes from studies in which attention has been isolated and studied independent of eye movements in reaction time tasks. Reaction time studies measure the speed with which a response (usually pressing or releasing a switch or the space bar on a computer) follows the presentation of a stimulus (usually a flash of light, an illuminated shape, or an auditory signal). Typically, patients with neglect are slower to respond to leftward stimuli than to rightward stimuli in reaction time tasks. It is assumed that they perceive the targets once they are located and that the delay is the result of impaired orienting of attention. In such studies, the movement of attention is assumed to precede and to be independent of eye movements. A now-classic paradigm designed by Posner and his colleagues demonstrated that this was so (Posner, Walker, Friedrich, & Rafal, 1984; Posner, Walker, et al., 1987). In their studies, a subject faced a computer screen on which a target would appear to the right or left of the center of the screen. Subjects fixed their gaze on a central fixation dot and a visual cue (e.g., an arrow or highlighted area) would signal the possible location of a target. Cues could be valid or invalid and served to shift attention to the cued location in anticipation of the target. Faster reaction times to validly cued locations indicated that a covert shift in attention had occurred toward the cued location and had improved response efficiency. Slower reaction times to invalidly cued locations indicated that attention had shifted to the wrong location, thus reducing response efficiency. The performance of patients with left neglect in such tasks confirms that, after an invalid cue to the right, shifting attention in relative leftward direction is more difficult than shifting attention rightward after an invalid left cue (Posner et al., 1984; Posner, Walker, et al., 1987; Farah, Wong, Monheit, & Morrow, 1989; Ladavas, 1993).

Based on their results, Posner et al. (1984, 1987) suggested three types of operations that are involved in covert attentional orienting: (1) *disengage,* which involves disengaging attention from its current focus; (2) *move,* which moves attention to a new location; and (3) *engage,* which focuses attention on the novel target or at the new location. They found that patients with parietal damage and neglect had particular problems *disengaging attention from an ipsilesional focus* and problems in *moving attention in a contralesional direction.* They also found that ipsilesional targets had an attentional advantage or a "capture effect," independent of their visual field or hemispace location. These results have been replicated with auditory stimuli (Farah et al., 1989) and with visual attention in the vertical dimension (Ladavas, 1993).

These findings help to explain the occurrence of neglect in non-neglected or ipsilesional space. Recall that, *when neglect occurs in the environmental frame of reference, the relative rightward position of a target will increase its saliency and the relative leftward position*

will decrease its saliency, regardless of its absolute hemispace location. In reaction time studies, subjects with left neglect not only are slower to respond to relative leftward targets, they also have been found to respond even *faster* than NBD controls to relative rightward targets, suggesting that their attention is automatically and consistently drawn rightward (Ladavas, Petronio, & Umilta, 1990). Attention in left neglect patients appears to be preset to the most rightward position so that any leftward shift of attention requires a correction of the directional bias and delays reaction times for leftward targets while shortening them for rightward targets (Ladavas, 1990). The results also suggest that the presence of rightward stimuli may have a deleterious effect on neglect because attention is drawn to or captured by them.

The finding that patients with neglect focus attention to the right even within ipsilesional space has been called "hyperattention" (Ladavas, 1993, p. 196), the "magnetic attraction" of the right (De Renzi, Gentilini, Faglioini, et al., 1989, p. 232), and the "attentional capture process" (Riddoch & Humphries, 1987, p. 170). Clinically, patients with neglect appear to have difficulty disengaging attention from rightward stimuli in a variety of tasks. They may, for example, overdraw rightward letters and numbers in writing tasks and right-sided details in drawing tasks. They may cancel individual items in right hemispace more than once in cancellation tasks.

There is some question as to whether attention is automatically drawn to the extreme right or whether a right-sided stimulus is necessary to evoke the hyperattraction. Mark, Kooistra, and Heilman (1988), for example, found that neglect was significantly reduced when subjects were asked to erase rather than draw over the lines in a cancellation task. The erasure condition obviously reduced the amount of right-sided stimuli, which seemed to help them more readily disengage and move attention leftward. When subjects were asked to color over lines in the second condition,

TABLE 2–6. Aspects of neglect explained by orienting deficits.

1. Automatic orienting toward rightward stimuli
2. The capture effect of right-sided stimuli
3. The occurrence of neglect in ipsilesional space
4. Narrowed focus of attention in ipsilesional space
5. Extinction of right-sided stimuli
6. The facilitatory effects of cueing attention to the left

they often did so several times, suggesting that they had trouble disengaging from a completed response. The authors also noted that some subjects colored over a line, colored over a more leftward line, and then colored over the original line again, as if their attention was drawn back again to the more rightward line. In neither condition was neglect eliminated, suggesting that not only is attention captured by rightward stimuli, but it also fails to be captured by leftward stimuli.

When confronted with bilateral visual stimulation in extinction tasks, some patients shoot their gaze in a sharp rightward direction. These immediate and deviant rightward eye movements have been called "magnetic gaze attraction" (Cohn, 1972). Patients with this problem generally look down and to the right during conversation and other forms of interaction, and it is difficult to get them to look forward on request. Rightward gaze attraction may be due to the *attentional* capture effect of right-sided stimuli. It tends to occur only in cases of severe neglect following RHD, and it

rarely, if ever, occurs following LHD (Gainotti, D'Erme, & Bartolomeo, 1991).

Studies of covert attentional orienting suggest that, in left neglect: (a) *attention is automatically oriented rightwards,* (b) *rightward stimuli attract attention even further,* and (c) *disengaging attention from rightward stimuli is particularly difficult when attention must be moved in a leftward direction.* Thus, attention theories of neglect offer a powerful explanation of ipsilesional neglect, for the stronger impairment subsequent to RHD versus LHD, and even for impaired construction of internal images. Table 2–6 lists aspects of neglect explained by orienting deficits. Underlying attention theories is the fact that neglect is sensitive to manipulations of attention independent of sensory and motor responses.

Impaired Directed Attention

Directed attention operates in the spatial domain, but it can also operate in the nonspatial, abstract domain of ideas and communication of those ideas. Orienting is considered just one aspect of directing attention. The term "directed" in directed attention refers not to the left-right direction of attentional focus, but rather to the multiple operations involved in directing or focusing attention toward a particular target. Table 2–7 identifies aspects of neglect that can be explained by an impairment in directed attention. For the most part, attentional orienting is considered an automatic process that is driven by primitive stimulus characteristics (i.e., shape, novelty, texture, line orientation, etc.) that

TABLE 2–7. Aspects of neglect explained by a deficit in the directed attention network.

1. Exploratory and scanning behavior in all sectors of space
2. Problems assessing stimulus significance in all sectors of space
3. Interaction of reduced attentional resources with attentional operations (arousal, vigilance, selective attention)
4. Relationship between types of neglect and site of lesion (frontal, parietal, subcortical)
5. Facilitatory effects of attentional cueing attention to the left

capture attention. Directed attention, on the other hand, encompasses arousal and the other, less automatic, attentional processes involved in aiming attention, such as the recognition of stimulus significance, expectations, motivation, and intention.

Proponents of attentional theories of neglect suggest that there is an interactive network of directed attention that has both a neurological and behavioral reality. Selective aspects of this attentional network may be impaired with differing consequences for and patterns of neglect behavior (see Heilman, Valenstein, et al., 1984; Heilman et al., 1987; and Mesulam, 1981, 1985 for reviews). Identification of this network and the impact of damage to it lends strong support to impaired attention as the underlying disturbance in neglect.

The proposed network includes cortical and subcortical areas and their interconnections. Accounts of it are based on extensive investigations of (a) single unit recordings of neurons in the primate brain, (b) behavior following circumscribed lesions in primates (ablation studies), (c) lesion localization in neglect patients, and (d) reaction time studies and various physiologic measures of arousal in non-neurologically impaired and brain-damaged adults. *Subcortical areas* in the network include (a) the reticular activating system, (b) the thalamus, and (c) the cingulate cortex in the limbic system. *Cortical areas* include (a) the posterior and inferior parietal lobe, and (b) the frontal lobe, particularly the frontal eye fields. Components of the network are outlined below to elucidate their impact on directed attention and on neglect.

The *reticular activating system* is considered crucial for arousal and overall readiness to respond. Bilateral lesions to the reticular activating system result in coma, whereas unilateral lesions result in contralateral inattention, which, according to Heilman et al. (1984), is likely the result of unilateral hypoarousal of the ipsilesional hemisphere. Reticular activating system damage may affect attention directly by reducing the readiness of the cortex to respond to input or it may affect it indirectly by reducing thalamic transmission to the cortex.

The *thalamus* is considered a relay station between the reticular formation and the cortex. Damage to various thalamic nuclei can result in a primary sensory loss. Damage to other thalamic areas (i.e., the nucleus reticularis) can result in impaired regulation or selective control over sensory input (Heilman, Valenstein, et al., 1984, 1987; Mesulam, 1981, 1985), which may be the source of neglect from thalamic lesions (Heilman, Valenstein, et al., 1984, 1987; Mesulam, 1981).

The *cingulate cortex* is part of the limbic system, which regulates affective behavior. Data from primates suggest that, via its connections to parietal cortex, the cingulate gyrus may specifically influence the perception of the motivational relevance of sensory events and the regulation of the spatial distribution of expectations for events (Mesulam, 1981). Medial frontal lesions in the cingulate area have been found to produce neglect in humans, possibly by interfering in limbic input to parietal areas where sensory information is further processed (Heilman & Valenstein, 1979; Mesulam, 1981).

Parietal lobe damage has long been associated with neglect. Certain areas in the parietal lobe, particularly the inferior parietal lobe, are considered areas of polymodal sensory integration. Neurons in these association areas respond to input from more than one modality. It is thought that these areas are important not only in detecting stimulus novelty, but also in detecting stimulus significance (Heilman, Valenstein, et al., 1984). For example, single unit recordings of neurons in these areas in primates have established that neurons in this area fire *prior* to reaching when the animal detects a motivationally relevant object such as food (Mesulam, 1981). This area also has extensive efferent projections to limbic and frontal areas. The frontal lobes may help establish the significance of stimuli to goal states while limbic connections may help establish biological needs. As Heilman, Valenstein, et al. (1984) stated, "these connections may provide an anatomic substrate by which motivational states (e.g., biological needs, sets, and long-term goals) may influence stimulus processing" (p. 211).

The *frontal lobes* may help to establish the significance of stimuli based not on stimulus characteristics per se, nor on biological needs, but on more abstract goals and objectives. In addition, certain areas in the frontal lobes are considered crucial for visual exploratory behavior. The frontal eye fields (Broadman's area 8, just rostral to premotor cortex), for example, by virtue of their reciprocal connections to the superior colliculus and sensory association areas in the parietal lobes, may play a considerable role in visual search, in the motor aspects of visual scanning and orienting, and possibly also in reaching (Mesulam, 1985). The superior colliculus in the midbrain is involved in detecting stimuli in the periphery of the visual fields and is heavily connected to the frontal eye fields. These connections may help to establish the motor plan within the area of space to be scanned.

Interestingly, according to Mesulam (1985), the inferior parietal lobule is considered one of the few cortical areas that has direct projections to both the frontal eye fields and the superior colliculus, suggesting that these areas are part of a network that is hard-wired in the brain for directing visual attention. Frontal lobe lesions have been found to produce a type of directional motor neglect in which there is reduced spatial exploration of the contralesional side and slowness and reduced amplitude of contralesional limb movements (Bisiach et al., 1990; Coslett et al., 1990; Ladavas et al., 1993).

Thus, neglect could arise from damage to areas of the thalamus, reticular activating system, the limbic system, and the frontal and parietal lobes. Together these areas may serve as a network for directing or guiding attention. Because of their exten-

sive interconnections, damage to any one of these areas may interfere in the operations of other areas. Thus, readiness to respond (arousal), responsivity to novel stimuli (stimulus detection), recognition of stimulus significance (selective attention), and the ability to orient toward a relevant stimulus may all be affected at various levels of severity following damage to a given area in the directed attention network.

Evidence of the existence of a functional and anatomically based attention network with an impact on neglect behavior offers strong support for the concept that neglect is a deficit in attention. In addition, attention theories offer explanations for a wider range of neglect behaviors than do representational theories. Behaviors addressed by attentional theories include: (a) *neglect in the environmental frame of reference*, (b) *ipsilesional neglect*, (c) *problems in moving attention in a contralesional direction*, (d) *excessive attraction of ipsilesional input*, and (e) *the predominance of left versus right neglect*.

SUMMARY

1. *Left neglect reduces responsivity toward leftward information and movement toward the left as defined by the body midline, the coordinates of the environment, and/or the stimuli within that environ ment.* It can occur in various frames of reference including viewer- and environment-centered, and in personal and extrapersonal space.

2. Neglect of the left half of the environment in ipsilesional space suggests that *neglect is dynamic, not static, and shifts with the focus of attention and the amount of effort required to disengage and move attention in a leftward direction.* The amount of rightward stimuli can help predict the focus of attention to the right in any set of spatial coordinates.

3. *Left neglect can occur in the auditory, tactile, olfactory, and visual modalities* and is

most commonly observed in the visual modality.

4. *Left neglect can occur in motor performance either by inhibiting leftward movements or by reducing movements of the left limbs.* In some cases, neglect can masquerade as or further reduce movement in hemiplegia.

5. *Neglect has been estimated to occur in anywhere from 30% to 90% of RHD patients.* Estimates of incidence vary with the type and number of tests used to establish its presence. It can last anywhere from several months to many years.

6. *Neglect is a negative predictor for recovery of independence in daily living.* It can interfere with reading, writing, self-care activities, navigating through space, and attention to significant information in ipsilesional as well as in contralesional space. Patients with neglect are often hypoaroused and less responsive in general, a factor that may impair cognitive as well as spatial skills.

7. Patients with left neglect often have *unconscious perception of left-sided input* in that they are aware of, but fail to fully process, neglected information.

8. Patients with left neglect *deny the deficit, and some may deny ownership of their left-sided body parts in a disorder called anosognosia.* Anosognosia may occur independently of neglect, but usually occurs in concert with other signs of neglect. Patients with anosognosia may experience *unconscious perception* in that they are aware of left-body parts on an intellec-

tual level, but fail to connect to them on an emotional level.

9. *Lesion sites associated with left neglect include areas in the frontal and parietal cortex as well as the basal ganglia, internal capsule, and the thalamus.* The most common cortical site is the parietal lobe, and the most common subcortical site is the thalamus. Neglect does not appear to depend on size so much as on site of lesion.

10. The two main explanations of the mechanism underlying neglect are the *representational theory* and the *attentional theory.* Representational theories suggest that neglect is the result of faulty internal representations of external spatial input. Attentional theories hold that neglect is the result of decreased capacity to direct and sustain attention toward left-sided input, as measured by studies of overt and covert attention. Attentional theories explain more neglect behaviors than do representational theories.

11. Attentional theories suggest that in patients with left neglect, *attention is automatically oriented to the right, that right-sided stimuli anchor attention, and that disengaging attention from right-sided stimuli is particularly problematic if attention must be moved in a leftward direction.* Attentional explanations are supported by the ameliorative influence of cueing and the presence of neglect in ipsilesional as well as in contralesional space. *Some attentional explanations suggest that neglect is but one aspect of a more general attentional deficit.*

CHAPTER

3

Attention Deficits

Chapter 2 explored deficits in the spatial distribution of attention subsequent to RHD. It was proposed that spatial attention is one aspect of an attentional network and that spatial attention deficits are often part of a more general attention disorder. This chapter explores the wide-ranging attentional impairments that can affect cognitive and communicative performance in RHD patients. Before addressing attentional defi- cits subsequent to RHD, some basic issues in the study of attention will be reviewed.

ASSUMPTIONS ABOUT ATTENTION

Attention is fundamental to cognitive processing and, hence, to cognition and communication. It enables us to detect sensory events and to monitor internal states. It allows us to be responsive to, but not overwhelmed by, the external environment and to be aware of, but not distracted by, internally generated thoughts and states. Its role in cognition is so fundamental that it has been difficult to identify its unique properties. Although the study of attention has a history almost as long as that of scientific inquiry in the field of psychology, only in the latter part of this century have investigators examined its neuroanatomical underpinnings. From these beginnings its identity as a separable system that operates independently of other systems (e.g., sensory or motor) and that can be selectively impaired has begun to be clarified (Heilman, Valenstein, et al., 1984; Mesulam, 1981; Posner & Petersen, 1990; Posner, Walker, et al., 1987; Rizzolati & Berti, 1993).

Several basic assumptions have guided inquiry into the nature of attention. They are outlined in Table 3–1 and are reviewed briefly here. Few would argue about the first three assumptions, but there is some controversy about the last two (Alloport, 1993).

The first assumption, that *there are limits to cognitive processing and to the brain's capacity to represent events,* is self-evident. Human beings have limited capacity to process the millions of bits of information that impinge on their sensory apparatus. The second assumption, that *attention protects the brain's limited capacity through the processes of selection and habituation,* identifies how we are able to process some events, but not others. For example, while driving,

TABLE 3–1. Assumptions about attention.

---
1. The brain's capacity to represent events is limited.
2. Attention protects the brain's limited capacity through attentional selection and habituation.
3. Attention itself is a limited resource.
4. Various forms of processing require different degrees of attention.
5. Attention is unitary/attention is not unitary.
---

you could have an accident if your attention is focused on irrelevant sensory experience (e.g., the texture of the upholstery on the seat, the color of the steering wheel, the buzzing sound in the dashboard, the leaves on the trees) or by internal experience (e.g., the content of a recent conversation, unfinished work to be done, images of an upcoming event). We are, of course, often distracted by one or more events as we drive, but if too many impinge at one time or if we become too focused on any one of them, we will not be able to represent more immediately relevant information like the sudden stop by the car ahead or the green light turning red.

The third assumption is that *attention itself is a limited resource* and, thus, is selectively allocated. The fact that the brain's cognitive and perceptual resources and attentional resources are limited sometimes has resulted in confusing attention with mental activity in general. However, attention appears to be independent of the systems dedicated to processing information. For example, the perceptual and cognitive resources one brings to bear on the activity of driving can be considered independently of attention. One must be able to distinguish colors to tell red from green lights. One must be able to judge distance to avoid hitting the car ahead. One must be able to synthesize information across modalities in order to recognize and accurately interpret a siren and flashing lights as a police car. However, this sort of perceptual and cognitive processing cannot occur if the signals have escaped one's attention. The siren and flashing lights may make no more impact on awareness than the stop sign you just passed through if your attention is focused elsewhere.

The fourth assumption follows from the third: *Some types of processing require more and others require less attention.* Processes requiring attention have been called controlled or focused attention, while processes that do not require full and conscious attention are called *automatic.* Sometimes, controlled and automatic attention are contrasted by the amount of conscious awareness brought to bear on the process. For example, you can usually drive a car and carry on a conversation without driving off the side of the road. Participating in the conversation may take more focused attention; following the road occurs more automatically and requires less attention. If something unexpected occurs on the road, however, attention to driving will be less automatic and more focused, at the expense of the conversation.

The fifth assumption, that *attention is unitary,* suggests that there is a central, sort of all-purpose, system of attention. Proponents of this view suggest that attentional operations at the level of adjustments to goals and priorities operate under a supervisory attentional system or "central executive" (Baddeley, 1986; Norman & Shallice, 1986). Those who dispute the idea of a central unified system propose separable attentional systems serving different processing purposes (Alloport, 1993; Posner & Petersen, 1990; Rizzolatti & Berti, 1993; Rizzolatti & Camarda, 1987). For example, spatial attention might be considered distinct from attention serving other purposes. Recent research supports the existence of anatomically distinct neural networks for attention, although more work needs to be done to specify these networks at the cellular level (Posner & Petersen, 1990). According to Alloport (1993), however, the effects of focal brain damage on various types of executive functions and the results of neuroimaging studies of attentional control, "make the idea of a general-purpose, functionally undifferentiated central executive (or attentional control system)—responsible for all aspects of nonspatial, voluntary, attentional control— highly implausible" (p. 202). The assumption that attention is unitary is very controversial. It appears more reasonable to conceive of attention as separable systems, rather than as unitary. However, it is rarely the case that attentional networks are independently disrupted in brain damage. For example, damage to the spatial at-

tention network (as in neglect) may, and very likely does, affect other attentional processes.

CATEGORIES OF ATTENTION

Attention has been categorized in numerous ways, resulting in somewhat confusing terminology. The same terms are sometimes used to refer to different operations and/or functions. The categories of attention reviewed below help to conceptualize attention in general and the attentional deficits that can occur with RHD, in particular (Table 3–2).

Attentional Operations

Perhaps the most familiar way of categorizing attention is to subdivide it into various operations. These attentional operations are defined below and will be discussed in more detail in subsequent sections.

1. **Arousal:** the neural and behavioral readiness to respond; considered fundamental to all other attentional operations
2. **Orienting:** directing of attention toward a stimulus or toward a location
3. **Vigilance:** a state of alertness necessary to processing intermittent stimuli; con-

TABLE 3–2. Ways of categorizing attention.

1. *Operations*	Arousal, orienting, vigilance, maintenance, selective attention
2. *Type*	Phasic versus tonic Voluntary versus involuntary
3. *Regulation*	Habituation Selection
4. *Systems*	Arousal Activation
5. *Domains*	Spatial Nonspatial
6. *Distribution*	Narrow Broad

sidered a pre-stimulus mode of attentional activation

4. **Maintenance:** sustaining attention over time; can occur without a state of vigilance
5. **Selective Attention:** the capacity to selectively attend to some, but not other, stimuli

Phasic Versus Tonic Attention

Attention also can be divided into phasic and tonic modes of operation. *Tonic attention refers to a steady state* whereas *phasic attention is intermittent.* Vigilance, for example, is characterized by a tonic state of readiness to respond, whereas orienting is phasic, and thus episodic, in nature. Phasic attention occurs in response to changes in the environment and can be considered stimulus-driven. Tonic attention, on the other hand, refers to undifferentiated readiness for action, which occurs independently of external events. It is driven more by internal motivation than by external events and is an active state. Phasic attention, in contrast, is more receptive. Tonic attention is tied more closely to the motor system in that it engenders a state of motor readiness (e.g., for fight or flight).

Arousal Versus Activation

Attention has also been categorized by dividing it into two broad systems of control. Neuroanatomical and neurochemical research has suggested two broad systems of control over attention and action that incorporate phasic and tonic attention. They are the *arousal system* and the *activation system* (Pribram & McGuiness, 1975; Tucker & Williamson, 1984). The arousal system regulates attentional readiness and phasic responsivity to sensory input. The activation system regulates tonic readiness for motor activation. Attentional orienting is controlled by habituation, which inhibits attention to repetitive, uninteresting, and in-

significant stimuli. The activation system exerts control by a form of self-limiting motor control. That is, at the same time that the activation system prepares an organism for action, it also limits the number of actions available in the repertoire. In a state of vigilance, the organism is prepared to act, but only in a limited, routinized way. For example, there is a stereotypic set of actions that enable rapid escape or flight. It should be noted that the premotor theory of attention suggests that both orienting attention and the actual programming of subsequent motor movements for a response are linked to attentional mechanisms (Rizzolatti, Riggio, Dascola, & Umilta, 1987; Tassinari, Alioti, Chelazzi, Marzi, & Berlucchi, 1987).

The arousal and activation systems have a neurochemical basis that is particularly relevant to issues of hemispheric specialization for attention. Although neurotransmitters are interdependent, experimental manipulations have suggested that noradrenergic pathways support the arousal system (Aston-Jones & Bloom, 1981; Bloom, 1979; Foote, Freedman, & Oliver, 1975; Posner & Petersen, 1990) and that dopaminergic pathways support the activation system (Iversen, 1977; Tucker & Williamson, 1984). Increased levels of dopamine in animals result in an increasingly narrowed set of actions that are performed over and over and eventually dissolve into behavioral stereotypies (Iversen, 1977). Increased levels of norepinephrine, on the other hand, reduce habituation and result in excessive and unselected responsivity (Tucker & Williamson, 1984).

Although activation and arousal can be conceptualized as independent systems, they clearly work together to produce coordinated behavior, especially noted in states of vigilance. Consider, for example, a reaction time experiment in which subjects must press a button at the onset of a signal. Prior to the stimulus, subjects are in a state of vigilance in which the motor activation system prepares the system to respond with a programmed finger movement. The arousal system decreases responsivity to extraneous input through habituation. At the onset of the target stimulus, a subject orients attention toward the stimulus (arousal, orienting) and makes a motor response, the preprogrammed finger movement (activation). Pressing the button is automatic, having been preprogrammed, and is not interfered with by other unprogrammed or extraneous movements in the subject's repertoire (e.g., using the other hand or moving one's foot). In this simplistic review of events in a reaction time task, we can see that the arousal and activation systems coordinate behavioral responses to the environment under conditions of arousal and vigilance through the regulation of responsivity and the regulation of responses. The arousal system controls attention by episodic arousal (orienting) and habituation. The activation system controls the actions taken by generating a state of motor preparedness and by facilitating some and reducing other motor responses.

Spatial Versus Nonspatial Attention

Another way to categorize attention is by the domains in which it operates, both spatial and nonspatial. Spatial attention, explored relative to neglect in Chapter 2, involves detecting, orienting to, and selecting events that are distributed in either physical (external) or mental (internal) space.

Nonspatial attention operates in a more abstract domain in which adjustments are made to ongoing goals and priorities. Nonspatial attention allows us to follow the weave of a story by selecting to concentrate on the content, rather than on the individual letters on a printed page. It enables us to complete a task by attending to the steps involved, keeping them in sequence, and making necessary adjustments as we proceed.

Narrow Versus Broad Attentional Distribution

Attention can be either broadly or narrowly distributed in both the spatial and nonspatial domains. For example, one can focus on a specific object or location in the environment or widen the scope of attention to take in an entire scene. Arousal and orienting are considered operations that function within a broad-based, global distribution of attention. An expansive attentional scope is essential to exploratory and scanning behavior.

Narrowly focused attention is essential to certain types of concentrated mental activities like proof-reading a manuscript. It is apparent that patients with neglect have a restricted attentional focus, not only *to* right hemispace, but *within* right hemispace where attention may be narrowly fixed on one or two elements at the expense of a broad overview (Halligan & Marshall, 1994; Kinsbourne, 1993; Robertson & Delis, 1986).

Voluntary Versus Automatic Attention

Finally, attention can be broken down into voluntary and automatic processing. Automatic processing has been considered by some to operate independently of and in the absence of attention (Shiffrin & Schneider, 1977). It is thought to be fast, effortless, and unavailable to conscious awareness (Logan, 1988). Attentional orienting often occurs in just such a rapid, effortless, and unconscious manner.

Voluntary attention is thought to be initiated by the organism, rather than by external input (Pribram & McGuiness, 1975). It is considered to be under one's conscious control whereas automatic attention is less available to conscious awareness. However, the lines between awareness and automaticity are fuzzy. Consider, for example, the phenomenon of "unconscious processing" in neglect, discussed in Chapter 2. A patient with neglect who fails to read the left end of a string of letters "d w i w n o," may accurately read the left end letters when the string forms the word "w i n d o w." The patient's attention is drawn to the left side of the letter string only when meaningfulness enters the picture. Attention has been moved leftward in response to cognitive influences, but without conscious awareness. Examples in which meaningfulness influences attentional orienting through implicit processing have been attributed to voluntary attention (Humphreys & Riddoch, 1993). Thus, voluntary attention docs not always rely on conscious processing, but it does appear to rely on cognitively driven motivations.

Summary

The above categories of attention distinguish various attentional operations, differing systems of attentional control, differing domains in which attention operates, differing types of attentional focus and distribution, motivation and control. Although grounded in experimental evidence, these distinctions can be too finely drawn. As the following sections suggest, attentional mechanisms interact with one another and are interdependent. With that caveat in mind, the neurophysiologic, neurochemical, and psychological reality of various attentional operations may be differentially affected by focal brain damage. The following sections explore the specific effects of RHD on attentional operations and the role of the RH in attentional performance.

THE ROLE OF THE RIGHT HEMISPHERE IN ATTENTION

RH Dominance for Directional Orienting

Chapter 2 explained that the two hemispheres orient attention toward the opposite sides of space and that unilateral brain damage can disrupt the balance in attentional orienting achieved by the two hemispheres. It is assumed that RHD affects this balance and creates more problems for attentional orienting than does LHD, but theories differ about why that happens. One theory holds that the LH is dominant for attentional orienting. The more generally accepted hypothesis holds that the RH is dominant. Both are reviewed below.

LH Dominance Hypothesis

Proponents of the LH dominance hypothesis maintain that, *in the intact brain the rightward directional orienting tendencies of the LH are dominant.* Based on studies of infants and NBD adults, Kinsbourne (1987, 1993) suggested that rightward orienting by the LH predominates, and the opposing leftward bias of the RH is weaker. In his model, the dominant tendencies of the LH are kept in check by the RH until damage to the RH occurs. When that happens, the dominant LH becomes disinhibited, and once its stronger contralateral bias is unleashed, a profound left neglect occurs. When the LH is damaged, however, the ensuing right neglect is not severe because the power of the LH prevails, compensating for and to some extent overcoming the less powerful contralateral bias of the RH. Thus, neglect subsequent to LHD is never as prevalent nor as profound as it is following RHD.

Two predictions about the severity of left neglect can be made on the basis of the LH dominance theory. First, severity of left neglect should decrease in response to damage in the LH. That is, by inhibiting the LH, thus reducing its dominant orienting bias, left neglect from RHD should improve when the LH is also damaged. Second, severity of left neglect should increase as the LH recovers from mass effects subsequent to RHD. In fact, just the opposite has been found.

Studies of humans and primates counter the notion that the severity of left neglect is a function of the influence of the unopposed attentional dominance of the LH (Heilman, Bowers, Valenstein, & Watson, 1987; Perani, Vallar, Paulesu, Alberoni, & Fasio, 1993; Watson, Valenstein, Day, & Heilman, 1984). For example, Perani et al. (1993) used positron emission tomography (PET) to track recovery in two RHD patients with neglect. In one case, recovery correlated with metabolic recovery not only in the RH, but also in the undamaged LH. In the second case with a severe neglect at 4 months postonset, PET revealed severe and widespread metabolic reduction in the LH. In other words, recovery correlated with improved LH function in one case, and in the second case, persisting neglect occurred in the face of decreased LH function. Thus, the relative intactness of the LH indeed may be important to the severity of neglect, but in a way that is just the opposite to that suggested by the LH dominance hypothesis.

RH Dominance Hypothesis

Proponents of the RH dominance hypothesis consider the RH, not the LH, dominant for attention. In addition, they conceive of the nature of that dominance differently than that posited by the LH dominance hypothesis. As discussed in Chapter 2, the RH is considered superior, not because it has a stronger orienting bias to left hemispace, but *because it has the capacity to attend to stimuli in both left and right hemispace* (see Figure 2–12, page 46). That is, like the LH, the RH directs attention to contralateral hemispace, but unlike the LH, *it also has the capacity to distribute attention across hemispatial boundaries* (Heilman, Valenstein, et al., 1984; Heilman et al., 1987; Heilman & Van Den Abell, 1980; Ladavas et al., 1989; Mesulam, 1981). Heilman and Van Den Abell (1980), for example, found differences between the two hemispheres in response to right- and left-sided input as measured by EEG activity in NBD subjects. Results showed increased left parietal activity in response to right-sided stimuli. The right parietal lobes, however, showed the same

level of activity to both right and left-sided input, suggesting that, unlike the LH, the RH responds to stimulation across *both* the right and left sectors of space. Thus, when RHD occurs, the unopposed LH directs attention rightward. But when LHD occurs, the RH not only directs attention leftward, but is able to overcome LH inhibition and direct attention rightward as well.

Proponents of RH dominance also suggest that the RH is dominant for a wide variety of attentional functions, not just orienting. In right neglect subsequent to LHD, impaired orienting may be an isolated symptom, but in left neglect following RHD, it may be but one of many equally important attentional deficits. Neglect in LHD patients may be less severe not only because the dominant RH can compensate to some extent by directing attention into right space, but also because orienting may be the *only* aspect of attention affected. In left neglect, however, the intact LH is not able to compensate, and other attentional operations may be affected, not just orienting.

One of the predictions of the RH dominance hypothesis is that RH lesions could disrupt attention in ipsilesional as well as contralesional space. Indeed, that is what happens in left neglect (Caplan, 1985; Feinberg et al., 1990; Weintraub & Mesulam, 1987, 1988). The RH dominance hypothesis has greater credence than the LH hypothesis because there is such a wealth of experimental evidence to support it.

RH Dominance for Arousal and Orienting

Arousal is more global in nature than other attentional operations and can be considered the backdrop against which other attentional operations take place. The broad-based attentional function of the arousal system "allows the perceptual system to maintain a continuously revised and maximally comprehensive map of the external context (Tucker & Williamson, 1984, p. 197). Deficits in arousal directly affect orienting and may indirectly affect vigilance, attentional maintenance, and selection, each of which, of course, impact on cognitive performance. Arousal facilitates registration of input by increasing neural readiness to respond to relevant input and by reducing responsivity to irrelevant or repetitive input through habituation.

At the most basic level, arousal separates conscious from unconscious states. In conscious states, there are varying degrees of arousal. Fatigue and/or brain damage, for example, may reduce the degree to which the brain is ready to respond. Importantly, *the RH appears to be dominant for arousal* (Davidson, Fedio, Smith, Aureille, & Martin, 1992; Posner & Petersen, 1990). Patients with RHD and neglect, for instance, have been characterized as "hypoaroused" (Heilman, Schwartz, & Watson, 1978; Heilman & Van Den Abel, 1980). Arousal may be impaired as well in RHD patients who do not have signs of neglect. This characterization comes not only from behavioral observation, but from physiologic indicators of arousal and neurochemical evidence suggesting that the RH plays a dominant role in arousal and attentional orienting.

Neurochemical Evidence

Evidence from animal and human research suggests that arousal, orienting, and other attentional operations are regulated by specific neurotransmitter pathways (Clark, Geffen, & Geffen, 1987; Koella, 1982; Tucker & Williamson, 1984). There are differing neurotransmitter systems, releasing different neurotransmitter substances (e.g., acetylcholine, norepinephrine, dopamine) that are distributed in differing concentrations in the nervous system. The noradrenergic system (e.g., norepinephrine and serotonin) appears to be particularly important to the arousal system (Aston-Jones & Bloom, 1981; Bloom, 1979; Clark, Geffen, & Geffen, 1989; Foote et al., 1975; Harley, 1987; McGuinness & Pribram, 1980; Posner & Petersen, 1990). Dopaminergic (e.g., dopamine and noradrenalin) pathways are consid-

ered important to the activation system, which interacts with attention by maintaining a tonic state of readiness for motor action (Iversen, 1977; Tucker & Williamson, 1984). Both neurotransmitter systems influence attentional orienting, but may serve different functions. The activity of norepinephrine cells in animals is particularly attuned to stimulus novelty (Foote & Bloom, 1979; Watabe, Nakai, & Kasamatsu, 1982), which fosters orienting to novel events in the environment.

The dopaminergic system, on the other hand, aids in the motor aspects of overt orienting (e.g., shifting the eyes). Lesions in areas supporting the dopaminergic system can result in neglect, in an increase in stereotypic motor behavior, and appear to interfere with the capacity to alternate or switch attention (Clark et al., 1989, 1987). In addition, Clark et al. (1989) found that manipulations of both dopamine and noradrenalin affected covert attention. The speed of disengaging attention from its current focus in NBD subjects was facilitated by both clondine, which acts on the noradrenergic system, and by droperidol, which acts on the dopaminergic system. Both agents decreased attentional maintenance in a directionally cued reaction time task. The authors pointed out that their results are not surprising because both norepinephrine and dopamine occur in high concentrations in the inferior parietal lobule, an area important to disengaging attention (Posner et al., 1984; Posner, Walker, et al., 1987).

Both neurotransmitter systems also may be important in directional hypokinesia subsequent to RHD in which there is reduced leftward movement. According to Heilman et al. (1985), each hemisphere may be responsible for movements toward contralateral space, but the RH is able to activate areas for initiating movements into either right or left space, giving it a special role in directional motor activation and possibly in other motor aspects of directional orienting.

The noradrenergic system appears to increase responsivity specifically to *envi-*

ronmental stimulation (Robbins & Everett, 1982; Tucker & Williamson, 1984). The external orientation of the noradrenergic pathways is consistent with the environmental scanning and the broad distribution of attention in arousal. The control mechanism of habituation in the arousal system allows maximal responses to new and rewarding events that have significant motivational value. The cingulate gyrus and its connection to the parietal lobes is particularly important in determining the primary motivational significance of certain classes of stimuli (Mesulam, 1981). Interestingly, the cingulate cortex has been found to have especially dense noradrenergic innervation in rats (Decarries & Lapierre, 1973).

Important to our discussion is the suggestion that norepinephrine, although widely distributed throughout the brain, is to some extent asymmetrically distributed. Evidence from studies of pharmacological interventions, surgical ablations in animals, and autopsy and neuroimaging in humans suggests that norepinephrine plays a very important role in the alert state and that maintaining alertness depends on RH mechanisms (Posner & Petersen, 1990; Tucker & Williamson, 1984). For example, unlike left frontal lesions, right frontal lesions deplete norepinephrine pathways bilaterally in rats (Pearlson & Robinson, 1981; Robinson, 1985). The right hemisphere of the thalamus has been found to have higher concentrations of norepinephrine than the left hemisphere in both rats and humans (Oke, Keller, Medford, & Adams, 1978; Oke, Lewis, & Adams, 1980).

Neurochemical evidence suggests that both the noradrenergic and dompaninergic pathways are important to arousal and to overt and covert orienting. The evidence also suggests that *noradrenergic pathways are particularly important in arousal and that they are to some extent lateralized to the RH.*

Autonomic Evidence

Levels of arousal can be examined by measuring autonomic nervous system responses that are considered the physiologic correlates of increased neuronal activity in the brain. Two such measures used to explore asymmetrical levels of arousal are electroencephalography (EEG) and galvanic skin response (GSR). The EEG is a recording of electrical activity in the brain. The GSR is a recording of electrodermal activity, which is considered to be a reflection of arousal.

EEG measures have been used to demonstrate that the RH mediates attention across spatial boundaries and that it is dominant for arousal functions. Heilman and Van Den Abel (1980), for example, used warning signals to engage attention prior to the onset of a stimulus in a reaction time experiment in which subjects' EEGs were monitored. They found that the right parietal lobes of NBD adults showed activity in the right parietal lobe to both right- and left-sided stimuli whereas activity in the left parietal lobe occurred only in response to contralateral input. Finding the same bilateral field of attention in the RH of split-brain subjects, Magnun et al. (1994) stated that the RH "serves as a sentry that monitors the whole of extrapersonal space" (p. 273). Damage to the RH appears to reduce arousal and responsivity to external events bilaterally. The finding that the RH mobilizes attention across spatial boundaries resonates with the arousal system's broad distribution of attention.

Studies of GSRs in populations with brain damage have found reduced responsivity to novel and significant input in RHD patients compared to LHD patients (Davidson et al., 1992; Heilman et al., 1978; Morrow, Vrtunski, Kim, & Boller, 1981; Zoccolotti, Scabini, & Violani, 1982). Heilman suggested that RHD is associated with a bilateral reduction in arousal based on the finding that RHD patients had smaller GSRs to ipsilesional limb stimulation than LHD patients. Given that the limbs are contralaterally innervated, their findings indicate reduced levels of arousal in the left as well as the right hemispheres of RHD patients (although not in the right hemispheres of LHD patients). Morrow et al. (1981) and Zoccolotti et al. (1982) found that arousal to emotional input also was reduced in RHD compared to LHD patients. In fact, they found that GSRs in their RHD group were almost nonexistent. In addition, Zoccolotti et al. (1982) found evidence of rapid habituation after an initially clear GSR to the first stimulus. Overly rapid habituation may be indicative of reduced arousal signaled by failure to register and orient to novel input. Davidson et al. (1992) found the same pattern of rapid habituation in right (but not left) lobectomy patients and suggested that such hypoarousal subsequent to RHD "may, indeed, provide the physiological backdrop for such commonly observed behavioral patterns as inattention and denial" (p. 1061). Interestingly, their left lobectomy group had *higher* GSRs and a slower rate of habituation than normal (i.e., "*hyper*arousal"), providing further evidence of the importance of the RH to arousal functions.

Behavioral Evidence: Deficits in Arousal and Orienting Subsequent to RHD

Arousal prepares one to respond by increasing attentional and neuronal responsivity. Orienting, both covert and overt, is the outcome of that readiness to respond in that it guides attention toward novel or significant input in the environment. As discussed in Chapter 2, *overt orienting* is accompanied by motor movement toward a stimulus. *Covert orienting* is movement of attention *prior* to a motor response. Orienting is driven by the information characteristics of external stimuli. When stimuli are no longer novel and significant, when they are repetitive or unrewarding, habituation reduces the orienting response.

Orienting deficits specific to RHD have been documented in numerous types of studies. Certainly, orienting to the left is impaired in patients with left neglect. In addition, *there appears to be a more general decrement in the orienting response, across spatial boundaries* subsequent to RHD. It is important to remember in the ensuing discussion that arousal and orienting are

intimately connected and difficult to separate in experimental paradigms.

As mentioned earlier, reaction time studies measure the speed with which a response (usually pressing or releasing a switch) follows a stimulus (usually a flash of light, an illuminated shape, or an auditory signal). Reaction time, or RT, is considered a sign of general arousal and attentional orienting, particularly in what are called "simple" RT tasks in which subjects respond to a single target appearing in a single predicted location. More complex RT tasks consist of paradigms in which subjects must discriminate between targets and foils depending on the configuration or spatial location of the stimulus. Complex RT tasks also may include valid or invalid warning signals that alert the subject to the spatial location of the stimulus (see Chapter 2). It is generally accepted that information processing demands increase in complex RT tasks, and that other attentional operations (e.g., selective attention) are enlisted. Attentional maintenance is considered a factor in all types of RT tasks because the required statistical analysis of RT results necessitates the presentation of a great many trials.

In general, populations with brain damage, regardless of side of lesion, have slower RTs than normal. Some studies have shown RHD subjects are slower than those with LHD (De Renzi & Faglioni, 1965; Howes & Boller, 1975; Ladavas et al., 1989; Nagel-Leiby et al., 1990; Yokoyama, Jennings, Ackles, Hood, & Boller, 1987). Some have failed to find differences between RHD and LHD patients (Anzola & Vignolo, 1992; Benton & Joynt, 1959; Dee & Van Allen, 1973; Tartaglione, Bino, Manzino, Spadavecchia, & Favale, 1986; Tartaglione, Oneto, Manzino, & Favale, 1987). However, no simple RT study has reported slower RTs in LHD than in RHD subjects (Benton, 1986).

Several factors may contribute to the conflicting evidence of laterality effects in the RT literature. First, the hemispheric effects reported in studies conducted before the use of neuroimaging techniques are less convincing than those in studies that used these techniques to define lesion location. Second, studies have included subjects in which etiology and lesion size differ considerably. Size of lesion has been found to affect RT performance differentially. One study, for example, found that, in RHD subjects, larger lesions were correlated with RT slowing, whereas in LHD subjects, lesion size did not affect performance (Tartaglione et al., 1986). Finally, aphasia has been significantly correlated with slower RTs in LHD subjects (Tartaglione et al., 1986).

Recent studies that have identified neglect in RHD subjects have found that they had slower RTs than LHD subjects (Ladavas et al., 1989; Yokoyama et al., 1987). In studies in which subjects did not have neglect, some investigators still found RHD subjects slower than LHD subjects (Nagel-Leiby et al., 1990); others found no significant differences between the groups (Anzola & Vignolo, 1992). Results of several studies suggest that presentation of a warning stimulus prior to stimulus presentation is particularly facilitatory for RHD patients (Howes & Boller, 1975; Posner, Walker, et al., 1987). LHD subjects with presumably intact right hemispheres did not appear as dependent on a warning to mobilize attention. Similarly, Heilman and Van Den Abell (1979) found that, in the intact brain, the RH is particularly responsive to the attentional mobilization provided by a warning stimulus. They also found that warning stimuli projected to the RH of NBD subjects reduced RTs for the right hand even more than those projected to the LH, which innervates the right hand.

Neglect subsequent to RHD appears to reduce the spatial distribution of attention, preventing the broad-based overview that is critical for environmental scanning for which the arousal and orienting systems of attention are so important. Spatial distribution of attention not only is reduced, but sometimes is sacrificed for attention to a single item, rather than to a location or an area (Bisiach & Rusconi, 1990; Kinsbourne, 1993). An expected consequence of intensely focused attention is that responsivity would be faster to items within that focus than it would be if attention were distributed across the stimulus field. As mentioned in the previous chapter, that prediction was born out by Ladavas et al. (1990) who found RHD subjects had faster RTs than NBD subjects to stimuli in a relative rightward position. Their findings confirm the narrow versus broad distribution of attention in RHD patients with neglect. Neglect subsequent to RHD thus inhibits the environmental immersion, exploration, and scanning so crucial for adequate orienting and the perceptual awareness it engenders.

Summary

Although arousal and orienting affect the whole brain's capacity to interact with the environment, there is considerable evidence that the intact RH plays a specialized role in orienting to the environment, and that RHD has a deleterious effect on both arousal and orienting. Covert orienting of attention appears to be disrupted by parietal damage in both hemispheres, but patients with RHD and left neglect have particular problems in disengaging attention from a current focus. Rapid habituation has been found to be more pronounced under certain conditions in RHD than in LHD patients. There is some suggestion that neurotransmitter pathways supporting arousal and orienting may be asymmetrically distributed. Finally, there is evidence that the RH is dominant in orienting attention toward both right and left hemispace.

The potential consequence of impaired orienting is *reduced and restricted interaction with the environment.* The focus of attention may be narrowed, and it may be difficult to shift away from prominent stimuli in one sector to relevant stimuli distributed elsewhere. Such behavior is apparent in picture description tasks, for example, in which RHD patients overdescribe certain areas of a picture at the expense of the whole. It is also apparent in the reduced capacity of some RHD patients to respond to external cues such as facial expression, body language, and the prosodic aspects of speech that signal mood. The apparent inner focus of such patients may be partly the result of reduced arousal and orienting and may be responsible for some of the cognitive, communicative, and pragmatic deficits subsequent to RHD, issues that will be explored in subsequent chapters.

THE EFFECTS OF RHD ON OTHER ATTENTIONAL OPERATIONS

Although the RH is considered dominant for arousal and orienting, other attentional operations can be affected by RHD, including *vigilance, sustained,* and *selective attention* (see Table 3–3). These attentional deficits also impact on cognitive and communicative performance and may be among the underlying mechanisms of those disorders.

Deficits in Vigilance and Sustained Attention

Although many situations call for sustained attention, it is fundamental to a state of vigilance, and the two often are discussed together. Sustained attention is the maintenance of attention over time. Vigilance is a state of intense attentional alertness that is necessary for processing intermittent stimuli. Clearly dependent on the arousal system, vigilance differs in degree and type of attentional mobilization from a more general state of arousal.

Both arousal and vigilance may culminate in orienting to a stimulus. In an arousal state, the stimulus is not necessarily expected or anticipated whereas vigilance is motivated by stimulus anticipation and driven by internal drives. It has been defined as a "pre-stimulus input state" which, by definition, assumes expectation on the part of the organism (Whitehead,

1991, p. 331). Because expectations are internal, a state of vigilance is less automatic and more under voluntary control than arousal. Whereas vigilance is tonic, arousal is phasic. As part of the activation system, vigilance is characterized by a motoric readiness to respond.

The postural and motor readiness for flight assumed by an animal sensing danger is a good example of what is meant by vigilance. A rabbit in the woods may be in a state of focused attention as he forages for food. Periodically, he will stop to monitor the surrounding scene, shifting attention from a narrow focus on the immediate area to the broad-based scope of environmental awareness. If the rabbit catches the scent of a predator, he enters a state of intense alertness or vigilance in which his motor system is prepared for flight. His attentional focus continues to be broad as he sustains the vigilant state. Any change in the scene, such as the snap of a twig, the movement of a shadow, or an increase of the scent, typically will result in rapid flight carried out by a preprogrammed motor response.

Similarly, in an RT task, humans not only are alert and aroused, but are in a state of vigilance until the appearance of an expected target. The onset of the target shifts attention toward it as orienting occurs, and the preprogrammed motor response (e.g., pressing a switch) takes place. A state of vigilance generally produces more rapid responding than a state of arousal alone, but speed comes at the expense of accuracy (Bub, Audet, & LeCours, 1990; Posner & Petersen, 1990). According to Posner and Petersen (1990), "In states of high alertness, the selection of a response occurs more quickly, based upon a lower quality of information, thus resulting in an increase of errors" (p. 36). So, too, for the rabbit in the woods. He may have run off at the sound of a mere mouse rustling the leaves, but he would probably think that the sacrifice of accuracy was very much to his advantage given the potential consequences.

One is in a state of vigilance in response to anticipated, but intermittent, events

TABLE 3–3. Attentional deficits specifically associated with RHD.

Attentional Deficit	Evidence
▶ **Arousal and orienting**	Neurochemical: noradrenergic pathways are important to arousal and somewhat lateralized to the RH
	Autonomic: reduced GSRs to novel/emotional input rapid habituation
	Behavioral: Slower RTs than LHD patients in some studies
▶ **Narrowed focus**	Faster than normal RTs to stimuli in a relative rightward position
▶ **Sustained attention**	Deteriorating performance of RHD subjects during RT tasks
	Reduced performance in RT tasks as ISIs increase
▶ **Vigilance**	Reduced autonomic signs of attentional mobilization (e.g., heart rate deceleration)
	Increased blood flow and metabolic activity in the RH of NBD subjects during vigilance tasks
▶ **Selective attention**	Slower RTs than LHD subjects in target-foil cancellation tasks
	Increased severity of left neglect in controlled, serial processing cancellation tasks

Note: GSRs: galvanic skin responses; RTs: reaction times; ISIs: interstimulus intervals.

even when the content of those events is unknown. In the laboratory, vigilance often is tested in RT paradigms in which the appearance of a target is expected, but its timing, location, or configuration is not known. In everyday life, one might assume a vigilant state while proofreading a manuscript, driving in city traffic, listening to a news bulletin, or when participating in a conversation in which one is uncertain of the veracity of the information communicated or the intentions of the speaker. In all of these situations one is ready to respond even though the content of the expected event is not known. Unlike a more general state of arousal, vigilance typically incorporates motor preparation that might take the form of reaching for the phone, leaning forward to catch a news item, or orienting attention toward a speaker's eyes during a conversation.

Vigilance Deficits and Reaction Time

The effect of vigilance in RT tasks is measured in subjects' performance over the duration of the task and across the inter-stimulus interval. Whitehead (1991) concluded that RH specialization in RT tasks is most commonly observed when a task requires continuous processing. Several studies have found that the RH is critical for maintaining performance levels over time in RT tasks. Bub et al. (1990) studied RTs to auditory stimuli and found that, whereas the RT performance of NBD and LHD subjects improved as the task progressed, the performance of RHD subjects deteriorated about 10 minutes into the task, indicative of impaired attentional maintenance. In NBD subjects, Diamond and Beaumont (1973) found that the intact RH was able to maintain its initial performance level longer than the intact LH. The isolated RH of split-brain subjects also has been reported to be better able than the LH to maintain performance in vigilance tasks (Diamond, 1976).

Although all RT tasks require vigilance, the importance of RH function and the impact of RHD on vigilance has been specifically demonstrated in paradigms in which the interval of time between stimulus presentations, or the inter-stimulus interval

(ISI), has been manipulated. Manipulating the ISI allows investigators to assess the potential drift of attention that may occur with longer intervals (i.e., with slower rates of stimulus presentation). Vigilance impairments should result in slower RTs to stimuli presented at longer ISIs. Most tasks use a short ISI of less than 1 second, but Whitehead (1991) reported a series of lateralized visual RT experiments with NBD subjects in which ISIs varied between 3 and 12 s. Longer ISIs resulted in an RH advantage whereas shorter ISIs produced an LH advantage. The results suggested that the intact RH is adept at maintaining attention across a longer inter-stimulus duration.

In subjects with brain damage, the results of ISI manipulations are mixed. Bub et al. (1990) used relatively long ISIs, averaging between 1 and 15 s. RTs of all of the subjects with brain damage were slower for longer ISIs, but there was no particular interaction between side of lesion and ISI length. Wilkins, Shallice, and McCarthy (1987), on the other hand, found that patients with right frontal lesions were specifically impaired with long ISIs, but not with short ones in a task in which subjects were required to count the number of clicks or pulses presented in a given time frame. The authors suggested that right frontal damage can impair the maintenance of voluntary attention in a monotonous task.

Finally, RHD patients have problems in attentional maintenance independent of their capacity to shift attention and independent of the presence of extinction (Ladavas et al., 1989; Posner, Inoff, Friedrich, & Cohen, 1987). In fact, Ladavas et al. (1989) found that slowed responses of RHD subjects relative to LHD subjects were independent of lesion site within the RH, suggesting a generalized reduction of attentional maintenance in RHD.

Neural and Autonomic Indicators of Vigilance

Studies of regional blood flow and metabolic activity in NBD subjects have re-ported increased RH relative to LH activity during vigilance tasks subjects (Cohen et al., 1988; Deutsch, Papanicolaou, Bourbon, & Eisenberg, 1987; Pardo, Fox, & Raichle, 1991). Cohen et al. (1988) used fluorodeoxy-glucose-positron tomography (FDG-PET) to study regions of brain activity during a continuous auditory discrimination task that required sustained attention and vigilance and in two tasks designed to decrease attentional requirements and invoke habituation. They found that areas of the prefrontal cortex demonstrated the most significant activity in the continuous discrimination task and that the RH showed more activity than homologous regions in the LH. Pardo et al. (1991) found similar results in a PET study of vigilance using somatosensory and visual input. Increased blood flow occurred predominantly in the right superior parietal and prefrontal cortex of their NBD subjects, regardless of the modality or laterality of sensory input.

Heart rate changes prior to orienting also are considered to be an autonomic indicator of vigilance. For example, during RT tasks, the heart rate of normal adults decelerates between the onset of a warning signal and the onset of the target stimulus. This slowing is considered a sign of attentional mobilization prior to the stimulus event that is then followed by heart rate acceleration during actual orienting (Jennings, 1986; Lacey & Lacey, 1974; Pribram & McGuinness, 1975; Yokoyama et al., 1987). Yokoyama et al. (1987) found that the heart rate deceleration of RHD subjects was significantly reduced compared to LHD and NBD subjects. LHD subjects had a stronger response than the NBD controls, indicating some disinhibition.

Posner & Petersen (1990) suggested that the posterior areas of the RH are particularly important to sustained attention and that norepinephrine may play a crucial role in maintaining attentional alertness. Heart rate studies in animals have shown that a drop in blood pressure and heart rate deceleration accompanies release of norepinephrine in brain pathways (Tackett, Webb,

& Privitera, 1981). Visual evoked potentials measuring cortical arousal in NBD adults have been found to be strongly lateralized to the RH during periods of low blood pressure and heart rate deceleration (Walker & Sandman, 1979).

Summary

Studies of vigilance suggest that the RH plays an important role in sustained attention and vigilance. Increased RH activity is demonstrated in neuroimaging studies of metabolic activity in the brain during vigilance tasks. The performance of RHD subjects deteriorates over time in RT tasks, suggesting problems with attentional maintenance. Finally, autonomic measures of attentional mobilization have shown that RHD has a negative effect on normally occurring anticipatory heart rate deceleration in vigilance tasks.

Thus, RHD appears to interfere with the capacity to maintain a state of increased attentional alerting in anticipation of expected stimuli. RHD patients may not be able to maintain attention for long periods of time and, even within short time frames, may be unable to sustain the level of attentional alertness required by cognitive and communicative events. Fluctuating levels of attention occurring in demanding situations can mean that they fail to process crucial information even when set to do so. Vigilance and sustained attention require effort, as anyone trying to concentrate while fatigued knows. Reduced arousal may disrupt the effortful mobilization that sustained attention and vigilance require.

Deficits in Selective Attention

The limited capacity of the brain to process information requires some form of gating or selectivity. Selective attention gives attentional priority to some information at the expense of less relevant or less significant information. It is difficult conceptually to separate selective attention from the selective gating that occurs in perceptual and cognitive operations. Cognitively motivated selective attention requires increased effort and attention. Increased attentional mobilization actually enhances the responsivity and selectivity of neurons, suggesting that selective attention has a neural as well as a behavioral reality (Spitzer, Desimone, & Moran, 1988).

Selective attention may occur *automatically* as it does in some types of orienting (e.g., hearing one's name in a crowd). It may occur with more *conscious awareness* when one is motivated to attend to a particular type of information or to extract specific content from background noise (e.g., listening for the temperature in a weather report, searching for a familiar face in a crowd, or trying to understand the main point of a narrative). Some have suggested that automatic selectivity does not require attention (Shiffrin & Schneider, 1977).

Like other forms of attention, selective attention interacts with other attentional operations. Cognitively motivated selective attention requires more effort than automatic selectivity, but both are dependent on the integrity of the arousal and orienting systems which alert one to the presence of novel or relevant input and enable attention to be directed toward it. Rapcsak, Verfaellie, Fleet, and Heilman (1989) suggested that decreased arousal subsequent to RHD reduces overall attentional capacity and interferes in selective attention in particular. Vigilance and sustained attention may be especially important to voluntary selective attention because the effort to extract significant information must be maintained over time and because there may be uncertainty about when or where this information will occur.

Because these other attentional operations interact with selective attention, anatomical areas important to these operations also play a role in selective attention. The posterior parietal lobes, for example, are important in spatial selection (Ladavas et al., 1989; Mesulam, 1981; Posner & Petersen, 1990; Posner, Walker, et al., 1987). The frontal lobes are important in maintaining attention during tasks requiring selective attention (Bench et al., 1993; Cohen et al., 1988; Deutsch et al., 1987) and in orchestrating spatial exploration (Mesulam, 1981). The cingulate gyrus has been implicated in difficult selective attention tasks that require the suppression of automatic responses (Janer & Pardo, 1991; Pardo, Pardo, Janer, & Raichle, 1990). In addition, it has been suggested that the cingulate gyrus may be implicated in the distribution of expectancy and the perception of the biological relevance of events.

Among the many controversies and uncertainties about the nature of selective attention is the issue of when or at what stage of processing it occurs. Does it occur before or after a stimulus has been identified? For example, does one need to identify an object before one rejects it for further processing? Proponents of early selection suggest there is a perceptual suppression in which some stimuli never enter the system for further processing because of perceptual constraints (Triesman, 1988; Triesman & Gelade, 1980). That is, selection occurs prior to information entry and independently of attentional constraints. Proponents of late selection suggest that all information enters the system after which attentional selection operates to suppress processing of irrelevant information (Shiffrin & Schneider, 1977). Two assumptions underlie theories of early and late selection. The first is that information processing is ordered in linear fashion. The second is that certain attributes such as spatial location are processed prior to semantic or other category features.

Much of the research on selective attention has centered on differences between automatic and controlled selection in hopes of determining where or when selective attention is required. The issue of early and late selection has not been settled and has itself been questioned as a point of theoretical departure for research in selective attention (Alloport, 1993). The issue is not particularly germane to our purposes. However, the effects of RHD on selective atten-

tion have been studied in the types of paradigms designed to address the issue of early and late selection.

In some of the most familiar paradigms, subjects must search an array of foils for targets that differ along varying dimensions (e.g., shape, category, color). Selective attention demands are measured by reaction times. More difficult discriminations result in longer response times. In Triesman's paradigm, for example, targets and foils may differ from each other by a single feature (shape) or by feature combinations or conjunctions (i.e., shape and color). In single feature detection tasks, the rate of target detection is rapid, and simultaneous or parallel processing is assumed to occur. Target detection is slower in feature conjunction tasks, presumably because each item must be processed individually in a serial manner. In feature conjunction tasks, attention must be directed to each item, whereas in single feature conditions targets tend to "pop out."

Targets and foils also may differ along the dimension of stimulus category (semantic or perceptual). A body of research has shown that RTs are slower when targets and foils are in the same category (e.g., a letter in an array of letters) than when they are from different categories (a number in an array of letters) (Ruff, Evans, & Light, 1986).

It has been suggested that the narrowed focus of spatial attention subsequent to neglect results in a slowed serial processing of each stimulus within the focus of attention. That is, for patients with neglect, targets do not "pop out" from distractors in a simple cancellation task because they focus on items within an area, rather than on the area itself. Broad-based attention is sacrificed and selective attention takes over as patients process each stimulus individually, one by one (Chaterjee, Mennemeir, & Heilman, 1992; Robertson, 1989). One can imagine the effects of imposing serial processing on situations calling for a more panoramic attentional scan. Not only would one be slower, but one also might have difficulty integrating information into a larger whole. This helps to explain not only the impaired cancellation performance in RHD patients with neglect, but also their slowed and overly precise descriptions of individual elements in scene description tasks or the extra strokes they make when writing or drawing.

The Stroop task also has been used to investigate selective attention (Stroop, 1935). It requires subjects to read the ink colors of printed color names that may or may not be congruent with the color name. When the word "blue" is printed in orange ink, for example, the correct response is "orange." The task requires selective attention to ink color and the selective suppression of an over-learned response (reading). As in other selective attention tasks, there is interference from competing signals. It is uncertain if the interference can be characterized as response competition (reading versus color naming) or as competition at the level of stimulus encoding (Bench et al., 1993; Pardo et al., 1990). In either case, it is considered an attention-demanding task.

Studies investigating anatomic correlates of selective attention have used positron emission tomography (PET) and have found asymmetric distribution of metabolic activity during selective attention tasks such as the Stroop task. Activation is particularly prominent in the right frontal cortex and the right anterior cingulate cortex in NBD subjects during Stroop tasks (Bench et al., 1993; Pardo et al., 1990). PET scans during other selective attention tasks have also revealed increased RH activity. Deutsch et al. (1987) conducted a retrospective study of 121 scans from NBD subjects performing a variety of visuospatial and auditory verbal tasks. They found that, regardless of modality or task category, frontal regions were active relative to the resting state, and in *all* conditions, right frontal regions showed greater activation than the left frontal areas. Equally interesting, a greater proportion of subjects had increased right compared to left hemisphere

activation on the tasks they ranked as most difficult, most of which taxed selective attention.

The importance of the right frontal cortex in selective attention and the impact of right frontal lesions on performance were demonstrated in a study investigating differences in serial and parallel processing by RHD and LHD subjects with lesions in the anterior and posterior regions of the brain (Ruff, Niemann, Allen, Farrow, & Wylie, 1992). Subjects were given 5 min to cancel numerical targets embedded in a series of distractors, which were either letters (different stimulus category—parallel processing) or numbers (same stimulus category—serial processing). RHD subjects, regardless of lesion site, were slower than LHD subjects in both conditions. Subjects with right frontal lesions performed more poorly than all other patient groups in both speed and accuracy. Accuracy in the LHD group, however, was no different from that in the NBD group.

In situations calling for controlled, serial processing, the severity of neglect in RHD patients often increases. As target-foil discriminations become more difficult in cancellation tasks or as the number of distractors increases, fewer targets are cancelled, severity of neglect increases, and reaction time increases (Kaplan et al., 1991; Rapcsak et al., 1989; Riddoch & Humphreys, 1987). Kaplan et al. (1991) found that the percentage of letters cancelled in left hemispace was almost directly correlated with the number of distractors present. Subjects in that study had a near-perfect performance in a baseline condition without distractors. In one condition, targets and distractors were placed on the right and targets without distractors were placed on the left. Neglect then occurred in right hemispace, and in 20% of the trials, neglect was more prevalent in right than in left hemispace. The increased effort required by selective attention can actually create a new area of neglect. Visual neglect thus shifts with the attentional demands of the situation, demonstrating once again the intimate tie between spatial and other forms of attention and the reduced cognitive performance that can occur in demanding situations as a result of neglect. As Robertson (1989) and Chatterjee et al. (1992) have suggested, there appears to be an attentional limitation in patients with neglect, which could be globally based or specific to certain types of attention. In addition, the narrowed focus of neglect in attention induces a slower, serial search even in tasks where that type of search is not enlisted by NBD subjects. Deficits in the broad-based attentional focus of the arousal system in RHD patients may induce an alternate attentional mode— selective attention—which requires more effort and stresses capacity.

Summary

Selective attention can be automatic, as demonstrated by both habituation and orienting to novel input. Studies of selective attention, however, typically focus on voluntary or cognitively driven selective attention, which is assumed to require effort and conscious control. For that reason, selective attention has almost become synonymous in the literature with controlled, serial processing.

Studies of both NBD adults and those with focal brain damage suggest that the RH plays an important role in voluntary selective attention. Neuroimaging studies of metabolic brain activity in NBD adults during selective attention tasks have demonstrated asymmetric activation. Right frontal areas, including the right cingulate gyrus, appear to be particularly active in tasks such as the Stroop task.

Studies of subjects with brain damage suggest that RHD interferes with selective attention. Selective attention demands appear to increase the severity of neglect, regardless of target location and can alter the spatial location of neglect. Taken together, these studies suggest that attentional resources are limited subsequent to RHD in some patients, and that increased attentional demands interfere with cognitive operations required by selective attention tasks.

As mentioned earlier, the segregation of attentional operations into discrete categories is somewhat artificial. It is difficult to know if RHD differentially affects selective attention or if impaired selective attention is the product of attentional deficits in arousal, orienting, and vigilance. Paradigms investigating selective attention deficits typically require multiple attentional operations. The increased attentional effort required by selective attention appears to interact with attentional impairments in overall arousal level, in orienting, and in vigilance. In particular, RHD appears to limit attentional resources so that attentional demands in one category such as arousal reduce attentional capacity in other categories. In some cases, patients may rely on selective attention to compensate for deficits in the broad distribution of attention characteristic of arousal. The result is a strategy that places even more demands on attentional resources, further limiting the distribution of attention.

SUMMARY

1. Focal damage anywhere in the brain can interfere with attention. However, *the RH appears to play a particular role in attentional operations.* Evidence from neurochemical, autonomic nervous system, neuroimaging, and behavioral studies suggests that: (a) *the arousal system is somewhat lateralized to the RH;* (b) *the RH is particularly engaged in orienting attention;* (c) *unlike the LH, the RH orients attention across spatial boundaries;* (d) *the RH plays a role in maintaining attention in states of vigilance;* and (e) *frontal areas in the RH are more active than comparable LH areas when selective attention and vigilance are required.*

2. Damage to the RH can result in a variety of attentional impairments, including *deficits in arousal, orienting, vigilance, and sustained and selective attention.*

3. Perhaps the *most fundamental attentional deficit that can occur subsequent to RHD is reduced arousal* (hypoarousal), which inhibits environmental awareness, restricts the focus of attention, and affects spatial and nonspatial attentional operations.

4. *RHD may make the sustained, internally driven attentional mobilization necessary for vigilance particularly effortful.* RHD patients may have difficulty maintaining the intensely alert state of expectancy required of certain activities such as monitoring a situation, printed material, televised broadcasts, or conversations for specific information.

5. *Selective attention impairments are apparent in patients with neglect.* Selective attention demands not only increase the severity of neglect, they can encourage neglect in previously non-neglected sectors of space.

6. *Patients with neglect appear to have a restricted focus of attention.* They may compensate for it by relying inappropriately on selective attention in situations calling for broad-based scanning and parallel, as opposed to serial, processing. As a result, these patients *may be slower to process what was once processed in a rapid, automatic, unconscious manner in both neglected and in non-neglected external space, as well as internally where spatial boundaries are not applied.*

7. *Attentional deficits subsequent to RHD can have a significant impact on cognitive and communicative performance and can affect the pragmatic aspects of communication as well.* Patients may be less alert and less able to mobilize voluntary attention required in vigilant states. They may be less aware of and less able to orient to, maintain attention toward, and select out important information in situations calling for complex levels of communication and cognitive effort.

CHAPTER

4

Prosodic Deficits

Prosody provides the melodic contour and rhythm of speech and facilitates in decoding syntactic and lexical meaning as well as the emotional content of spoken language. It helps speakers convey intended meanings and it helps listeners understand them. Research over the past 15 to 20 years has supported clinical observations of prosodic production and comprehension impairments associated with RHD. The speech of RHD patients may sound flat and monotonous, and they may have problems using prosody to decode the messages of others.

Prosody consists of variations among three parameters that are defined perceptually as *pitch, stress,* and *duration.* These same parameters are defined acoustically as *fundamental frequency, intensity,* and *timing* (Table 4–1). Prosodic variation occurs across single words and sentences and serves both linguistic and nonlinguistic functions.

Linguistic prosody contributes meaning to spoken language by disambiguating word and sentence types (Table 4–2). Alterations in stress and duration, for example, enable one to distinguish compound nouns

TABLE 4–1. Parameters used to describe prosody.

Perceptual	Acoustic
Pitch	Frequency
Stress	Intensity, amplitude, volume
Duration	Timing

TABLE 4–2. Linguistic and emotional prosodic functions.

Linguistic Prosody: Disambiguates words and sentences

Examples:

1. Alterations in word stress and syllable duration: distinguishes noun phrases from compound nouns

2. Alterations in frequency contour: distinguishes interrogatives from declaratives

3. Alterations in stress: clarifies sentence meaning

Emotional Prosody: Identifies emotional content and speaker attitudes

Examples:

1. Increased intensity: anger, surprise

2. Increased pitch: excitement, fear

3. Lowered intensity and lack of pitch variation: sadness

4. Reduced duration and pause time: excitement, surprise

(e.g., *light*house, *high*chair) from adjective/ noun phrases (e.g., light *house,* high *chair*). Alterations in terminal fundamental frequency help distinguish interrogative from declarative sentences. Interrogatives usually end in a rising pitch and declaratives do not. Placement of pauses and alterations in the duration and intensity of words in sentences can enhance their meaning. For example, stress on the initial word in the sentence, "Joe gave flowers to Ella," answers the question "Who gave flowers to Ella?" Stress on the third word answers the question, "What did Joe give Ella?" Stress on the final word answers the question "To whom did Joe give flowers?"

Prosody also helps identify the emotional content of spoken words and sentences and speaker attitude (Table 4–2). Prosody is associated most typically with a person's emotional state. For example, raised intensity or volume often is associated with anger. When someone is sad, pitch is usually less varied and lower than it is when someone is happy. Rapid rate within and between words can signal excitement.

Speaker attitudes not associated with a primary emotion also can be conveyed by prosody. For example, the single word "sure" in response to a request can indicate cheerful compliance, affirmation, or sarcasm depending on the intonation pattern and stress changes across the word. The prosody in the phrase "Yes, Sir" is quite different when used by a Marine at attention versus a waiter responding to a customer's request. Deference, formality, humor, and irony are just a few examples of the attitudes conveyed through prosody. Prosodic cues thus help us interpret what is meant from what is said, the emotional state of the speaker, and the speaker's attitude toward the listener and the situation. When these cues are absent, attenuated, or disrupted it takes more effort to determine and to convey the meaning of the spoken word.

OVERVIEW OF PROSODIC DEFICITS

Disturbances in emotional well-being and mental status, sensorimotor integrity, motor programming, and language formulation can disrupt normal control over the prosodic components of speech output. Prosodic deficits associated with RHD appear to be independent of these impairments, although the influence of motor deficits associated with certain types of dysarthria cannot be entirely ruled out. A sampling of prosodic impairments, including an overview of those associated with RHD, is presented below. As one reads down the list of prosodic deficits that can occur subsequent to neurologic damage, it is important to remember that brain-damaged patients may have more than one disorder or disease process. It is important, then, to distinguish RHD prosodic impairments from those caused by other neurologic problems and to be sure that a patient's prosodic impairment is not the symptom of some other deficit.

Motor Speech Disorders

Dysarthria and apraxia of speech are neurological disorders known to interfere with the fluid production of connected speech. Motor programming deficits can also affect prosody. Apraxia of speech can be characterized by inappropriate pauses and lack of variation in syllable duration, and by restricted or altered pitch and loudness (Duffy, 1995; Kent & Rosenbek, 1982).

A few examples of disturbed prosody resulting from impaired motor control in dysarthria include increased syllable and word duration and reduced speech rate associated in spastic dysarthria; disruption of timing and rhythm and disproportionate lengthening of unstressed syllables in ataxic dysarthria; and reduced stress, monopitch and monoloudness in the hypokinetic dysarthria characteristic of Parkinson's disease (Duffy, 1995).

Dysarthria is almost never addressed as a contributing factor in studies of RHD prosodic deficits. Ryalls et al. (1987), for example, found a nonsignificant trend for early postonset patients with RHD to have more prosodic problems than late postonset patients, suggesting the possibility of a "resolving dysarthric component" (p. 690). Cancelliere and Kertesz (1990) questioned the influence of dysarthria on their results in a study on lesion localization and prosodic deficits. Unilateral upper motor neu-ron dysarthria associated with stroke is not likely the cause of the prosodic deficits associated with RHD because it can accompany strokes in both the LH and the RH, but it may exacerbate prosodic production deficits in RHD patients.

It was once thought that prosodic comprehension deficits were restricted to RH lesions. However, prosodic comprehension deficits have recently been found to occur in patients with motor speech problems subsequent to Parkinson's disease (Blonder, Gur, & Gur, 1989; Scott, Caird, & Williams, 1984) and Huntington's disease (Speedie, Brake, Folstein, Bowers, & Heilman, 1990).

Language Impairments

Aphasia may result in inappropriate pausing during word retrieval, disrupting the timing, fluency, and normal prosodic pattern across sentences (Duffy, 1995). Agrammatic speech, characteristic of Broca's aphasia, may result in inappropriate word stress. The range (variation) of fundamental frequency may be restricted in some types of aphasia (Ryalls, 1982). Aphasic patients are sometimes included in studies of RHD prosodic impairments, and their performance often is impaired relative to NBD controls, not only in production, but in comprehension as well.

Psychiatric Conditions

Schizophrenia, depression, and mania are among the psychiatric conditions that may affect prosody. In schizophrenia, prosodic deficits vary with the phase and the variety of the illness. Some patients have rapidly alternating melody and pitch and abnormal stress patterns (Aronson, 1990). Others have flattened affect, and amplitude, and frequency patterns may show less than normal variation so that speech sounds flat and colorless (Aronson, 1990; Merewether & Alpert, 1990). In depression, the range of intensity and pitch may be reduced, pauses may be longer than normal, and intensity may decrease across a sentence (Aronson, 1990; Merewether & Alpert, 1990).

Right Hemisphere Damage

The clinical presentation of RHD prosodic production impairments is a flattened, monotone pattern that is characterized by *attenuated variation in stress, duration, and fundamental frequency* (Duffy, 1995). The overall effect may make patients sound depressed and give their speech a somewhat robotic quality. Patients often stress words by changes in amplitude, rather than by changes in pitch or duration. In addition, RHD patients may have difficulty with prosodic comprehension, particularly with emotional prosody. Their comprehension problems appear to be more severe than those associated with other neurogenic disorders.

The mechanisms of RHD prosodic deficits are not presently understood. More is known about what these disorders do not represent than about what they do represent. The impairments can exist in the absence of motor speech disturbances and, therefore, are not thought to be the result of impaired motor or sensory function (although presence of dysarthria is rarely reported in studies of RHD prosodic impairments). Because language is fundamentally intact following RHD, linguistic processing deficits are not considered the source of the problem. RHD prosodic deficits are not characterized by the false starts and groping attempts at self-correction characteristic of apraxia of speech, and they do not seem to represent a motor programming deficit as we typically think of it. Finally, because the deficits can occur in the absence of clinical depression, they are not considered part of a psychiatric condition.

Although research has distinguished emotional from linguistic prosody, the distinction represents hypotheses about prosodic processing and does not necessarily reflect psychological reality. The brain may not process emotional prosodic features any differently than it does linguistic pros-

ody. As pointed out by Joanette, Goulet, and Hannequin (1990), "There are no acoustic parameters enabling one to differentiate emotional from linguistic stimuli" (p. 113). Much of the early work on prosody in RHD patients was inspired by the hypothesis that RHD reduces emotional responsivity (see Chapter 7 on affective deficits), and much of the research on prosodic impairments has been conducted within this functional framework.

LABELING RHD PROSODIC IMPAIRMENTS

A number of terms have been used to describe prosodic problems secondary to RHD. In one of the first investigations of RHD prosodic deficits, Heilman, Scholes, and Watson (1975) used the term *auditory affective agnosia,* suggesting that RHD affected prosodic comprehension and occurred in response to emotional prosody. Subsequently, Ross (1981), widely recognized for associating prosodic production as well as comprehension deficits with RHD, used the term *aprosodia* to describe both comprehension and production problems. *Aprosodia* was originally coined by Monrad-Krohn (1947) to describe loss of the prosodic features of speech, although it now refers to *attenuation* rather than *loss* of prosody. As used by Ross and his colleagues, the term *aprosodia* is restricted to processing *emotionally based* paralinguistic information and includes deficits in emotional gesturing as well as prosody (Gorelick & Ross, 1987; Ross, 1981, 1985, 1988, 1993; Ross, Harney, deLacoste-Utamsing, & Purdy, 1981; Ross & Mesulam, 1979). He and his colleagues promoted a model in which RHD prosodic disturbances are categorized according to function (emotional versus linguisitic) and affective behavior is tied to the RH (Ross, 1993). As we shall see in this chapter, a better approach to prosody may be one in which its component *features*, rather than its *function*, are addressed. That is, certain prosodic features such as pitch appear to be more vulnerable to RHD than other features, and pitch may be particularly crucial in distinguishing among types of emotions. Thus, RHD prosodic impairments may be linked more by happenstance than by design to emotional processing.

Some researchers have used the term *dysprosody* with reference to RHD prosodic impairments (Behrens, 1988; Hird & Kirsner, 1993; Joanette et al., 1990; Ryalls et al., 1987; Shapiro & Danly, 1985). *Dysprosody* was also used by Monrad-Kohn (1947) in reference to the preserved, but abnormal, prosody in an LHD patient with pseudo-foreign accent. The term describes a variety of prosodic abnormalities, however, and does not elucidate anything in particular about RHD prosodic impairments.

Perhaps a label that uniquely identifies the range of RHD prosodic deficits and that is restricted to prosody independent of gesture must await a more precisely formulated operational definition and a clearer picture of the nature of the problem. Hence, in this chapter, prosodic dysfunction associated with RHD will be referred to simply as *RHD prosodic deficits* or *RHD prosodic impairments.*

RESEARCH ON RHD PROSODIC IMPAIRMENTS

Several characteristics considered unique to prosodic deficits in RHD patients have guided research in the area over the past 20 years. First, prosodic impairments associated with RHD may occur in the face of intact sensorimotor and linguistic processes, just as it does in certain psychiatric conditions. Second, emotional prosody appears to be more disrupted than linguistic prosody, and some RHD patients may sound depressed. Third, RHD patients are known to have problems in interpreting emotional material in other domains such as facial expression and the emotional content of stories and scenes. Fourth, until recently, prosodic comprehension deficits

were thought to be unique to RHD. This combination of features raised the possibility that prosodic processing may be housed in the RH and may be related to a disturbance in the encoding and decoding of emotional behavior. As a result, the central themes driving research in this area have been: (a) *the relationship between prosody and hemispheric laterality and the possible superiority of the RH for prosodic processing,* and (b) *issues related to the categorization of prosody according to function (emotional versus linguistic).* Experimental work on these issues has in some ways elucidated and in some ways muddied our understanding of the clinical picture of RHD prosodic deficits.

Because laterality has been the focus of much of the experimental work, questions about the nature of those deficits were really questions about the role of the intact RH in prosodic processing. Was it dominant for prosody just as the LH is dominant for language? Was its role restricted to emotional prosody or did it include linguistic prosody as well? Much of what we know comes from studies in which the goal is to clarify hemispheric contributions to prosodic processing in the intact brain, rather than to explore clinical manifestations of prosodic deficits. As a result, in almost all of the experimental studies, subject selection has been based on the presence of unilateral hemispheric damage and not on the presence of prosodic deficits. This is a problem for those interested in the characteristics and mechanisms of RHD prosodic deficits because it is from these studies that most of our knowledge about the nature of RHD prosodic impairments has been derived, even though many subjects included in the data pool did not actually have prosodic deficits. Even when the goal was to describe the defining features of RHD prosodic deficits, studies typically have used unselected subjects. The situation is not unlike studying the nature and clinical presentation of aphasia from the pooled data of aphasic and nonaphasic LHD patients. Without a good definition of RHD prosodic deficits, it has been difficult to select patients accordingly. It is important to remember, then, that in almost every case *findings from group studies exploring the signs and underlying mechanisms of prosodic deficits secondary to RHD are based on patients who may or may not have prosodic deficits.*

Despite this shortcoming, research in the area has added to our knowledge base. First and foremost, it has heightened awareness of potential prosodic deficits in RHD patients. Symptoms that may have gone unrecognized before are now noted in medical charts and addressed by speech-language pathologists. Families, patients, and professionals are more aware of the impact of prosodic deficits on communication. Second, research has helped to establish that RHD can affect linguistic as well as emotional prosody and that certain prosodic features may be more impaired than others. This knowledge can help guide remediation efforts. This chapter explores prosodic comprehension and production deficits that can occur subsequent to RHD. We do not know the incidence of prosodic deficits, in part for lack of a solid definition. However, the clinical picture suggests that prosodic impairments occur in some, but certainly not in all, RHD patients.

PROSODIC PRODUCTION DEFICITS

The flat, robotic prosodic production of RHD patients with prosodic impairments is not difficult to recognize. Understanding its nature is more problematic. Clinical observations and single-case reports of reduced prosodic expression subsequent to RHD (Gorelick & Ross, 1987; Ross, 1981; Ross & Mesulam, 1979) have been supported by experimental group studies (Borod, Koff, Lorch, & Nicholas, 1985; Hird & Kirsner, 1993; Shapiro & Danley, 1985; Tucker, Watson, & Heilman, 1977).

Emotional Prosodic Production Deficits

Clinically, prosodic production problems are evident in both emotional and non-emotional conversational contexts. In experimental work, these problems have been found to be more pronounced in the service of emotional communication (Table 4–3). Tucker et al. (1977), for example, compared the ability of RHD and NBD subjects to produce neutral sentences with a specified emotion and found that judges had significant problems determining the emotion conveyed by RHD subjects. RHD subjects have been found to be more impaired than patients with unipolar depression and those with Parkinson's disease in the accuracy and intensity of emotional prosodic production produced on command (Borod et al., 1990). RHD patients with prosodic deficits may rely more on word choice than on prosody to convey their emotions (Borod et al., 1985).

The apparent similarities between the prosodic production of RHD patients and patients with depression at first led to the hypothesis that these expressive deficits were the outcome of alterations in subjective emotional experience. For example, in a study of prosodic production in patients with stroke, patients under psychiatric care for depression, and physically ill patients, judges could not differentiate the stroke patients from the clinically depressed group, despite the fact that the stroke patients were free of depression on clinical rating

TABLE 4–3. Characteristics of emotional prosodic production deficits in RHD.

1. Flat, robotic, monotone prosodic contour
2. Problems in matching prosodic contour to emotional content
3. Reduced reliance on pitch variation to signal emotions
4. Increased reliance on semantic information, rather than prosody, to convey emotions

scales (House, Rowe, & Standen, 1987). However, the self-reports of RHD patients with prosodic production deficits suggested that attenuated prosody is at odds with their experience of emotions. The two patients described by Ross and Mesualm (1981), for example, complained of difficulty making their tone of voice match their mood. Ross and Rush (1981) described a patient whose impaired prosody coexisted with depression. However, her flattened prosodic production remained even when the depression was successfully treated with antidepressants.

A second hypothesis is that prosodic production impairments reflect a general disturbance in *encoding* emotional behavior, but not necessarily in the subjective experience of emotions (Borod et al., 1985; Borod, Koff, Lorch, Nicholas, & Welkowitz, 1988; Ross, 1985). That is, *the display of emotions, rather than the emotions themselves, is impaired* and is reflected in prosodic production as well as in other forms of emotional expression. Disturbances in encoding emotional behavior subsequent to RHD have been noted in the reduced expressive output in other channels such as gestures and facial expression. Individual case reports suggest that more than one form of spontaneous emotional gesturing may be compromised by RHD (Ross, 1981; Ross & Mesulam, 1979) and that other signs of emotional behavior in these patients (i.e., pathologic crying) can be dissociated from internal emotional states (Ross, 1981). For example, RHD patients have been found to show less facial expression than LHD patients in response to emotionally evocative pictures (Borod et al., 1985; Borod et al., 1988; Buck & Duffy, 1980) and to be less expressive in a variety of ways than LHD patients when interviewed about their disability (Blonder, Burns, Bowers, Moore, & Heilman, 1993).

Reduced prosodic expressivity may be the outcome of a "dominant role for the right hemisphere in emotional expression" (Borod et al., 1985, p. 348), but it appears that factors other than those involved in encoding emotional behavior play a role in prosodic production impairments. That is, prosodic processing may be compromised, independent of affective behavior and encoding. Use of prosody is more apparent when conveying emotion, but it has been found that RHD patients may have difficulty using prosody for linguistic purposes as well. The clinical impression that patients with prosodic production deficits sound abnormal in conversational speech, regardless of the emotional content of their discourse, has been supported to some extent by experimental work as described in the following section.

Linguistic Prosodic Production Deficits

Although prosodic production deficits may be more apparent and more dramatic in emotional situations, they also can occur in nonemotional conversations. Table 4–4 outlines some of the linguistic production deficits reviewed below.

Emphatic Stress: Phrase Level

In normal production, stressed syllables generally are greater in amplitude and duration and have a higher fundamental frequency than unstressed syllables (Behrens, 1988). In general, RHD does not appear to affect the ability to produce the contrastive stress necessary to distinguish between com-

TABLE 4–4. Characteristics of linguistic prosodic production deficits in RHD.

Phrase Level:

1. Over-reliance on intersyllabic pause and duration to distinguish nouns from noun phrases

Sentence Level:

2. Minimally impaired use of emphatic stress on words in sentences

3. Some deficits in the use of fundamental frequency to distinguish sentence types

pound nouns (redcoat) and noun phrases (red coat) (Behrens, 1988; Emmory, 1987). Behrens (1988) found, however, that RHD patients use fewer of the cues available to signal contrastive stress. Intersyllabic pause was the most commonly used cue and syllabic duration the least used cue by NBD subjects. However, no RHD subject used intersyllabic pause. This finding mirrors the impression of the somewhat robotic production in RHD in which spacing between words and syllables seems uniform and consistent, rather than varied as it is in normal production. When we think of computerized speech, for example, one of the striking characteristics is the uniform pausing between words and syllables, giving its characteristic robotic or mechanical sound.

Emphatic Stress: Sentence Level

Emphatic stress helps to convey intended meaning and can distinguish differences in meaning between sentences with the same content (e.g., "The *horses* are racing from the barn," versus, "The horses are racing from the *barn*"). RHD patients may not use emphatic stress normally in spontaneously elicited sentences (Wientraub, Mesulam, & Kramer, 1981), although they may be able to do so on command (i.e., when asked to stress the initial or final word in sentences) (Behrens, 1988). Behrens, however, found that, even on command, some RHD subjects occasionally increased the amplitude of the final unemphasized word in sentences in which the initial word was meant to be stressed. This pattern was the opposite of that produced by the NBD subjects. However, in other ways, the pattern of productions on command was like that of the NBD subjects in that they (a) *relied most often on changes in pitch and least commonly on changes in intensity to stress words in sentences,* (b) *produced stressed words with longer syllabic duration than they did unstressed words,* and (c) *produced the same patterns of fluctuation in fundamental frequency for words*

they did stress. Behrens concluded that prosodic production of stress in both phrases and sentences is affected minimally, if at all, by RHD. The clinical impression, however, is that patients with prosodic production deficits seem to rely more on an increase in volume than on alterations in pitch or duration in both spontaneous and elicited sentences.

Distinguishing Sentence Types

Declaratives and interrogatives differ principally in frequency contour, and for that reason, pitch has been the parameter most typically investigated. A fall in frequency contour is associated with declaratives whereas a rising pitch is associated with yes-no interrogatives. Not surprisingly, Hird and Kirsner (1993) found no differences between the productions of RHD and NBD adults on measures of *duration* in distinguishing interrogatives from declaratives. On measures of *fundamental frequency,* however, RHD patients have been found to have difficulty producing differences between declaratives, interrogatives, and imperatives (Behrens, 1989; Shapiro & Danly, 1985; Weintraub et al., 1981). Among the abnormalities noted are: (a) *an abnormally flat pitch pattern in declaratives,* and (b) *less than normal variability and fluctuation in pitch in interrogatives* (Behrens, 1989).

Ryalls et al. (1987), on the other hand, found no significant differences between NBD and RHD subjects on measures of fundamental frequency and frequency fluctuations. However, as noted by the authors, differences between their results and those of other investigators may have occurred because their subjects were asked to imitate rather than spontaneously generate different sentence types. This difference was important because the authors noted that the prosody in the spontaneous speech of their RHD patients sounded abnormal to the authors and even to some of the patients themselves. Patients' spontaneous productions seemed lower in overall pitch and reduced in range of intensity and pitch.

In general, it appears that prosodic impairments secondary to RHD may have an impact on linguistic prosodic production at the sentence level. Patients may not have normal levels of pitch variation and may use fewer and less salient cues to signal emphatic stress.

Acoustic Analysis

Acoustic analyses of prosodic production impairments support the hypothesis that production deficits are related to reduced use of frequency information. These analyses suggest that: (a) *pitch variation and control is a significant factor in the impaired prosodic production that can accompany RHD,* and (b) *pitch variation is a key factor in distinguishing the emotional tone conveyed by prosody.*

An early acoustic analysis of the production of a neutral declarative sentence elicited from subjects by Kent and Rosenbek (1982) revealed that the productions of RHD subjects had reduced energy in the mid and high frequency ranges and strong energy in the low frequencies consistent with nasalization and inadequate articulation. All three of their subjects were judged to have mild dysarthria with left-sided facial weakness, which may have contributed to their prosodic deficits.

Hird and Kirsner (1993) investigated duration in patients with RHD, multiple sclerosis, Parkinson's disease, and in NBD controls. They found that, although the mean duration of emotionally intoned sentences was shorter for RHD than for any other group, the results were not significant.

Pitch variation and pitch range seem to be critical variables for differentiating the emotional prosodic productions of RHD, LHD, and NBD subjects (Shapiro & Danly, 1985). When variability is normalized for the mean fundamental frequency, RHD patients have less variation in pitch than normal (Colsher, Cooper, & Graff-Radford,

1987; Ryalls, 1986). At first, this did not seem to be the case. Shapiro and Danly (1985) found that patients with right anterior and right central damage had restricted pitch variation and range compared to LHD and NBD subjects. Surprisingly, however, their right posterior patients had *more* pitch variation, *greater* range and a higher mean fundamental frequency than all other subjects. This finding of "hypermelodicity" in the posterior patients was challenged by Colsher et al. (1987) (see also Ryalls, 1986), who explained that, because the overall mean pitch level in some patients might be higher, mean pitch should be taken into account when analyzing acoustic results. Normalizing the variability measure, they found the direction of differences between anterior and posterior RHD patients in the Shapiro and Danly data reversed. Patients with posterior damage had slightly lower pitch variability and patients with anterior damage had slightly higher pitch variability than NBD subjects. To prove their point, Colsher et al. (1987) also tested two RHD and three NBD subjects on a sentence reading task. Prior to normalizing for mean fundamental frequency, they found that the RHD subjects had higher mean fundamental frequencies and more pitch variability than normal. However, when the variability was normalized for the mean fundamental frequency, the RHD subjects demonstrated reduced variability compared to the NBD subjects.

Pitch information also appeared to be a key acoustic parameter in a Wada test study of emotional intonation patterns in NBD subjects (Ross, Edmondson, Seibert, & Homan, 1988). During a Wada test, sodium amytal is introduced into one of the two hemispheres, thereby reducing its function. Test results showed a flattening of the intonation pattern after injection in the RH of NBD subjects, a pattern reflected principally in various measures of fundamental frequency rather than in duration or intensity. Thus, the perceptual impression of reduced use of pitch variation as a key factor in the impaired prosodic production of RHD patients has been substantiated by acoustic measurements.

PROSODIC COMPREHENSION DEFICITS

There is no doubt that RHD can interfere with prosodic comprehension as well as production. These deficits are particularly evident in identifying emotional prosody. Research suggests that RHD prosodic comprehension impairments, including those in emotional prosodic comprehension, may be *perceptually* based. That is, *prosodic comprehension deficits may exist independently of the function prosody serves (linguistic or emotional).* These problems may be more evident in emotional than in linguistic prosodic processing because certain acoustic or perceptual features (i.e., pitch variation) are critical to emotional prosody and are more vulnerable to RHD than others.

Emotional Prosodic Comprehension Deficits

Emotional prosodic comprehension has been investigated in a variety of ways, but the most common paradigm isolates prosody from content by asking subjects to identify the mood with which a nonemotional sentence is spoken. Typically, subjects listen to sentences with neutral semantic content, such as, "He went to the store," said with a given emotion and then choose the emotion best represented by its the prosodic contour. The emotions tested are those considered to be universal across cultures and thus part of the human condition (e.g., happiness, sadness, anger, surprise) (Alpert & Rosen, 1990; Ekman, 1973).

This type of task often is used in informal evaluation of patients as well as in experimental work. Regardless of the goal, clinical diagnosis or controlled study, it is important to validate the stimuli prior to presentation as even normal subjects can disagree on the emotional valance of pro-

sodic productions. For example, in preparing a set of stimuli, Tompkins (1991) found that judges could only agree on the emotional tone of 64 out of 192 sentences. In many studies, the protocols are not as carefully controlled, and in some cases, stimuli are not tape-recorded in advance for standardized presentation, but instead are produced in live voice by the investigator at the moment of testing (e.g., Gorelick & Ross, 1987; Ross, 1981).

Case reports of impaired ability to identify the mood conveyed by prosody have been supported by experimental studies of individual subjects (Cancelliere & Kertesz, 1990; Starkstein, Federoff, Price, Leiguarda, & Robinson, 1994), in group studies (Blonder, Bowers, & Heilman, 1991; Borod et al., 1990; Tompkins & Flowers, 1985; Van Lancker & Sidtis, 1992), and in studies comparing performance to LHD subjects (Blonder et al., 1991; Bowers, Coslett, Bauer, Speedie, & Heilman, 1987; Heilman et al., 1975; Tompkins & Flowers, 1985; Tucker, Watson, & Heilman, 1977) (Table 4–5). In the few studies that have failed to find differences between the performance of LHD and RHD subjects (e.g., Schlanger, Schlanger, & Gerstman, 1976; Van Lancker & Sidtis, 1992), it appears that severity of aphasia in the LHD subjects and lack of neglect in the RHD subjects may have influenced the results. Schlanger et al. (1976), for example, found that the mean scores of RHD subjects fell between those of severely and mildly impaired aphasic subjects. Severity of aphasia may not affect prosodic processing per se, but it may in-

TABLE 4–5. Characteristics of emotional prosodic comprehension deficits in RHD.

1. Reduced use of prosodic contour to discriminate and identify mood in neutral sentences presented without supporting context

2. Reduced ability to identify mood in sentences in which the meaning is incongruent with prosodic contour

fluence performance on prosodic identification tasks in other ways. For example, Tompkins and Flowers (1985) found that, as task difficulty increased, the performance of aphasic subjects fell to that of the RHD subjects. It has been suggested that cognitive demands and impaired verbal comprehension may have a negative influence on the performance of aphasic subjects (Ross, 1993; Seron, van der Kaa, & van der Linden, 1982; Tompkins & Flowers, 1985).

RHD patients with neglect also tend to have more trouble in prosodic identification tasks than those without neglect, possibly because they are less aroused, less attentive, and less responsive to extralinguistic information. Starkstein et al. (1994), for example, found a significant correlation between severity of neglect and prosodic deficits. Prosodic comprehension deficits have been associated with posterior parietal lesions, an area known for its association with neglect (Cancelliere & Kertesz, 1990). Finally, neglect was present in 70% to 100% of the subjects in studies finding prosodic identification deficits in RHD patients (Blonder et al., 1991; Heilman et al., 1975; Ross, 1981; Tucker et al., 1977). None of the RHD subjects in the Schlanger et al. (1976) study that failed to find differences among aphasic and RHD subjects had neglect.

Identifying the emotional prosody in neutral sentences that are said without accompanying context is a somewhat artificial task and does not necessarily reflect performance in conversational speech in which semantic content and prosody usually match one another. It does, however, suggest that without supporting context, RHD patients have problems comprehending the emotional tone conveyed by prosody alone.

What happens to prosodic identification if, instead of neutral sentences, sentences have emotional content? Is performance improved when the content matches the emotional tone? Is it further disrupted when it does not? RHD patients appear

able to interpret emotional semantic content in simple stories and sentences when prosody is not a factor (Laland, Braun, Charlebois, & Whitaker, 1992; Tompkins, 1991). Blonder et al. (1991), for example, found that RHD patients were able to identify the emotion in sentences that were read without inflection such as, "You are thrilled with the gift," or "Your spouse may not survive surgery." However, they found that these same subjects had problems judging emotions in sentences that *described* facial, prosodic, and gestural information such as, "She smiled," or, "He spoke quickly and breathlessly" (Blonder et al., 1991, p. 1119). Thus, RHD patients may have more difficulty identifying emotions when their interpretation rests strictly on decoding paralinguistic information that signals internal emotions even when this information is verbally conveyed.

The influence of semantic content has been tested in paradigms in which verbal content was either congruent or incongruent with the prosodic pattern in which the sentence was said. In conversational, speech incongruency between content and tone is present when something is said but not really meant as in sarcastic comments. Not surprisingly, identifying prosody is more difficult for everyone when it does not match the verbal content, but it appears to pose more problems for RHD than for LHD or NBD subjects (Bowers et al., 1987; Starkstein et al., 1994; Tompkins, 1991). Attentional deficits in general, and vigilance deficits in particular, may play a role in the performance of RHD patients on such tasks. Faced with incongruent stimuli that are taken out of context, subjects must suppress attention to the semantic content while focusing on prosody. The paradigm is not unlike a Stroop task in which one feature of a stimulus (e.g., the meaning of the printed word) must be ignored in favor of another feature (the ink color in which the word is printed). As discussed in Chapter 2, vigilance deficits may impair the performance of RHD patients on such tasks. Hence, it is difficult to know the source of

RHD deficits in determining the emotion conveyed by prosody in incongruent stimuli. Specific prosodic deficits may be exacerbated by attentional demands.

From the research, it appears that RHD patients have trouble interpreting the mood conveyed by prosodic contour when prosody is isolated from or is incongruent with semantic content. The same patients who have difficulty interpreting emotional prosody typically are able to interpret the emotional valance of linguistic information in simple sentences and stories (Blonder et al., 1991; LaLande et al., 1992; Tompkins, 1991), suggesting that their problems are specific to the interpretation of prosodic and other paralinguistic information as opposed to the interpretation of emotions, per se.

Linguistic Prosodic Comprehension Deficits

Studies of linguistic prosodic comprehension have tended to support the notion that prosodic comprehension deficits are independent of the function (emotional versus nonemotional) that prosody serves. RHD subjects have been found to be impaired relative to NBD subjects in the following tasks: (a) *distinguishing compound words from noun phrases* (e.g., green *house* from *green*house), (b) *discriminating nouns from verbs based on syllabic stress* (e.g., con*vict versus convict*), (c) *determining if two identical sentences were said with the same stress pattern* (e.g., *Steve* is driving the car versus Steve is driving the *car*), (d) *identifying stressed words in sentences,* (e) *discriminating correct from incorrect use of stress in a sentence,* and (f) *discriminating imperative and interrogative from declarative sentences* (Bryan, 1989; Weintraub et al., 1981) (Table 4–6). In most of these tasks they are impaired relative to aphasic patients as well as NBD controls, although they may be better than aphasic patients in discriminating compound words and sentence types (Bryan, 1989; Emmory, 1987).

It appears that the two hemispheres cooperate in decoding linguistic prosodic in-

formation. In a dichotic listening study, for example, NBD subjects were asked to identify stress placement in filtered, unfiltered, and nonsense words (Behrens, 1985). A shift in laterality occurred as the linguistic significance of the stimuli was reduced through filtering. Subjects demonstrated a right ear/LH advantage with real words and a left ear/RH advantage when the same words were filtered to remove phonemic information. Finally, there was no advantage when nonsense words were used. That is, when phonemic information was available but not significant, neither hemisphere predominated.

The data on linguistic prosodic comprehension deficits is limited, but the fact that RHD can interfere with nonemotional prosodic processing suggests that prosodic comprehension deficits are not restricted to emotional processing. It further suggests that the function of prosody as either a linguistic or emotional marker may be less important than its acoustic and perceptual characteristics. That possibility is explored in the following section on prosodic perception.

PROSODIC PERCEPTION DEFICITS: THE IMPORTANCE OF PITCH INFORMATION

The fact that studies have found RHD subjects impaired relative to both NBD and LHD subjects in prosodic discrimination suggests that they have deficits in making purely perceptual judgments about prosodic information. Further evidence of a perceptual level deficit comes from studies in which phonemic information is markedly reduced or eliminated. For example, RHD patients were more impaired than LHD and NBD control subjects in discriminating the emotions conveyed by a single vowel projected with differing emotional prosody (Denes, Caldognetto, Semenza, Vagges, & Zettin, 1984). Similarly, they had problems relative to LHD and NBD subjects in determining the prosody conveyed

TABLE 4–6. Characteristics of linguistic prosodic comprehension deficits.

Problems:

1. Distinguishing parts of speech from one another based on stress patterns:
   a. nouns from noun phrases
   b. nouns from verbs

2. Determining whether two sentences are identical based on stress patterns

3. Distinguishing correct from incorrect use of stress in sentences

4. Determining sentence type from prosodic contour: declarative versus interrogative versus imperative

by a prolonged humming sound produced with different intonational contours (Laland et al., 1992).

In filtered speech paradigms in which spoken sentences are acoustically filtered in such a way as to render the semantic content unintelligible while preserving the intonation pattern, RHD patients have been found to be impaired in identifying the emotions conveyed by prosody relative to both NBD subjects (Bowers et al., 1987; Heilman, Bowers, Speedie, & Coslett, 1984; Tompkins & Flowers, 1985) and relative to LHD subjects (Bowers et al., 1987; Heilman, Bowers, et al., 1984). However, they were no more impaired than LHD patients in determining sentence types by prosodic contour (Heilman, Bowers, et al., 1984). Heilman, Bowers, et al. (1984) concluded that, although RHD may affect both linguistic and emotional prosodic perception, the LH appears to contribute to linguistic prosodic perception, even when phonemic information has been filtered out. Emotional discrimination may be more difficult than linguistic because certain acoustic prosodic parameters may be particularly important to emotional prosody whereas others are more important to linguistic prosody. That is, each hemisphere may be more adept at processing unique prosodic features, and those features for which each

hemisphere predominates may be more or less important to processing linguistic versus emotional prosody.

Not surprisingly, given the importance of pitch variation deficits in RHD prosodic production impairments, the results of several types of studies have suggested that *pitch perception* also may be selectively impaired by RHD. For example, nonlinguistic auditory stimuli that are dependent on frequency information such as melodies and chords, and laughing and crying have been found to be processed more efficiently in the intact RH compared to the LH (Gordon, 1970; Kimura, 1964; King & Kimura, 1972). Sidtis and Feldman (1990) described a case of isolated pitch perception impairment in a man who, in the course of several ischemic attacks, lost his ability to perceive pitch and intonational contour. Approximately three weeks later, he developed a left hemiplegia subsequent to RHD. The patient characterized the first 20-min episode leading up to the stroke as a loss of the vocal variety in the speech of people at a party. Voices sounded flat and monotone, although semantic content was not disrupted. He characterized the second episode as a loss of the melodic contour of music on the radio. Loudness and rhythm was retained, but not the melody. The authors suggested that, "The patient's subjective reports of perceptual alteration suggest that the selective loss of complex-pitch discrimination observed after right hemisphere damage is an important component of the more general syndromes of amusia, dysprosody, and aprosodia" (p. 470).

In addition, dichotic listening studies have demonstrated the importance of pitch in hemispheric processing of acoustic input. Sidtis (1980), for example, found that a left ear/RH advantage in a pitch discrimination task increased with the number of overtones contained in the stimuli. Sidtis and Volpe (1988) found RHD subjects were impaired in pitch, but not in speech discrimination, whereas LHD subjects were impaired in speech, but not in pitch discrimination. Chobor and Brown (1987) found a similar dissocation among brain-damaged subjects in a phoneme and timbre monitoring task. LHD subjects were more accurate at monitoring timbres than phonemes whereas the opposite was true for RHD subjects.

Rather than a verbal/nonverbal or linguistic/emotional dichotomy, laterality effects seem to be based on the degree to which properties such as temporal order, timing, duration, and frequency come into play. The LH may be more involved when material is time-dependent and sequential processing is required. The RH may be more prominent when material is time-independent (Carmon & Nachson, 1971; Chobor & Brown, 1987; Robin, Tranel, & Damasio, 1990). Nontemporal properties include spectral information such as pitch and harmonic structure. Temporal properties include temporal order, sequence, and duration of sounds and of intervals between sounds (Robin et al., 1990). RHD patients appear to be selectively impaired on time-independent spectral tasks (Divenyi & Robinson, 1989). Robin et al. (1990), for example, found that RHD patients were more impaired than LHD subjects in spectral tasks such as frequency discrimination and pitch matching, whereas LHD subjects were significantly impaired relative to RHD subjects in temporal pattern perception and gap detection. The authors concluded that spectral processing impairments contribute to RHD prosodic comprehension problems by creating a perceptual impairment that specifically affects the capacity to judge frequency changes. All of their RHD subjects had prosodic production and comprehension deficits. The three subjects whose prosodic productions were acoustically analyzed were found to have problems using fundamental frequency, but not durational cues. The results suggested that prosodic impairments subsequent to RHD may be "related to an inability to perceive frequency-related information rather than a higher level disability in assigning a meaningful representation to a normal acoustic trace" (p. 552).

A study by Van Lancker and Sidtis (1992) provides further evidence that individual prosodic parameters may be differentially affected by unilateral brain damage. They found that both LHD and RHD subjects were impaired relative to NBD controls in comprehending emotional prosody, but for different reasons. Fundamental frequency variability was found to be the most significant factor distinguishing the affective sentence types from one another. Error analysis revealed that RHD subjects relied more on durational cues than on frequency information to make their judgements, whereas LHD subjects relied more on fundamental frequency. In addition, RHD subjects had a greater tendency to confuse positive emotions with negative ones. The authors concluded that, "receptive dysprosody can be accounted for at the level of perceptual deficit without invoking additional deficits in affective or cognitive processes" (p. 35).

The evidence from acoustic, dichotic, and other types of studies strongly suggests that comprehension deficits begin at the level of perception and that pitch perception and other aspects of nontemporal, spectral information are particularly important in: (a) the impaired performance of RHD patients, and (b) distinguishing emotions. This body of research suggests that the problems RHD patients have in comprehending prosody in both emotional and nonemotional contexts may be the result of a deficit in aspects of pitch perception. Perhaps the problems RHD patients have in prosodic production are also related to pitch perception problems (e.g., problems in their ability to distinguish frequency cues as they speak).

LOCALIZATION

Intact prosodic production depends on the integrity of various cortical and subcortical structures, each of which may contribute differently to prosodic processing. Lesions in the temporal, frontal, and parietal lobes as well as lesions involving the basal ganglia, the internal capsule, and the insula have all been associated with impaired prosody secondary to RHD. Ryalls and Behrens (1988) remind us of Luria's admonition that complex functional systems are not likely to be localized "in narrow zones of the cortex or in isolated cell groups," but must be organized into systems that work in concert with one another and may be located at some distance from one another (Luria, 1973). We know so little about the nature of the disorder, the degree to which it relates to motor control, to attention, to neglect, to acoustic perception, and to automatic and voluntary control over emotional expression that the role of various structures in prosodic processing is difficult to determine. In addition, few studies have specifically addressed lesion location. Site of lesion has been reported for individual subjects in a number of group studies, but individual performance has not, so it is difficult to match performance to lesion site. Other methodological problems include failure to fully describe subjects in terms of accompanying deficits such as dysarthria and neglect. Despite these limitations, some recurring themes appear in the literature.

Prosodic comprehension deficits have been associated with both anterior and posterior cortical lesions, with an emphasis on posterior lesions. The majority of the subjects in studies by Heilman et al. (1975), Heilman, Bowers, et al. (1984), Tucker et al. (1977), and Van Lancker and Sidtis (1992) (reported in Van Lancker & Sidtis, 1993) had parietal lobe involvement.

A variety of lesions have been cited in studies of prosodic production deficits. Areas of involvement in linguistic prosodic deficits include frontal, temporal, and parietal areas as well as the caudate nucleus, the internal capsule, and the thalamus (Behrens, 1988; Weintraub et al., 1981). Some studies have found frontal areas particularly important (Borod et al., 1985); others have found the right parietotemporal area particularly significant in producing

linguistic prosodic production and comprehension deficits (Bryan, 1989).

The association of prosodic production deficits with frontal lesions and of prosodic comprehension deficits with posterior lesions stems largely from a model proposed by Ross and his colleagues in which prosodic deficits are mapped in the RH in a mirror image of language deficits in the LH, according to the model of Benson (1979) and Kertesz (1979) (Gorelick & Ross, 1987; Ross, 1981, 1985, 1993; Ross et al., 1981). For example, a "motor aprosodia" would consist of poor prosodic production and repetition with preserved comprehension and would be associated with frontal lesions in areas considered the anatatomic counterpart of Broca's area (Gorelick & Ross, 1987; Ross, 1981). "Transcortical sensory aprosodia" would stem from lesions in temporoparietal areas that would result in preserved production and impaired comprehension. The model has been criticized for methodological reasons and for problems in attempted replication of findings. Most of the investigations on which the model is based used a bedside technique to test prosody in which the examiner was both the source of prosodic imitation and the judge of performance. Basically a clinical tool, this method, as outlined by Ross (1981), involves few stimulus presentations, no stimulus validation, and a broad classification of impairments into "normal, abnormal, or moderately impaired" (Ross, 1981, p. 554).

The Ross model may be accurate in that patients may have isolated deficits in either production, comprehension, or repetition, or may have combinations of deficits. However, the localization of these deficits to anatomic sites has been challenged by the findings of other investigators interested in localization (Bradvik et al., 1991; Cancelliere & Kertesz, 1990). Bradvik et al. (1991) investigated localization of prosodic deficits in RHD patients who were given a battery of tests emphasizing linguistic prosody. Impairments included identification of contrastive stress, sentence type, and emotional prosody, and the production of emphatic stress and differing sentence types. Interestingly, RHD subjects were able to produce emotional prosody with accuracy (note that none of their subjects had neglect). Lesion location assessed by a combination of CT scan, EEG, and regional cerebral blood flow (rCBF) did not support the anatomic model proposed by Ross. Unfortunately, individual subtest scores were not reported, but subjects with quite disparate lesions produced the same scores on the test protocol. The extent of brain damage appeared to play a role in comprehension deficits. The performance of several patients with lesions restricted to subcortical areas was similar to or worse than those with large cortical lesions, and results of rCBF suggested that subcortical structures may be "directly involved in neuronal circuits guiding prosodic performance" (p. 123).

According to Cancelliere and Kertesz (1990), the basal ganglia appear to play a significant role in prosodic impairments. They classified the emotional prosodic production and comprehension of LHD and RHD subjects according to the aphasia classification system used by Ross (1981) in an effort to replicate the Ross findings. Lesions were classified into central cortical, frontal, central deep, and posterior areas. The basal ganglia was the most frequent site of lesion in subjects with prosodic deficits. Other areas included the anterior temporal lobe, insula, and perisylvian regions. There was no association of lesion site with *type* of prosodic deficit.

The main functions of the basal ganglia are related to motor control. For example, the basal ganglia help regulate muscle tone and the movements that support goal-directed movements such as swinging the arm when walking, and they influence the motor aspects of speech by modulating the cortical output of the motor cortex (Duffy, 1994). Cancelliere and Kertesz (1990) discussed evidence of possible nonmotor functions of the basal ganglia which include a circuit with limbic connections and circuits with frontal lobe connections that may be involved in "effecting emotion into action" and the expression of emotional communication. The relationship between emotional communicative functions and the basal ganglia is speculative, and is based on neuroanatomical connections to limbic structures involved in mediating emotions and on connections to frontal structures that are involved in emotional blunting associated with prefrontal syndromes. On the other hand, there is a well-established association between basal ganglia dysfunction and motor speech impairment, specifically in hypokinetic dysarthria as manifested in Parkinson's disease, which is directly linked to basal ganglia dysfunction (Duffy, 1995). Some features of hypokinetic dysarthria, such as lack of normal pitch variations, variation of intensity, and reduced stress, are shared by RHD prosodic production disturbances. Spectrographic analysis of the speech patterns of RHD subjects has been found to strongly resemble that of Parkinsonian subjects (Kent & Rosenbek, 1982). Thus, the frequency of basal ganglia involvement in prosodic production deficits found by Cancelliere and Kertesz may be related to hypokinetic dysarthria or to impaired ability to modulate pitch at the laryngeal level. Damage to the basal ganglia may interfere with emotional prosody either via limbic and frontal lobe connections or through motor circuits that may have a direct effect on motor control over pitch variation.

The basal ganglia also have been associated with deficits in emotional prosodic comprehension. Prosodic comprehension deficits have been found in patients with diseases of the basal ganglia such as Parkinson's disease (Blonder et al., 1989; Scott et al., 1984) and Huntington's disease (Speedie et al., 1990). Starkstein et al. (1994) found temporoparietal and basal ganglia lesions more frequent than other lesion sites in RHD subjects with impaired emotional prosodic comprehension. These patients also were more likely to have anosognosia and extinction on tests of neglect.

Lesions in the basal ganglia have been associated with neglect as well (Damasio et al., 1980; Ferro et al., 1987; Fromm et al., 1985; Vallar & Perani, 1986). Based on a variety of experimental evidence, LeLand et al. (1992) speculated that the basal ganglia may be involved in certain attentional functions that could interfere in prosodic processing, specifically attentional switching and processing simultaneously occurring events. They suggested that deficits in divided attention may partly account for impaired performance on semantic/prosodic congruency tasks. One could speculate further that most emotional prosodic comprehension tasks involve some form of divided attention in that the semantic content of sentences, even neutral ones, must be ignored in favor of the prosodic information. Attentional impairments may then also contribute to the connection between basal ganglia damage and emotional prosodic comprehension deficits.

Ultimately, the association of lesion site within and between the hemispheres depends on more precise and more universally accepted definitions of prosodic comprehension and production deficits associated with RHD. The role of a motor speech component cannot yet be ruled out. One of the main findings in the localization study by Cancelliere and Kertesz (1990), for example, was that although 75% of their RHD subjects had prosodic deficits, 78% of their LHD subjects were also classified as aprosodic. A number of the LHD patients were characterized as "hypoprosodic" on measures of prosodic variability. As the authors suggested, their findings could have been more precise if they had had information on motor deficits, depression, and dysarthria in their brain-damaged groups. In particular, given the localization data, they speculated that dysarthria may have played a role in the performance of both RHD and LHD subjects. As Ryalls and Behrens (1988) suggested, "An attempt must be made to articulate the manner in which 'speech prosody' of the right hemisphere (both of the affective and linguistic do-

main) is 'joined up' with ongoing segmental production (in almost all accounts, clearly a left hemisphere activity)" (p. 113).

SUMMARY

1. *RHD is one of many neurological disorders that can result in prosodic impairments.*

2. *The fact that there is no universally accepted working definition of prosodic impairments associated with RHD has impeded efforts at understanding the nature of those impairments.* In addition, most studies have focused on issues of hemispheric specialization, and as a result, *most of our knowledge comes from studies in which subjects with and without prosodic deficits are included in the same data pool.* Future research on the nature of RHD prosodic deficits should screen subjects for the presence of identified impairments.

3. *Aspects of prosodic production and comprehension may be impaired simultaneously or independently of one another.*

4. Prosodic production and comprehension deficits can occur in both *linguistic* and *emotional* prosody, but *emotional prosodic disturbances are more prominent in RHD.*

5. Impaired prosodic production associated with RHD is characterized by a *flattened, monotone production in which pitch variation is particularly attenuated and between-word pausing may be abnormally uniform.*

6. *Emotional prosodic production deficits have been dissociated from internal emotional states* (i.e., depression), and patients have been known to be frustrated with the discrepancy between emotional experience and the ability to convey it through prosody.

7. *Linguistic prosodic production deficits may interfere with modulating fundamental fre-*

quency and intersyllabic and inter-word pause time. RHD patients also may use fewer of the available prosodic cues to stress words for linguistic meaning in sentences. Data are limited, but support the hypothesis that prosodic impairments are not restricted to the emotional domain.

8. Emotional prosodic comprehension deficits appear to be related to *reduced responsivity to paralinguistic information signaling affect* (gesture, facial expression) *and to problems in prosodic perception, specifically pitch perception.*

9. *Prosodic perception studies suggest that individual parameters of prosody can be selectively impaired by both RHD and LHD.* Specifically, the LH appears to be dominant for time-dependent features such as temporal order and duration. The RH appears dominant for time-independent features such as spectral information.

RHD appears to disrupt the ability to perceive spectral information.

10. *Frequency (pitch information) may be more impaired than duration and timing in RHD and may be more important in distinguishing type and valance of emotions.*

11. The relationship between emotional prosodic deficits and emotional encoding and decoding may be important, but perhaps less significant than *the relationship between emotional prosody and the perception of and control over frequency information in understanding the nature of emotional prosodic deficits.*

12. *Prosodic deficits have been linked to a variety of cortical and subcortical lesions.* The particular importance of the *basal ganglia* may be related to their involvement in motor control in general, laryngeal control in particular, and to their role in attention.

CHAPTER

5

Linguistic Deficits

Chapter Outline

The speech of adults with RHD is not typically characterized by word finding problems, paraphasias, circumlocutions, or impaired phonological processing. When RHD adults do circumlocute, it seems to be around a concept, not a word. That is, they may not be able to tell you why they are in the hospital, not because they cannot access the word "stroke" or other words appropriate to their situation, but because of discourse level deficits and cognitive impairments that interfere with their ability to get to the point and convey their intent. These discourse and cognitive problems are covered in detail in Chapter 6.

In general, RHD patients use syntax that is accurate and varied, seem to understand the literal meaning of most utterances, and do not seem to have word retrieval problems. In other words, they are not aphasic. In spite of these abilities, they still may not perform normally on tests of aphasia. Although their errors may be attributable to non-linguistic deficits in attention, it appears that they may have additional semantic processing problems unique to RHD.

These semantic processing problems are the primary focus of this chapter.

In one of the first investigations of the linguistic performance of RHD patients, Eisenson (1962) noted a certain "looseness of verbalization." He suggested that RHD appears to affect "relatively abstract language formulations," and that the RH might be involved in "super- or extra-ordinary" language function. By "extra-ordinary" language function, Eisenson probably was referring to deficits that occur at the level of narrative or conversational discourse as opposed to straightforward language tasks. More recently, however, it has been reported that the RH contributes to lexical and semantic processing even at the single word level (Burgess & Simpson, 1988; Chiarello, Burgess, Richards, & Pollock, 1990; Gazzaniga, 1983a; Zaidel, 1985). Because the RH is involved in certain types of semantic processes, certain semantic deficits may be part of the overall communication impairment secondary to RHD.

This chapter is divided into two sections, one on *convergent* semantic processing and one on *divergent* semantic processing. For our purposes, *convergent processing refers to relatively straightforward linguistic tasks in which the number of responses is limited* (Table 5–1). In convergent processing, response possibilities converge to a single point. Convergent tasks elicit the most dominant and familiar word meanings. For example, the expected response when naming a picture of a dog, is "dog," not "mutt," or "pet," or "buddy," or "member of the animal kingdom." Conversely, the word "dog" is expected to evoke a protoypical concept of a furry four-legged creature.

Divergent tasks, on the other hand, *elicit a wide range of meanings which may diverge from a single semantic concept to include non-dominant meanings that are alternate, connotative, and/or less familiar* (Table 5–1). For example, the connotative meanings of the word "dog" might be "loyal" and "friend." Alternate and more colloquial meanings for "dog" in various parts of the United States include something that is not pleasing or not up to one's expectations. In some regions of the country, "dogs" refers to feet. Divergent tasks activate meanings that are less frequently used and that may be at the periphery of the dominant meaning of a word. Word fluency tasks in which patients are asked to produce as many members of a semantic category as possible are a good example of a divergent task at the single-word level. Other types of divergent tasks, such as open-ended questions, require a narrative level response, and will be discussed in Chapter 6 on discourse deficits. Although the division between convergent and divergent linguistic processing is somewhat arbitrary, it should enhance the

TABLE 5–1. Convergent versus divergent semantic processing tasks.

Elicitation Tasks	
Divergent	**Convergent**
Confrontation naming	Verbal fluency
Yes/No questions	Open-ended questions
Definitions	Resolving ambiguities

Types of Responses Elicited	
Divergent	**Convergent**
Denotative meanings	Connotative and denotative meanings
Dominant, familiar meanings	Alternate, less familiar meanings

reader's understanding of linguistic deficits subsequent to RHD.

CONVERGENT SEMANTIC PROCESSING

Auditory Comprehension

Single Words

Linguistic comprehension problems in RHD patients surface at the single word or sentence level, but not at the phonemic level of processing. Phonological discrimination is almost always intact subsequent to RHD (Cappa, Papagno, & Vallar, 1990; Chiarello & Church, 1986; Gainotti, Caltagirone, Miceli, & Masullo, 1981; Lesser, 1969; Vallar, Papagno, & Cappa, 1988). Some studies find RHD patients perform normally in single word comprehension (Kertesz & Dobrowolski, 1981; Myers, 1979; Van Lancker & Kempler, 1987) and others find them impaired (Adamovich & Brooks, 1981; Eisenson, 1962; Gainotti et al., 1981; Lesser, 1974). For the most part, however, comprehension of the dominant meanings of single words does not appear to pose problems for RHD patients in conversational speech.

Sentences

A number of studies have demonstrated normal sentence comprehension by RHD subjects on aphasia batteries including the *Boston Diagnostic Aphasia Examination* (Goodglass & Kaplan, 1983); the *Minnesota Test for Differential Diagnosis of Aphasia* (Schuell, 1965), and the *Western Aphasia Battery* (Kertesz, 1982) (Kertesz, 1979; Kertesz & Dombrowolski, 1981; Lesser, 1974; Myers, 1979). Sentence comprehension has been tested in various studies by asking subjects to follow commands, answer yes-no questions, and match sentences to pictured scenes in a multiple choice paradigm. Performance on these tasks is varied, but it does seem that RHD can affect sentence comprehension under certain conditions. For example, some RHD patients may have problems matching pictures to simple sentences (Hier & Kaplan, 1980; Huber & Gleber, 1982; Van Lancker & Kempler, 1987).

Multi-Stage Commands

Multi-stage commands without supporting context may present problems, especially if syntactic structure is complex. Various versions of the *Token Test* (DeRenzi & Vignolo, 1962) have been presented to RHD patients with mixed results. The test was designed to test auditory comprehension of sentences without supporting context. It requires patients to scan and manipulate colored shapes in response to commands (e.g., "touch the large blue circle" or "touch the small red square with the large green circle"). The commands increase in syntactic complexity and crucial information is contained in adjectives, prepositions, and conjunctions. In several studies, RHD subjects have performed normally on this test (Cappa et al., 1990; Huber & Gleber, 1982; Vallar et al., 1988). However, in reviewing their normative data for the *Revised Token Test,* McNeill and Prescott (1978) reported that, although RHD subjects were more accurate and faster than aphasic subjects, they did not perform as well or as quickly as normal controls. Swisher and Sarno (1969) also found that RHD subjects made errors on portions of the test that involve particularly complex syntactic structures. It is unlikely that impaired performance on tests like the *Token Test* is the result of disordered syntactic comprehension. RHD subjects have performed normally on other tests of complex syntactic comprehension (Parisi & Pizzamiglio, 1970). The effects of brain damage per se, versus a deficit unique to RHD, may impair performance. Other likely sources of deficit specific to RHD may be reduced vigilance and attention to detail and poor visual scanning.

Reduced arousal also may interfere with a patient's ability to mobilize the effortful attention required for comprehension of complex commands and sentences presented without supportive context. RHD patients may not be able to muster the vigilance required in situations in which every functor word and adjective is crucial to accurate performance as it is on the *Token Test*. If they are not sufficiently aroused, they also may have problems sustaining attention over the course of a test. When context is provided, comprehension problems that do occur appear to be cognitively, not linguistically based, an issue that is addressed in Chapter 6.

Word Retrieval

RHD adults do not seem to have problems with word finding in conversational speech nor with defining familiar words or naming objects that are described to them (Eisenson, 1962; Hier & Kaplan, 1980; Rivers & Love, 1980; Vallar et al., 1988). A number of studies have found that they also perform within the normal range on confrontation naming tasks (Myers, 1979; Myers & Brookshire, 1995; Rivers & Love, 1980; Vallar et al., 1988). Others have found problems with confrontation naming (Diggs and Basili, 1987; Gainotti, Caltagirone, & Miceli, 1983; Joanette, Lecours, Lepage, & Lamoureaux, 1983), but in most of these studies the deficits were mild. For example, Diggs and Basili (1987) found a difference between the average scores of NBD and RHD subjects on a 20-item naming test of only 1.6 points.

Several investigators have analyzed RHD naming errors to understand the contribution of visuoperceptual, cognitive, and/or semantically based effects. It appears that errors on confrontation naming are not necessarily the result of visual confusions and that semantic problems may play a role. For example, Gainotti et al. (1983) classified errors into three categories: (1) *visual and nonsemantically related errors* (e.g., "ball" for "apple"), (2) *semantically and nonvisually related errors* (e.g., "pear" for "apple"), and (3) *visually and semantically related errors* (e.g., "peach" for "apple"). Subjects who scored poorly on a mental status battery made most of the errors, and most of

their errors were either visual or semantic. The rest of the subjects made predominantly visuo-semantic errors. The authors felt that their results pointed to semantic, as opposed to purely visual, confusions as the source of impaired confrontation naming. Diggs and Basisli (1987) came to the same conclusion. Most of the errors committed by their RHD subjects on a shortened version of *The Boston Naming Test* (Kaplan, Goodglass, & Weintraub, 1983) were semantic rather than visual. Myers and Brookshire (1995) found that although subjects with severe neglect had more visual confusion errors than did those whose neglect was mild, even in the severely impaired group there were very few errors based on visual confusion. Thus, it is a mistake to assume that naming errors among RHD patients are influenced by visual perceptual impairments alone. In fact, it appears that in many cases, even among those with neglect, RHD naming errors that do occur can be attributed to impairments in semantic processing.

DIVERGENT SEMANTIC PROCESSING

Hemispheric Differences in Semantic Processing

Divergent semantic processing emphasizes sensitivity to relationships among items. Relationships can be made by category membership (e.g., a dog is an animal) or by other forms of association. For example, words may be related by antonymic contrast (e.g., top/bottom), metaphoric meaning (e.g., warm/loving), membership in a common category (e.g., bank/building), common functional association (e.g., bank/money), or uncommon or less familiar association (e.g., bank/river). Semantic concepts may be strongly or weakly associated (e.g., suits/articles of clothing versus suits/men in upper management).

There is some evidence that the right and left hemispheres process semantic relation-

TABLE 5–2. Proposed hemispheric differences in semantic processing.

Differences in Types of Semantic Concepts Activated	
Left Hemisphere	**Right Hemisphere**
Familiar, dominant	Less familiar, connotative, alternate
Tightly connected	More loosely connected
Strong semantic overlap	Weaker semantic overlap

Differences in Activation	
Left Hemisphere	**Right Hemisphere**
Operates in conditions of automatic processing	Operates in conditions of controlled processing
Rapid, strong activation of dominant meanings	Slower, weaker activation of alternate meanings

ships differently. The RH is thought to be *more adept at maintaining multiple meanings that may be weakly connected (i.e., have less semantic overlap).* The LH is thought to be *more likely to focus on a single meaning or on several meanings with strong semantic overlap* (Beeman, 1993; Brownell, Potter, Michelow, & Gardner, 1984; Brownell, Simpson, Bihrle, Potter, & Gardner, 1990; Burgess & Simpson, 1988; Chiarello et al., 1990) (Table 5–2). The model of differences in semantic processing across the two hemispheres proposes that the LH engages in *fine semantic coding* by rapidly selecting a single dominant meaning while suppressing other less immediately related meanings of a given word. The RH, on the other hand, is thought to engage in *coarse semantic coding* in which it slowly produces multiple meanings that are weakly activated and weakly linked together. Thus, the word "dog" may rapidly evoke the common meaning of four-legged furry animal in the LH, whereas in the RH, associated meanings ("companion") and related concepts ("cat") may be evoked. Connotative and metaphoric meanings like "companion" or "friend" for the word "dog" are considered to be more distantly related to the word than the denotative or literal representation.

Many of the studies investigating the unique semantic processing capacity of the

RH have focused on subjects' responsivity to the relationships among words. Some have asked subjects to group words together based on a perceived semantic relationship. Others have used a priming paradigm in which word recognition is facilitated (occurs faster) when a target word is preceded by a semantically related word. In general, this body of work suggests that the intact RH is important to aspects of single word processing in which alternative, less frequent, and less central meanings are important.

Clues about how the two hemispheres work together in semantic processing have come from lateralized lexical priming research with NBD subjects. In these studies, stimuli are presented to either the RH or to the LH by positioning the primes and targets within the right or left visual field. In such a task, Burgess and Simpson (1988) found that, in situations calling for consciously controlled and attentive processing, the less frequent or subordinate meanings of words were facilitated when the stimuli were presented to the RH, whereas facilitation of the more dominant meaning declined. That is, *under conditions in which processing was not automatic, the RH appeared to be more responsive than the LH to less familiar aspects of word meaning.* This finding not only supports the notion that damage to the RH could interfere in processing alternative and connotative meanings, but also suggests that semantic processing by the RH is called upon *when focused attention is required.* The LH may predominate in automatic processing such that it rapidly processes familiar, denotative meanings. The semantic information in the RH, on the other hand, may be activated only when controlled attention is required—that is, in situations in which the dominant meaning does not appear to be a good fit and effort must be made to substitute an alternate meaning.

It seems logical then that damage to the RH might interfere with the production of less dominant alternative meanings, and thus have an impact on divergent semantic processing. Indeed, RHD patients tend to be less sensitive to connotative (versus denotative) meanings. Brownell et al. (1984) presented subjects with sets of three words and asked them to group together the two that were closest in meaning. Words could be grouped according to their denotative or connotative meanings. In the set "deep/wise/shallow," one could group "deep" with "shallow." A less familiar, more figurative or connotative connection is shared between "deep" and "wise." They found a double dissociation in their results. LHD subjects tended to group words according to their connotative meanings while RHD subjects tended to group them according to their more common denotative meanings. NBD subjects, on the other hand, tended to respond to both connotative and denotative meanings with equal frequency. In another study, Brownell et al. (1990) used a similar paradigm to demonstrate that RHD patients were insensitive not only to metaphoric meanings in particular, but to less familiar or alternate meanings in general. Thus, it seems that damage to the RH does interfere in accessing non-dominant semantic concepts.

There is also evidence that the RH is particularly sensitive to semantic as opposed to other types of relationships (Chiarello et al., 1990). That is, it may be especially attuned to relationships that specify category membership. For example, the word

"hat" and "pants" are members of the same category "clothes," and thus are semantically related by *category.* The words "wool" and "suit" are associated with one another, but are not related by category because they belong to different categories (e.g., "fabric" and "clothing"). They are related by *function* rather than semantic organization. In a lateralized priming study, Chiarello et al. (1990) found that priming directed to the RH facilitated the recognition and naming of categorically related words, but not of associated words. The authors reasoned that the intact RH has the capacity to activate word meanings that are not necessarily associated in everyday situations, but that happen to fall in the same semantic category. They proposed that the intact RH activates multiple meanings that appear to have minimal overlap with one another whereas the meanings activated in the LH have a great deal of overlap and are tightly connected. The LH appears to be highly selective, while the RH is both slower and less selective, allowing many meanings to surface and remain in a holding pattern in case they are needed to clarify or disambiguate intended meaning. If one meaning does not fit in a given context, the LH then may select one of the alternate meanings that has been activated and maintained by the RH.

RHD Deficits in Divergent Semantic Processing

Differences between the hemispheres in divergent semantic processing are supported by investigations of divergent processing in RHD patients. Deficits in divergent processing associated with RHD and their potential effect on the communication ability of RHD are reviewed in the following sections and are summarized in Table 5–3.

Accessing Semantic Relationships in Collective Noun Naming

Given the data on the intact RH and semantic processing, one might reasonably

TABLE 5–3. Divergent semantic processing deficits found in RHD patients.

Problems in Accessing Semantic Relationships

- Collective noun naming:
  reduced ability to produce category names for groups of objects
- Lexical judgment tasks:
  reduced ability to determine if two items are related
- Verbal fluency tasks:
  increased production of central, prototypical, dominant items
  increased production of items sharing common attributes within a semantic category
  more difficulty with goal-derived than semantic categories
  initial activation of dominant category members with decreasing production of items

---

Potential Effects of Deficits in Activating Semantic Relationships

---

- Reduced ability to apply less central, less familiar, less dominant meanings when needed
- Reduced ability to move beyond tightly connected semantic categories
- Reduced ability to resolve lexical ambiguity

---

predict that RHD would interfere in the ability to apprehend relationships among items within a given semantic category. Such problems were apparent in the naming study by Myers and Brookshire (1995). They found that, compared to NBD subjects, RHD subjects had particular problems in naming pictures of collective (versus single) nouns. Collective nouns were divided into those that were concrete (e.g., beverages, fruits) and those that were more abstract (e.g., transportation, communication). Both NBD and RHD subjects had more trouble with collective than single nouns, particularly abstract collective nouns. Patients with severe neglect were significantly less accurate than controls on both types of collective nouns and contributed the majority of the errors by the RHD group. Almost none of their errors could be attributed to either visual confusion or neglect of the left-sided objects. Analysis of errors suggested a relationship between neglect and cognitive factors that may have influenced performance. Most of the NBD errors on collective nouns were semantically related to the category name (e.g., "tools" for "measuring instruments"). However, most of the RHD errors consisted of listing items (e.g., "plane, car, truck, train") without producing the category name ("transportation"). All subjects understood the task, and named some categories accurately. Generating a list of objects rather than a group name suggests a problem in appreciating how items are related, possibly because of a deficit in deducing an organizing semantic principle to link them to a superordinate category. RHD patients also had problems in determining whether two items were related (e.g., apple and pear) in a lexical judgment task (Chiarello & Church, 1986).

Accessing Semantic Relationships in Verbal Fluency Tasks

The performance of RHD patients on certain types of verbal fluency tasks also suggests impaired recognition of semantic relationships. A verbal fluency task requires people to generate members of a given category within a time limit (usually 1 minute). The categories may be *alphabetic* (i.e., words beginning with a given letter) or *semantic* (e.g., "animals," "vegetables"). *Semantic categories* also may be *common* (e.g., "animals" "vegetables"), *uncommon and less familiar* (e.g., "modes of communication," "uses for a brick"), or *goal-derived* (e.g., "things to take on a camping trip," "things that roll"). Responses are scored for the number of accurate exemplars and the number of errors or items named that are unrelated to the category. Sometimes, responses are scored for prototypicality, which refers to how central a category member is considered to be to the defining qualities of a category ideal or prototype. For example, *sparrow* could be considered more central to the category "bird" than *puffin*.

Unlike picture naming and other convergent tasks that limit the response set, verbal fluency tasks are designed to activate a broad semantic field. For this reason, they also are a good measure of sensitivity to semantic relationships. Subjects must search for multiple object concepts that are related to one another by virtue of their membership in a given semantic category. Compared to NBD subjects, patients with RHD have reduced verbal fluency in response to *common* semantic categories (Diggs & Basili, 1987; Hough, Pabst, & Demarco, 1994; Joanette & Goulet, 1986), but are less impaired than LHD subjects (Diggs & Basili, 1987) and than LHD subjects with aphasia (Grossman, 1981). LHD and aphasia may interfere in different aspects of word retrieval in word fluency tasks. Aphasic patients, for example, may have the semantic concept in mind, but have problems accessing the word to match it, thereby reducing the number of items named.

In RHD patients, the number of responses is of less interest to investigators than their quality. Prototypicality of accurate responses, quality of errors, and the time frame in which reduction of fluency occurs have been assessed in an effort to understand the contribution of the RH to semantic processing and the effects of RHD on semantic access. Grossman (1981), for example, found that RHD subjects seemed to draw on the strengths of the intact LH in generating responses. Their responses consisted of items that were more tightly connected to one another and more central or prototypical than those listed by NBD subjects who presumably relied on both hemispheres when generating responses. The lists of RHD subjects had more instances of objects that shared common attributes as well as category membership compared to those generated by NBD subjects. For example, spinach, cabbage, and lettuce all share the attributes of "green and leafy" in addition to membership in the category "vegetables." Similarly, in the category "sports," sailing, swimming, and water ski-

ing all share water in common. Whereas NBD subjects listed more loosely connected category members or members that have only semantic category in common (e.g., "basketball," "sailing," "tennis" for sports), subjects with RHD tended to list category members that had other attributes in common as well. Their responses were also more central or protoypical than those of fluent aphasic patients (although not more so than those of nonfluent aphasic patients).

In addition to relying on more tightly connected meanings (a LH function) in word fluency tasks, RHD patients also have more difficulty generating responses for goal-derived than for semantic categories (Diggs & Basili, 1987; Hough et al., 1994). This is not surprising, given that goal-derived categories (e.g., "things that float," "things to take on a camping trip") are thought to require an organizing strategy and the integration of concepts that are from disparate semantic categories (i.e., "tent," "water," "bug spray" for camping trip). Response production in goal-derived categories is thought to be more effortful and less automatic than generating members of a common category such as "vegetables." Interestingly, aphasic and NBD subjects tend to name more items for goal-derived than for semantic categories (Hough et al., 1994; Hough & Pierce, 1988; Hough & Snow, 1989). Hough et al. (1994) suggested that the relatively poor performance of RHD subjects on goal-derived categories might reflect a particular type of semantic processing deficit. That is, subjects must be sensitive to intersections among concepts that do not ordinarily overlap with one another, a task for which the RH might be particularly well suited. Items taken on a camping trip are linked by utility and function, not by semantic category. The link may be less obvious until one generates the concept of camping and accesses memories of those experiential associations that connect "tent" and "flashlight" together. This is just the sort of loose overlap of meaning for which the RH is thought to be superior and which RHD may disrupt. As the model predicts, connections such as these that are not organized by common category might be less available to RHD than to LHD patients. It is not surprising that aphasic subjects find it easier to name items for goal-derived than for semantic categories and that the opposite has been found in RHD patients.

Finally, data from a verbal fluency study by Joanette, Goulet, and Le Dorze (1988) supports the possibility that RHD adversely affects the effortful activation of less central members of a given semantic category. RHD subjects produced a normal number of responses in the first 30 seconds of a 2-minute time frame. However, unlike the NBD subjects, their responses decreased significantly after that. The authors speculated that initial productivity may reflect automatic activation of the most obvious and most dominant members of a category (enlisting the intact LH). Subsequent productions may involve less automatic, more effortful processing in which the less central members of a semantic field are activated. Thus, once the first 30 seconds have passed and the most familiar exemplars have been named, attentive processing is needed to search the lexicon for less dominant category members. RHD seems to impair this process either because it inhibits generation of more loosely connected meanings or because the process requires effortful and sustained attention, or both.

SUMMARY

1. *For the most part, RHD patients perform adequately on tests of linguistic performance that stress convergent processing.* Given their unimpaired phonological processing abilities and their performance on most tests of auditory comprehension, it appears that linguistic comprehension is not an issue for RHD patients.

2. *Performance on tests of complex semantic and syntactic processing in which there is no supportive context may present problems due to the effect of hypoarousal and impaired vigilance.*

3. Word retrieval skills may be mildly impaired in some situations and in some cases. However *conversational speech of RHD patients is not characterized by paraphasic errors or circumlocutions, and most patients do well on confrontational naming of single objects.*

4. *Divergent language tasks present more problems for RHD patients than do convergent ones.*

5. Performance on divergent tasks such as verbal fluency *support a model of semantic processing in which the RH is superior in generating multiple, loosely connected meanings with little overlap.* The intact RH appears to be particularly active in resolving ambiguity, apprehending metaphoric and other secondary word meanings, and responding to less frequent and connotative meanings.

6. RHD appears to have a negative impact on divergent language operations such that *RHD patients may be less facile in understanding intended meaning because they have problems generating, maintaining, or inhibiting additional, alternate, and related meanings when the dominant meaning is inappropriate to the context.* Needless to say, the impact of such deficits extends beyond tests of verbal fluency and laboratory tasks into conversational discourse. These effects are explored in the next chapter.

CHAPTER

6

Discourse Deficits

Discourse deficits are at the heart of the communication problems associated with RHD. *Discourse consists of communicative events in which information is conveyed by a speaker to a listener or among participants in conversational speech.* Discourse can take various forms, including procedural, expository, narrative, and conversational (Hough & Pierce, 1994; Ulatowska, Allard, & Chap-

man, 1990). *Procedural discourse* describes the procedures involved in performing an activity. *Expository discourse* conveys information on a single topic by a single speaker. *Conversational discourse* conveys information between a speaker and listener or among several speakers and listeners. *Narrative discourse* is a description of events. Whether one is explaining how to fry an egg, expounding on the pros and cons of eggs in the diet, having a conversation about what to have for breakfast, or telling a story about a chicken and an egg, information is being exchanged in a process called discourse. What is exchanged is not just words and ideas, but a wealth of additional information that helps us establish our connections with others, our limits, our boundaries, our group identity, and our self-definition. Thus, discourse is a means by which we convey not only facts and fiction, but our self-concept to others.

Discourse involves a speaker, listener, and a situational context. To be successful, discourse participants must be aware of the general topic, the purpose of the exchange, the limits of shared knowledge, the cultural mores for expressing ideas and emotions, and the means of repairing communicative breakdowns that may occur in the process. Running through the fabric of verbal interaction is the ability to draw on the inferential components of communicative interaction, so that the true meaning of that which is said, and that which is left unsaid, is understood and conveyed.

RHD patients may retain linguistic proficiency, but many of them are impaired in negotiating the extralinguistic aspects of communication that are so important in discourse. They may be insensitive to the cues that help establish the communicative context, the intentions of the speaker, the nuances and shades of meaning behind the words. They may be able to recall the facts of a story, but have trouble integrating the facts to arrive at the overall theme. They

may have problems assimilating new information and revising original interpretations. They may be less sensitive to social conventions for starting, continuing, and ending conversations. Finally, they may have difficulty conveying their own intended meanings, thus shutting off one of the most effective means of updating and communicating their individual identities to those around them. Table 6–1 lists broad categories of discourse deficits associated with RHD.

Discourse deficits occur in both comprehension and expression (Tables 6–2 and 6–3). Indeed, it is often difficult to distinguish between the two. Impaired *comprehension* of general themes, speaker intentions, and inferred meaning naturally has an impact on verbal *expression* in conversational speech. As one patient said, he could

TABLE 6–2. Discourse comprehension deficits associated with RHD.

Reduced Sensitivity to

1. The gist of written and spoken narratives
2. Intended and implied meanings
3. New information and revision of old information
4. Emotional content
5. Paralinguistic information (body language, facial expression, prosody)
6. Shared knowledge
7. Conversational rules and conventions
8. Communicative setting, purpose, and role of the participants

---

TABLE 6–1. Major problem areas underlying discourse deficits associated with RHD.

---

1. Reduced ability to generate inferences
2. Reduced ability to comprehend and produce main concepts and central themes
3. Reduced level of informative content
4. Reduced ability to manage alternative meanings
5. Reduced sensitivity to communicative context

TABLE 6–3. Discourse production deficits associated with RHD.

---

1. Impaired ability to generate a macrostructure
2. Reduced level of informative content
3. Reduced specificity
4. Reduced flexibility
5. Reduced capacity to generate alternative meanings
6. Reduced use of conversational conventions
7. Excessive speech output
8. Unelaborated speech output

---

no longer understand, "the complex mosaic of meaning that is language, even though I understand the words" (Beeman, 1993, p. 104).

It is important to remember that not all RHD patients have discourse deficits, and among those that do, not all discourse situations are problematic. When information is highly redundant or straightforward and explicit, RHD patients may be quite able to negotiate main ideas and details (Brookshire & Nicholas, 1984). However, more complex discourse may present problems. When it does, most patients have deficits in more than one of the underlying discourse processes discussed in subsequent sections of this chapter. There appear to be connections among RHD discourse impairments and, as discussed in the remainder of the chapter, discourse deficits can be attributed to impairments in specific cognitive operations, some of which may be related to reduction of underlying attentional resources, and some of which may be independent of attentional disorders.

Finally, as mentioned in Chapter 1, some of the deficits associated with unilateral RHD have been found in patients who have bilateral and/or unilateral prefrontal lesions in both the right and left hemispheres, particularly those patients with extensive lesions or small lesions in association with more widespread cortical dysfunction (McDonald, 1993). Disorders associated with prefrontal lesions include problems in managing inferences, attending to communicative context, integrating information, managing some of the pragmatic aspects of communication, and generating a theory of mind. The fact that these disorders may be seen in patients with left, right, and/or bilateral prefrontal lesions does not minimize the impact that these deficits have on patients with unilateral RHD or on patients with more diffuse damage that includes the RH, nor does it suggest that these disorders are exclusive to patients with prefrontal lesions, as they have been found as well in patients with unilateral posterior or fronto-posterior dam-

age that does not include prefrontal areas. As stated in Chapter 1, the RH may be more diffusely and less precisely organized compared to the LH so that lesions in a variety of areas within the RH may result in similar types of deficits by virtue of interruption to larger, more interconnected and less focally organized operational systems.

INFERENCE DEFICITS AND RHD

Because the success of discourse rests on adequate interpretation, this first section reviews inference deficits. *An inference is an interpretation that is based on earlier interpretations and beliefs.* The brain expends much of its energy interpreting incoming sensory signals. Visual signals, for example, are integrated at some stage of processing into patterns that are interpreted as discrete objects. Auditory signals are integrated and interpreted as environmental sounds or as words and sentences. In the context of communication and cognition, inference occurs when previously processed input is further interpreted so that objects and words are integrated into a larger pattern of meaning. Instead of fabric and wood, the visual pattern becomes a chair and sofa; instead of a chair and sofa, the object patterns suggest a living room. Instead of individual words, word strings are synthesized into patterns that represent ideas and feelings. Simple inferences, like interpreting a collection of furniture as a living room, are not a problem for most RHD patients, but more complex inferences may prove difficult.

Level of inferential difficulty rests in part on how ambiguous the information is or on the degree to which it does or does not jibe with previously presented information. For example, many RHD patients have trouble interpreting the scene in Figure 6–1 as the waiting room of a hospital or doctor's office (Myers & Brookshire, 1996). The only indications that it is a waiting room are the bandage around one man's head, a partial view of a sign on the wall saying, "quiet

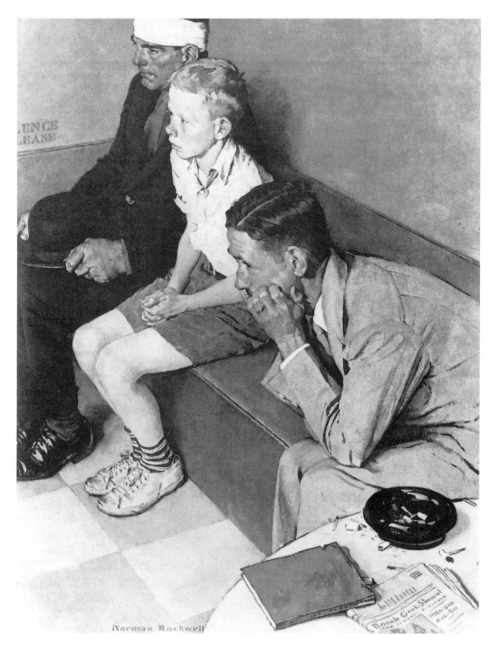

Figure 6–1. Norman Rockwell illustration depicting a "waiting room" scene. (From the *Saturday Evening Post*, October 16, 1937. Reprinted with permission from the Norman Rockwell Family Trust.)

please," and a magazine-laden table. RHD patients have interpreted the picture variously as three people, "watching a baseball game," "three boys sitting in a church pew," "people looking at television or a movie," or "returned from a war." One man said that it could be a house or doctor's office, but he was not too sure if the people pictured, "were waiting for something or just daydreaming." Although it took them a moment to figure out the picture, age-matched controls did not have problems recognizing the setting as a waiting room.

Operations Involved in Inference

How does one conclude or infer that the scene in Figure 6–1 is a waiting room? Assuming adequate sensory and perceptual ability, inference is a complex process involving a number of operations. Among the most obvious are: (a) *attention to individual cues,* (b) *selection of relevant cues,* (c) *integration of relevant cues with one another,* and (d) *association of those cues with prior experience or world knowledge.* Although listed sequentially, these operations probably operate in parallel.

Attention to individual elements in a narrative, conversation, pictured scene, or ongoing situation is, of course, a crucial first step in interpretation. RHD patients may miss important information because they are hypoaroused and/or have problems sustaining attention. For example, their attention to prosody or nonverbal information signaling mood in facial expression and body language may be reduced. They may not attend to important verbal information that sets up a topic in conversational exchange. Scene descriptions by RHD patients often are clogged with irrelevant detail, as in the following explanation of the events depicted in Figure 6–1:

> There are three people waiting, sitting on a bench. An older man. It looks like he has a bandage on his head. And the boy in the middle has his hands clenched in his lap. He's wearing blue shorts, white shoes with striped socks. And the man on the end of the bench is wearing leather shoes. And the boy on this end of the bench, I guess he's between the two of them in age. And he has a cigarette tray right by him. And he looks a little anxious. He's got his elbows on his knees. He's got his chin in his hand. He's wearing a khaki suit. The boy's wearing a short sleeved shirt, blue shorts. The man's wearing a dark suit with a tie, and the man has a bandage on his head.

In the preceding description, the "quiet sign," a key clue to the picture's meaning, is not mentioned (possibly because it is not attended to) whereas almost every piece of clothing is. Focus on irrelevant information at the expense of that which is relevant inhibits building appropriate inferences.

Not only must one attend to and recognize significant information, one must integrate elements with one another. The man with the bandage on his head might look like someone just returned from a war, as more than one patient has suggested. However, in combination with the young boy, the "quiet" sign, the magazine-laden table, the bandage suggests a doctor's office or local emergency room more than a field hospital or war zone.

Finally, accurate inferences depend on associating significant features with one's experience or world knowledge. One must call on prior experience with doctor's offices or hospitals to reach an interpretation of the "waiting room" scene. Even on an item-by-item basis, previous experience helps inference generation. For example, the interplay between the overall context of the picture and familiarity with hospitals enables one to reach the conclusion that one man has a bandage, not a hat or towel, on his head.

Inference in Discourse

The concept *waiting room* was an inference about the overall theme of the scene in Figure 6–1. A central concept or thematic inference is sometimes referred to as a *macrostructure.* There are other types of inferences that operate in discourse as well. *Bridging inferences,* sometimes called *coherence inferences,* are those that link ideas to one another (Clark and Haviland, 1977). According to Brownell and Martino (1998), listeners make bridging inferences as they listen to conversational speech even when ideas do not seem to fit with the central theme of the conversation. The level of comprehension difficulty depends in part on the amount of effort required to link pieces together into a single interpretation. The less explicit information is, the more important the bridging inferences are. For example, as they leave for a vacation, Ella might say to Joe, "Oh, I hope the weather is good at the resort. They have two sailboats there!" Understanding that Ella hopes they can go sailing requires a bridging inference between her reference to the weather and her reference to the fact that the resort has sailboats. The connection or bridge is made by virtue of Joe's knowledge of Ella and her love of sailing.

Overview of Inference Deficits Associated with RHD

Clearly, not all inferences present problems for RHD patients. Most RHD adults are perfectly capable of making simple inferences (Joanette et al., 1990; McDonald & Wales, 1986). Just as aphasic adults have not lost the knowledge of language, but rather experience interference and language breakdowns, so, too, patients with RHD have not lost the capacity to draw inferences. For example, McDonald and Wales (1986) found that given the premise that, "the woman held the little girl's hand," followed by the premise, "her daughter was only three years old," RHD subjects were able to make the inference that the woman was holding her daughter's hand. In a study by Myers and Brookshire (1994), most, although not all, RHD subjects were able to deduce that the people seated around the table in Figure 6–2 are gathered for a Thanksgiving dinner. Other studies have found RHD subjects capable of drawing inferences from straightforward verbal material as long as the inferences to be drawn were internally consistent (i.e., the propositions presented were consistent with one another) (Brownell, Potter, Bihrle, & Gardner, 1986). For example, it might be easy for RHD patients to conclude that Ella was trying to catch a flight from the proposition, "Ella grabbed her bag and rushed to the gate." However, the original interpretation of rushing to the gate would have

to be revised if a second sentence stated, "Once there, she pulled out her key and unlocked it." At first glance, the second sentence is inconsistent with the first and the accurate inference requires more effort to reach. Although simple inferences are managed, inference deficits tend to occur when implicit information is somewhat ambiguous, open to more than one interpretation, unfamiliar, requires revision, or requires integration on several levels. Those specific problems are discussed in the next several sections.

MACROSTRUCTURE DEFICITS

A macrostructure is an overarching inference about the theme or central message of a narrative, conversation, procedure, explanation, essay, pictured event, situation, film, TV show, news story or any other communicative event. According to Van Dijk and Kintsch (1983), we generate inferences about the global themes in discourse from individual sentences. Initial macrostructures enable us to understand subsequent sentences in a top-down fashion. The degree to which individual sentences fit with the macrostructure we have generated helps establish its validity. Thus, a macrostructure enables us to "extract meaning from individual sentences and integrate that meaning into the context supplied by the other sentences in the narrative" (Hough, 1990, p. 253). The relative difficulty of macrostructure generation depends on how explicit the links between individual sentences are or how unexpected the central theme is, as well as on how explicitly the theme itself is stated (Hough, 1990). It is obviously easier to apprehend the essential message of a passage when it has a title or heading, than when it does not. It is harder to understand the gist of a conversation if one enters in the middle of it than if one is present when the topic of conversation has been introduced.

RHD adults may have trouble generating macrostructures both as listeners and as speakers. That is, they may miss the

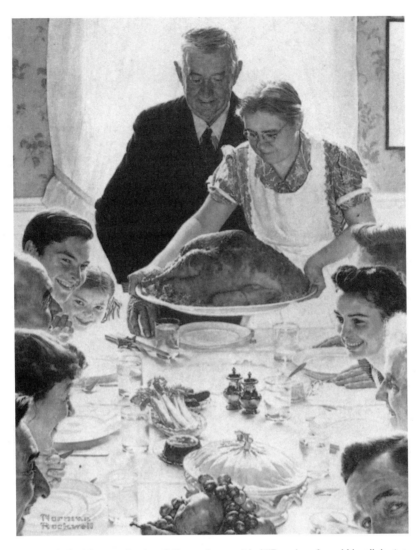

Figure 6–2. Norman Rockwell illustration, entitled "Freedom from Want," depicting Thanksgiving dinner. (From the *Saturday Evening Post*, March 6, 1943. Reprinted with permission of the Norman Rockwell Family Trust.)

main point of what someone is saying to them and, when they speak, they may have difficulty getting the gist of their message across to their listeners. Numerous studies have found RHD patients impaired in apprehending and/or maintaining central concepts in narrative and conversational discourse and in pictured stories and events (Benowitz, Moya, Levine, & Finklestein, 1990; Gardner, Brownell, Wapner, & Michelow, 1983; Hough, 1990; Joanette, Goulet, Ska, & Nespoulous, 1986; Lojek-Osiejuk, 1996; Mackisack, Myers, & Duffy, 1987; Myers & Brookshire, 1994, 1996; Rehak, Kaplan, et al., 1992; Wapner et al., 1981). Myers and Brookshire (1994) found that, when describing the scene in Figure 6–1, the term "waiting room" or its equivalent (e.g., E.R., emergency room, hospital, doctor's office) was mentioned by over 80% of the NBD subjects but by less than 29% of the RHD subjects.

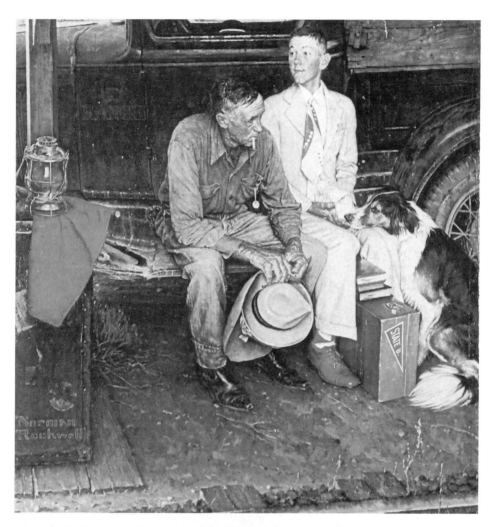

Figure 6–3. Norman Rockwell illustration, "Breaking Home Ties," depicting a young man leaving home for university. (From the *Saturday Evening Post*, September 25, 1954. Reprinted with permission of the Norman Rockwell Family Trust.)

Figure 6–3 depicts a young man leaving home for university. The father, dressed in overalls, farmer's hat in hand, looks dejected. The son, dressed in an ill-fitting suit is looking down the tracks with the bright and eager expression of anticipated adventure on his face. The picture takes some effort to interpret. To fully understand the picture, one needs to attend to subtle cues, such as the state university pennant on the boy's suitcase, and to more obvious features, such as the clothing, body language, and facial expressions of the people depicted, as well as to the overall setting. Although RHD subjects figured out that the two men were on the running board of a car or truck, they were not always sure what they were waiting for. Several suggested that the men had had a flat tire or that the boy was hitching a ride on his way to college or across the country. Some suggested that they had stopped to fix the car. One said, "I think that is one of the real old tank horses. And I think they ran over a chicken. They have some suitcases. Maybe he's saying, 'I told you not to drive so fast.'" Several elderly NBD subjects also thought at first that the car had broken down, but 80% still identified the scene as one of leaving home and going to college. Whereas 63% of the NBD subjects identified the older man as a father or grandfather of the younger man, only 37% of the RHD subjects made that inference. None of the RHD subjects accurately interpreted the sad emotion in the father's face and body language, and most of them did not appreciate the central concept of leaving home. What is particularly striking is that RHD subjects were accurate in identifying the individual elements in this and other pictures, but they often were unable to understand the central ideas conveyed. Their problems were not perceptual, but conceptual. They perceived the contents, but did not conceive the theme. For example, one subject said,

> It appears like somebody got picked up for a free ride. Got his suitcase and dog along. He's probably going to a state university. He doesn't look too happy about the whole affair. Neither does the dog.

Other studies have also found RHD patients impaired on tasks requiring the appreciation of the macrostructure. They have trouble giving titles to simple stories (Benowitz et al., 1990), extracting story morals (Gardner et al., 1983), and choosing a statement summarizing story contents (Rehak, Kaplan, et al., 1992). Joanette et al. (1986) found they produced significantly fewer "core" concepts compared to NBD subjects when formulating a story based on a picture sequence.

A central theme sentence helps to set up the macrostructure of paragraph length stories. Hough (1990) found that RHD subjects had problems interpreting narratives in a study in which a central theme sentence was placed either at the beginning or at the end of simple stories. When the theme sentence was delayed until the end of the story, subjects were forced to develop their own macrostructure. Neither NBD

nor LHD subjects were affected by the location of the theme sentence, whereas the performance of RHD subjects deteriorated when themes were delayed until the end. Even when the theme sentence appeared first, the accuracy of RHD subjects' interpretations was inferior to that of the NBD group.

Levels of difficulty in developing a central theme were demonstrated by Myers, Linebaugh, and Mackisack-Morin (1985) in a study investigating categorization skills in brain-damaged adults. Subjects were given nine pictures to sort into three categories based on the underlying theme of the pictures. They were not told the categories, but had to generate them on their own. Only one RHD subject made an error in sorting pictures of objects (i.e., toys, animals, clothing). RHD subjects, however, did not fare as well in sorting action pictures (i.e., cleaning, playing, construction/builiding), although they still were not significantly worse than NBD controls. However, in sorting pictures scenes by theme (mistrust, work, joy, love), they were significantly impaired. The three pictures representing the theme "mistrust" from the study are depicted in Figure 6–4. At the end of the sorting tasks, subjects were asked to explain their groupings. Whereas responses from 96% and 66% of the NBD and LHD subjects, respectively, reflected the implicit meaning of the pictures, only 33% of the RHD subjects' responses did so. Many of their explanations showed an appreciation, but inaccurate assessment, of the implied themes. Some explanations suggested that subjects sorted the pictures based on concrete interpretations that missed the implicit meaning altogether. For example, some RHD subjects explained their groups as "families," "soldiers," or "parks." The LHD group, on the other hand, tended to use labels like "poverty," "curiosity," and "hugging," which, although not necessarily accurate, reflected less concrete conceptualizations.

RHD deficits in macrostructure formulation reduces patients' ability to follow con-

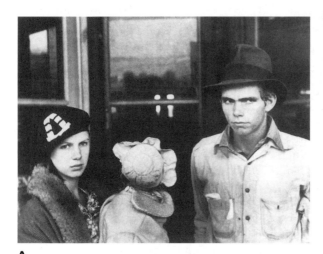
A

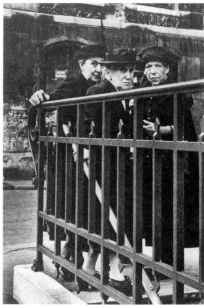
B

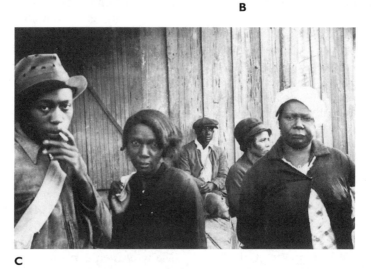
C

Figure 6–4. Pictures depicting the theme "Mistrust/Suspicion" (Myers, Linebaugh, & Mackisack-Morin, 1985). Pictures from the Farm Security Administration and Office of War Administration (FSA/OWA). Courtesy of U.S. Library of Congress, Washington, DC. Reprinted with permission from BRK Publishers, Minneapolis, MN.

versation and other forms of discourse. It may impair their understanding of the gist of nonverbal material as well. In some situations, the effort of formulating a macrostructure may interfere with other aspects of discourse processing. Possible factors involved in macrostructure impairments include *impaired appreciation of discourse structure, impaired integration of discourse fea-tures,* and *attentional impairments.* Each is reviewed in the following sections.

Appreciation of Discourse Structure

Discourse structure is the framework around which conversational, procedural, narrative, and other forms of discourse are organized. Deficits in the knowledge and use of various types of discourse structure have been investigated as a possible source of macrostructure impairments. "Script knowledge," for example, is the knowledge of a stereotyped sequence of events, or "script," for activities such as mailing a letter or eating in a restaurant (Shank & Ableson, 1977). Scripts also may function in narrative and conversational discourse as a structure or schemata for the organization of concepts (Lojek-Osiejuk, 1996; Roman, Brownell, Potter, Seibold, & Gardner, 1987). A script of a common activity is activated by the mention of it in a conversation (Roman et al., 1987). For example, if, in the course of conversation, one mentions eating at a restaurant, the listener need not be told all that is entailed in dining out to appreciate the setting and events because he or she can call up a familiar script of eating out. That is, the speaker does not have to make the actions involved in dining out explicit. Knowledge of scripts helps prepare us for that which is and is not familiar, helps us determine what is and is not plausible, and helps conversation move along in an efficient manner. If a conversational partner states that their food appeared before they had a chance to order, for example, the listener would be immediately attuned to the unusual nature of that occurrence.

Problems with script knowledge could adversely affect macrostructure generation by interfering in the construction of and access to a narrative framework. It appears, however, that script knowledge of routine activities is preserved in RHD adults (Lojek-Osiejuk, 1996; Purdy, 1997; Roman et al., 1987). In addition, there is evidence that RHD does not impair basic social and emotional script knowledge. For example, although they tended to be biased toward positive emotions, RHD subjects were able to figure out what a character would say or do next in simple stories with familiar emotional content such as the birth of a child (Ostrove, Simpson, & Gardner, 1990). They also are able to construct narratives given a story framework and appear to have control over story structure (Lojek-Osiejuk,

1996; Rehak et al., 1992). Thus, *deficits in scripts knowledge and narrative framework do not appear to be a factor in macrostructure deficits in this population.*

Integration of Discourse Features

Another possible explanation for macrostructure deficits is an impairment in the ability to integrate information into a larger whole (i.e., macrostructure). The macrostructure provides a "conceptual anchor" that relates individual concepts to one another (Brownell, Gardner, Prather, & Martino, 1995). In a sort of chicken-egg situation, the macrostructure helps make the relationship among individual concepts clear, but concepts must be related to one another in the process of generating a macrostructure. Not only must abstract concepts be related to one another, they must be integrated with the setting, purpose of the exchange, role of the conversants, prosodic contour, and facial expression and body language of the speaker. Even individual inferences require appreciation of relationships. For example, whereas "waiting room" is the macrostructure of the picture in Figure 6–1, the word "patient" to describe the man with a bandage is an instance of an *individual* inference. Inferring that the figure is not only a person, but also a patient depends on the ability to relate his bandage to the overall setting. The term "man" can be considered a literal or concrete interpretation, whereas the term "patient" is inferred.

Several studies have found that, as a group, RHD subjects are significantly impaired in generating inferences about individual elements of pictured scenes (Mackisack et al., 1987; Myers, 1979; Myers & Brookshire, 1996). Myers and Brookshire (1996), for example, found that although RHD subjects and NBD controls did not differ in the number of literal concepts produced in describing pictured events, RHD subjects produced significantly fewer inferred concepts. Similarly, Myers (1979) found that they produced fewer inferred concepts when describing the "Cookie

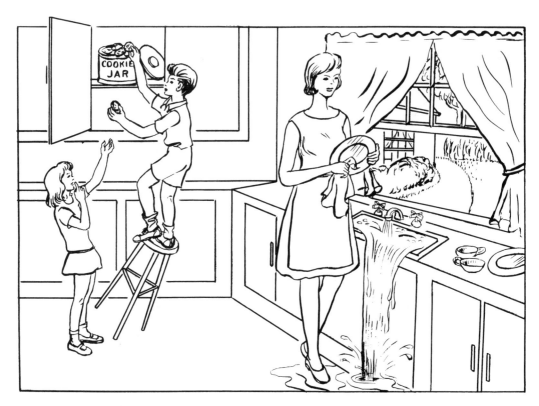

Figure 6–5. The "Cookie Theft" stimulus picture. (From Goodglass and Kaplan [1983], *Boston Diagnostic Aphasia Examination,* copyright © 1979 by Lea & Febiger. Reprinted by permission of the publisher, Williams and Wilkins, 351 West Camden Street, Baltimore, MD 21201-2436.)

Theft" picture from the *Boston Diagnostic Aphasia Examination* (Goodglass & Kaplan, 1983) (Figure 6–5). The following quote from a patient describing the picture illustrates the effect of integration impairments on inference generation and macrostructure formulation. Asked what was happening in the picture, the patient replied:

> I see a woman holding a plate. I see a boy standing on a small stool. I see shoes. The boy is opening a jar—feeling cookies, I guess. He might fall. The woman is mother. I see a girl. Her left arm is upraised. The boy—presumably his sister.

It appears as if the patient is processing each item in isolation. For example, it is not until he is nearly finished that the patient recognizes that the "woman holding a plate" is likely a "mother." "Washing dishes," an inference based on integrating the woman, the plate, the sink and towel was never drawn. The girl stands alone in the patient's eyes with her "arm upraised." Understanding that she is reaching for a cookie requires integration of her posture with the boy reaching in the cookie jar. Although the patient recognizes that the boy might fall, he never connects his activity to the vacant look on the mother's face, the overflowing sink, and other signs of a kitchen disaster. Thus, he concludes he is "feeling," rather than "stealing," cookies.

Similar integration problems surface in responding to verbal material. One patient in a study by Beeman (1993) complained that, even though he was able to read straightforward texts, he no longer read multi-character novels, "because I can't put it all together" (p. 104). Hough (1990) noticed that, when interpreting paragraphs,

RHD subjects "retained isolated pieces of paragraph data rather than integrating this information to deduce the meaning of the narrative. . . . This often resulted in 'listing' of information, rather than generating an overall narrative theme" (p. 271). Myers and Brookshire (1995) found in a naming study that, when asked to give the superordinate category name for a group of objects (i.e., "transportation" for the objects: car, plane, truck, and train), the majority of the errors made by RHD subjects were characterized by listing isolated objects without arriving at the overall category name, indicating problems in appreciating the relationships among the objects. This type of error did not occur on easy, familiar object categories such as fruits or drinks, suggesting that it is not integration per se, but effortful integration that poses a problem.

RHD patients also may have problems ordering sentences into paragraphs, even when the macrostructure is provided by an initial theme sentence (Delis, Wapner, Gardner, & Moses, 1983; Schneiderman, Murasugi, & Saddy, 1992). As Hough (1990) found, the performance of RHD subjects, unlike that of NBD and LHD subjects, was not facilitated by the provision of a central theme sentence in the Schniederman et al. (1992) study, suggesting to the authors that RHD patients have problems in *recognizing* a macrostructure when it is provided as well as problems in *generating* one when it is not provided.

Finally, there may be a relationship between problems in organizing spatial relationships and problems in integrating and abstracting information from narrative material (Benowitz et al., 1990; Moya, Benowitz, Levine, & Finklestein, 1986). Benowitz et al. (1990) asked subjects to select a title and answer inferential questions about narratives (e.g., information about character motivations that was not explicitly provided). They found a robust correlation between performance on these tasks and the presence of neglect and impairments in visuospatial organization as measured by tests of visual construction (copy drawing and drawing from memory). In addition to

neglect of left-sided detail, the drawings of RHD patients often show a disorganization of overall form and apparent disregard for internal integrity or schema as shown in the example in Figure 6–6. Not surprisingly, preservation of details from the stories did not correlate with inference deficits, appreciating relationships among the characters, or abstracting the macrostructure. Just as they included detail in their drawings, but had problems organizing the elements into a coherent whole, patients were accurate in recall of factual information, but had trouble integrating the facts into a macrostructure. The authors stated that the relationship between spatial organization and comprehension and integration of the relationships among elements in a narrative "may to some extent require a common mechanism that relies upon the integrity of particular right hemisphere structures" (p. 240).

Thus, it appears that problems in integrating information and apprehending relationships among pictured objects and abstract concepts in discourse can be a problem for some RHD patients. It is worth remembering that the scope of attention in patients with RHD, particularly in those with neglect, may be narrowed. The narrowed focus of attention inhibits integration by highlighting isolated elements at the expense of "seeing the whole picture." Integration deficits across modalities play into problems in drawing individual inferences and in generating thematic inferences or macrostructures. They may be related to deficits in integrating information in the spatial domain or, as Benowitz et al. (1990) suggested, to some common mechanism that allows us to appreciate relationships across domains. Although integration deficits may not be a complete explanation, they offer one viable clue to the mechanism underlying macrostructure deficits.

Attentional Impairments

Few studies of either macrostructure impairments in particular, or discourse defi-

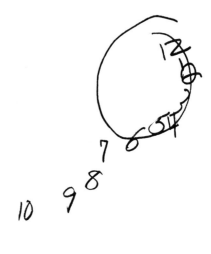

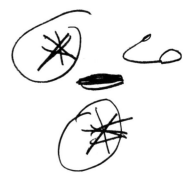

Figure 6–6. Sample free-hand drawings of a clock and a bicycle by a patient with RHD and neglect. Note the lack of internal structure in the patient's renditions.

cits in general, have examined the influence of neglect on performance. This is probably because neglect is so often considered a perceptual, rather than an attentional, problem. It's relationship to more generalized attentional impairments with consequent impact on cognition is often overlooked, despite evidence of a strong relationship between severity of neglect and more general attentional deficits. For example, impaired performance on nonvisual tasks such as digit span and paced auditory serial addition abilities have been found to correlate with degree of neglect (Robertson, 1990; Weinberg, Diller, Gerst-

man, & Schulman, 1972). Discourse studies that have measured neglect have found that, when describing inferentially complex scenes, RHD subjects with severe neglect produce fewer main concepts than those with less neglect (Myers & Brookshire, 1994) and make fewer accurate inferences than those with less severe neglect (Myers & Brookshire, 1996). Subjects in these studies were cued to the left when necessary, and they accurately labeled as many items in the pictures as did NBD controls. Thus, *perceiving* the elements was not the problem. Interpreting and integrating them into the larger whole was. Of note is the fact that RHD subjects *without neglect* tend to produce descriptions of the "Cookie Theft" picture (Figure 6–5) that are not that different from normal elderly subjects (Tompkins et al., 1992). Trupe and Hillis (1985) found that RHD subjects who produced normal descriptions of the picture also performed normally on tests of memory and attention.

Attentional deficits may interfere in macrostructure generation at a number of levels. *Hypoarousal* may make patients less aware of important contextual information, and reduce the resources available for complex inferential processing. *Selective attention deficits* may make it difficult to distinguish significant from insignificant information. *Reduced vigilance and attentional maintenance* may cause attentional fluctuations during conversation such that key points and significant clues to macrostructure are missed. Finally, as mentioned earlier, a *narrowed focus of attention* may interfere in integration of multiple elements. Just as they may lack insight and seem unconcerned about their other deficits, patients with inference deficits may deny their problems and be unable or unwilling to engage in the cognitive effort required. Attentional deficits, thus, may be another factor in macrostructure impairments in the RHD population.

Summary

Of the three factors discussed, deficits in attentional and integration operations appear to be reasonable candidates for interfering with macrostructure generation. These deficits have a negative effect on generating individual inferences and probably disrupt the appreciation of overall themes. That is not to say that these are the only factors relevant to macrostructure deficits. Other possibilities include deficits in managing alternate meanings, reduced capacity to adopt the perspective of the communicative partner, and problems in revising old information, each of which is discussed later in this chapter. The reader

should keep in mind that, although these deficits disrupt discourse in specific ways, they also may have an indirect and more general influence on generation of and appreciation of macrostructures.

REDUCED LEVEL OF INFORMATIVE CONTENT

Given the difficulty RHD patients may have in appreciating the main concepts and macrostructure in discourse, it is not surprising that the level of informative content in their discourse may be substandard (Apel & Pospisil, 1997; Bloom, Borod, Obler, & Gerstman, 1992; Bloom, Carozza, Berg, & Curran-Curry, 1997; Cherney & Canter, 1993; Gardner et al., 1983; Joanette et al., 1986; Lojek-Osiejuk, 1996; Mackisack et al., 1987; Myers & Brookshire, 1994, 1996; Rivers & Love, 1980; Urayse, Duffy, & Liles, 1991; Wapner et al., 1981). They may produce just as many words, no more and no less, than their NBD counterparts, yet convey less information.

The conversational speech of RHD patients has been characterized as *verbose and excessive* in some patients and as *abrupt and perfunctory* in others (Brownell et al., 1995; Gardner et al., 1983; Kennedy, Strand, Burton, & Peterson, 1994; Myers, 1994, 1997; Roman et al., 1987; Sherratt & Penn, 1990; Trupe & Hillis, 1985). In either case, RHD adults may not provide an appropriate amount of information. As a result, their conversational speech can be inefficient and may burden the listener with having to sift for relevant information to fill in the missing pieces and bridge the gaps. The following sections describe characteristics of unelaborated as well as excessive output.

Impoverished/Unelaborated Output

Unelaborated output is a characteristic of the discourse of some, but certainly not all, RHD patients. Trupe and Hillis (1985), for example, found that only 10 of their 62 RHD subjects had speech characterized by low output. Many of the patients that have reduced output seem *hypo-responsive and lacking facial expression and physical animation.* However, others appear attentive, but *impatient and abrupt.* They may seem unresponsive to and disinterested in the intent behind questions. In explaining the Thanksgiving dinner scene (Figure 6–2), one patient said, "They're about to have dinner. She's got the dinner." Another said, "Looks like the mother's got turkey. That's it." Looking at the "waiting room" scene in Figure 6–1, this same patient said, "They're sitting on a bench is all." Although we often admire "men of few words," in the case of RHD patients, fewer words often means less content. They produce fewer content units and fewer episodes in picture description and story re-telling tasks, even when their answers to factual questions suggest a grasp of the material (Trupe & Hillis, 1985; Urayse et al., 1991).

The patient's perfunctory manner of interaction may seem negative and may perplex family and friends. "He just seems so angry and talks so kind of short," one spouse said. We do not know the cause, lesion location, or much about the affective changes that may contribute to paucity of verbal output. We do not know if these patients become more elaborative over time. Nonetheless, it is important to recognize and explain to families that alterations in the speech output of the type described here may be a consequence of damage to the right side of the brain, and not necessarily idiosyncratic to the patient.

Excessive/Overelaborated Output

More typical of disturbed verbal expression accompanying RHD is excessive output, characterized by *digressions, tangentiality, intrusions, and a kind of "looseness" of expression* (Cherney & Canter, 1993; Eisenson, 1962; Gardner et al., 1983; Hough, 1990; Mackisack et al., 1987; Myers, 1994, 1996; Roman et al., 1987; Schneiderman et

al., 1992; Sherratt & Penn, 1990; Trupe & Hillis, 1985; Wapner et al., 1981). For example, Mackisack et al. (1987) found that RHD subjects used twice as many words as NBD subjects in describing pictured scenes, even when tangential comments were excluded from the count. In a detailed study of the discourse of a single patient, Sherratt and Penn (1990) found that the subject produced over four times as many words in narrative discourse as an age-matched control subject. Although the speech of many older adults can be tangential (usually in the form of personalization), Roman et al. (1987) found that RHD subjects made an average of seven intrusive comments compared to about three for normal elderly subjects when describing how to change a flat tire or order a meal in a restaurant. Intrusions consisted of opinions, jokes, tangential remarks, or references to other activities. Apel and Pospisil (1997) found that, whereas NBD, LHD and RHD subjects produced an equal amount of tangential information in telling stories, the nature of that information differed among the groups. The extraneous remarks of LHD subjects were usually related to their task performance, whereas those of RHD subjects were unrelated to the story topics all-together. Patients with verbose output *may wander off the topic* or *bury the topic in an avalanche of unnecessary detail.* As one patient said, "My mind, like a vacuum cleaner, sucks up every thought along the way and spews them out."

The irrelevant comments that occur subsequent to RHD often reflect problems in apprehending the gist or macrostructure of a conversation. As Gardner et al. (1983) stated, "Without an organizing principle, the patients are consigned to undirected rambling, unable to judge which details matter, and what overarching points they yield" (p. 187). The following explanation by an RHD patient of what is happening in Figure 6–3 illustrates excessive detail:

> Well, collie or Lassie—looks like they're
> going to take him back to college. That's

State U, or U State. State U. And they've had car trouble somewhere. Old Dad's still puffin' on cigarettes. This is before cigarettes went out of fashion. They better watch out about that porch they're sitting on there. Isn't that a mess? It's all rotted away. Termites must be at it. Look at those bumper shoes that kid—he's a collegiate. Look at the socks. Striped socks and he's got those snub-nosed kickers on. Must be gonna be the kicker for the team. He's got a yellow handkerchief in his shirt—coat jacket—and he thinks he's very dapper. You'll find this hard to believe, but that is an Atlas tire and I sold those stinkers for 20 years. Now how do I know? I know because of the figuration on the side of the tire. That's an Atlas Junior, sold by Atlas TBA Company to Exxon, and American Oil, and Chevron on a wire wheel and that tire is probably a 475 by 17. I mounted many of those. That's a Model A Ford truck.

It is evident that the patient understands that the boy is leaving home for college, but he is easily diverted and never develops the central theme. He makes no comment and draws no inferences from the emotional content of the picture (e.g., the contrast between the boy's expectations and the father's resignation, not to mention the dog's dejection). The quote is replete with intrusions and unnecessary detail, almost as if the patient is thinking out loud. Although he is taken by the boy's clothes, he fails to draw the inference from his appearance that the boy is a raw and naïve farm boy. He clearly is confused about the wood in the foreground, which represents a railroad bed, not a porch. However, this visual confusion does not seem to be of great import in understanding the central concept of the picture. Note how he appreciates small details such as the make of the tires. It appears that a general uncertainty about the theme contributed to the amount of unnecessary information, as this same patient was less verbose in describing pictures in which the macrostructure was more readily apparent. In those descriptions, he also included more detail than necessary, but

had fewer intrusive comments and was generally more efficient.

In conversation, verbose patients appear to have difficulty appreciating what the listener needs to know. As listeners, they respond to single ideas as isolated and unrelated, rather than as integrated into the main theme of a conversation. They may have a defect in the inhibitory mechanisms that function when the memory of an event is activated and retrieved (Sherratt & Penn, 1990), as illustrated by the references to personal history of mounting tires in the above quote. Discourse conventions require that tangential information be acknowledged as such by the speaker, a convention rarely followed by RHD patients with excessive output.

Occasionally, patients engage in *confabulatory behavior* which contributes to overall inefficiency. Typically, confabulations occur in situations in which the patient is uncertain of the meaning of events. For example, Gardner et al. (1983) found that, unlike aphasic and NBD subjects, RHD patients reacted to nonsensical or bizarre story outcomes without apparent surprise, laughter, or other acknowledgement that the stories made no sense. When re-telling a story, they often confabulated reasons to justify the odd elements (e.g., reasons why a lazy hired hand was given a raise).

The tendency to justify things that do not make sense can carry over into other situations. Neglect and anosognosia can contribute lack of insight into the nature of their impairments and may result in lengthy explanations as patients try to make sense of the world around them. Many have problems recognizing they have had a stroke, for example. Asked why he was in the hospital, one patient described in chronological detail the events leading up to his stroke, including a trip taken the day before and what he'd had for breakfast the morning it happened. His breakfast of, "egg beaters," he pointed out, was low in cholesterol—an irony lost on the listener because up to that point he had not mentioned his stroke. He ended his story quoting his wife saying, "Oh, John has had a stroke." He got to the point, but inefficiently and indirectly. Asked why she was in the hospital, another patient explained how she had fallen on the floor and went on to describe the deep texture and quality of the rug (possibly to signify that a blow to the head was not the cause of her hospitalization). She went on to explain that her husband called the doctor and told a few anecdotes about the doctor that led her to trust his diagnosis, but never once did she say what that diagnosis was. Another explained that he had fallen over, "because a couple of my arms and legs weren't working." Such patients rarely admit to lack of knowledge, but instead give detailed answers in what appears to be a desperate attempt to make the world fit their limited understanding of it. As one RHD patient with anosognosia said, after claiming he could move his paralyzed left arm:

> You see, doctor, the fact that the hand didn't move might mean that I don't want to raise it. My words may astonish you, but there are bizarre phenomena. My not moving my hand might be due to the fact that if I keep from performing this movement, I might be in a better position to make movements which would otherwise be impossible. I am well aware of the fact that this seems illogical and uncanny. Indeed, this obscurity is repugnant to my mind, which is very rational. I hope I am not boring you with my apparently odd talk. (p. 470) (Reprinted by permission of Oxford University Press from Bisiach, E., "Language Without Thought." In L. Weiskrantz, (Ed.), *Thought Without Language* (pp. 464–484). Oxford, UK: Oxford University Press).

GENERATING ALTERNATE MEANINGS

A central feature of discourse is the constant introduction of new information that must be mapped onto a previously formulated macrostructure. In some situations, this is an easy task because the new infor-

mation fits in readily or is easily predicted. In other situations, it is more difficult because the new information may seem at odds with that which has preceded it. Bridging inferences help make new input cohere with earlier input. Integrating apparently discordant or less predictable information takes more effort and draws more heavily on attentional and cognitive resources. The new information may require generating an alternate meaning or new interpretation for previously conveyed input.

As discussed in Chapter 5, the RH is thought to be important for processing less frequent, less central, or alternative meanings of single words. It is thought that whereas the LH focuses on meanings that are closely related to one another, the RH proposes multiple meanings with less semantic overlap (Beeman, 1993; Brownell et al., 1984, 1990; Burgess & Simpson, 1988; Chiarello et al., 1990; Tompkins, Baumgaertner, Lehman, & Fossett, 1997). Many discourse deficits also appear to reflect problems in processing alternate meanings. Patients may have difficulty revising original interpretations, accessing figurative or metaphoric meanings of idiomatic expressions, and/or adequately interpreting intended meanings in narratives and conversational speech. These difficulties are discussed in the next two sections. Possible mechanisms for them are presented in the final two sections.

Deficits in Appreciating Non-Literal Meanings

Figurative Language

Among the earliest observations of patients with RHD was that, under certain conditions, they appeared insensitive to the metaphoric meaning of idiomatic expressions (Myers & Linebaugh, 1981; Winner & Gardner, 1977). Most idioms, such as "tough row to hoe" or "hit the ceiling," carry two meanings—one literal and one figurative. For example, one could literally and physically "hit the ceiling," but generally the phrase refers to an explosion of anger. Typically, the figurative meaning of idioms is more familiar than their literal meaning (Brownell et al., 1995), and the figurative meaning, unlike the literal one, may act as a single lexical entry because it is so familiar as a unit (Huber, 1990; Schweigert & Moates, 1988; Swinney & Cutler, 1979).

Patients with RHD can be insensitive to figurative meanings when they must choose between literal and figurative pictorial representations of idiomatic representations (Bryan, 1988; Myers & Linebaugh, 1981; Van Lancker & Kempler, 1987; Winner & Gardner, 1977). For example, Winner and Gardner (1977) asked subjects to point to a picture representing isolated phrases like, "He had a heavy heart." RHD adults tended to point more often to literal depictions (e.g., a man bending under the weight of a large valentine-like heart) than to the figurative representation (a man crying). Myers and Linebaugh (1981) found the same tendency in a study in which idioms were presented in story contexts. Choices included literal and figurative (i.e., correct) depictions in both appropriate and inappropriate settings as well as a picture that depicted the opposite meaning of the story outcome. Figure 6–7 depicts the literal and figurative choices for the following story:

Jack and Mary found some leftover cake in the kitchen. But when Jack divided it up, Mary complained that he had taken the lion's share of the cake.

The majority of RHD subjects picked literal representations for the idioms (e.g., pictures with the lion), rather than the figurative one (e.g., Jack and Mary). This tendency was unique to the RHD patients, rather than the product of brain damage in general. Only 3% of the aphasic subjects' responses were literal choices compared to the 57% literal choices made by the RHD group.

There are no data on the use of figurative expressions in the conversational speech of RHD patients. The interest in their figurative language deficits originated not so much from their inadequate appreciation of idioms in discourse as from their performance on idiom-to-picture matching tasks and its relationship to a general tendency among RHD patients to respond to the most superficial and concrete meanings of verbal interaction. It appears that figurative meaning of idiomatic expressions *can* be accessed by RHD adults under certain conditions. For example, patients are able to define and explain idioms (with prodding), although this is a difficult task for both normal and brain-damaged subjects (Myers & Mackisack, 1986; Winner & Gardner, 1977). Also, it appears that they can access the metaphoric meaning of single words and idioms in automatic processing conditions (Tompkins, 1990; Tompkins, Boada, & McGarry, 1992).

Why, then, do they fail when asked to match text to pictured representations of idioms? Possible explanations are related to the nature of the task. First, they may have problems maintaining activation of both the literal and figurative meanings while determining which one is appropriate to the context (Tompkins et al., 1992). Second, the literal depiction may be easier to comprehend in pictured form than the figurative one for which subjects must draw a more distant or more difficult inference. Contrast the picture of Jack taking a large piece of cake with that of him taking the lion's cake in Figure 6–7. Because the physical representation of "lion" may be very salient, it represents a less effortful choice. Patients may see a lion and impulsively relate it to the phrase "lion's share" rather than making the effort to integrate it with the story context. How much easier to simply find a picture of a lion. In addition, patients may not hold onto the phrase as a unit by the time they have finished examining the pictured choices. Salient nouns like *lion* or *heart* (as in "heavy heart") may stand out in isolation from the complete

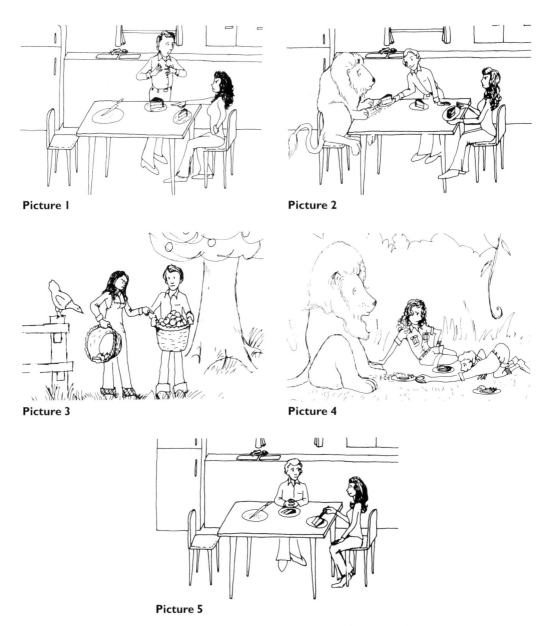

Figure 6–7. Set of pictures depicting literal and non-literal interpretations of the story, "Jack and Mary found some left-over cake in the kitchen. But when Jack divided it up, Mary complained that he had taken the Lion's share of the cake." Picture choices include, **Picture 1:** accurate interpretation/correct setting; **Picture 2:** literal interpretation/correct setting; **Picture 3:** accurate interpretation/incorrect setting; **Picture 4:** literal interpretation/incorrect setting; and **Picture 5:** inaccurate interpretation/correct setting.

phrase when the patient sees them in picture form. Finally, Huber (1990) suggests that the literal meaning is often easier to match to a picture because the range of possible depictions of the literal interpretation is more restricted compared to figurative depictions. That is, there are many representations and situations appropriate to "the lion's share," but all literal depictions must include an actual lion. What is apparent, is that under conditions of effortful processing, RHD patients tend to respond to the literal, not the figurative meaning of idiomatic expressions, suggesting some problems in coping with more than one (i.e., alternative) meanings, a deficit that can have considerable effect on discourse comprehension and production.

Indirect Requests

Indirect requests such as, "Can you open the window?" also have alternate meanings and can be taken literally or not, depending on the situation. Literally, "Can you open the window?" is an inquiry into a person's physical capacity to perform the act of opening a window. In a warm room it functions as a request to open the window, as in, "Would you open the window?" In the case of a fire, it perhaps should be interpreted literally. Requests can be more or less direct. For example, the statement, "I'm so hot," is less direct than, "Can you open the window?"

RHD patients have demonstrated reduced sensitivity to the non-literal meanings of such requests in paradigms using pictured representations (Foldi, 1987; Hirst, LeDoux, & Stein, 1984) as well as in studies in which stimuli and responses were verbal (Weylman, Brownell, Roman, & Gardner, 1989). In general, these studies have found that RHD subjects are not entirely insensitive to situational context in that they are able to distinguish situations that represent indirect versus direct requests. They are not, however, as good as NBD subjects in doing so (Weylman, Brownell, Roman, & Gardner, 1989), and they may have particular problems in processing requests that are extremely indirect and inexplicit.

Because the non-literal meaning of indirect requests is implicit, rather than explicit, their accurate interpretation requires an inference based on the preceding context. Context determines the intended meaning. One possible explanation for deficits in processing indirect requests could be problems in assimilating the verbal and physical contextual cues that suggest the non-literal meaning (Weylman et al., 1989). Reduced sensitivity to context has been posited for problems in interpreting whether or not characters in stories were being sarcastic (Kaplan, Brownell, Jacobs, & Gardner, 1990). Like indirect requests, sarcasm and irony have a literal meaning and another meaning that captures the pragmatic intent of the speaker. The non-literal meaning must be gleaned from the context in which the statement is made.

Aside from the physical and verbal context, other contextual features that help establish whether or not a request is direct include: (a) the relationship between the speaker and the listener (i.e., their familiarity with one another and their relative position of power), (b) the listener's sense of obligation to carry out the request, (c) the speaker's right to make the request, and (d) the estimated likelihood that the listener will comply with the request (Stemmer, Giroux, & Joanette, 1994). Stemmer et al. compared the capacity of NBD and RHD subjects to evaluate and to produce direct and indirect requests following short vignettes. Their in-depth analysis accounted for a wide variety of linguistic and situational contextual features. They found that, in many respects, RHD patients behave similarly to NBD adults. They investigated responsivity to direct requests, indirect requests, and extremely indirect requests or hints, which are the least explicit form of requesting. For example, if Sally were thirsty she might say to Bob, "Please get me some water" (direct). She might say, "I need some water" (indirect). Or she might say, "Boy, I worked up a thirst doing the gardening" (hint). Direct requests can be interpreted through linguistic decoding alone. Hints are totally dependent on comprehension of the situational context. Stemmer et al. (1994) found that RHD subjects processed direct and indirect requests normally, but had problems with hints. They were responsive to contextual variables in some situations, but less so in others. The authors suggested that their problems may have occurred at a conceptual level in which a mental model based on *contextual information is revised* or *a new representation of the text must be generated.* In the case of hints, the linguistic text does not match the intent, and a new representation for the words must be generated to produce a good fit between the hint and the preceding situation. Both the literal and non-literal meaning must be appreciated and one chosen. If the hint is not integrated with the context, it may be rejected.

Thus, problems in evaluating, interpreting, and producing indirect requests may be related to problems in several areas. Patients may be *less attentive to important contextual features.* They may have *trouble accessing and/or maintaining more than one representation for a set of words.* Finally, they may have *problems mobilizing the effort to map the words back onto the context to arrive at the accurate inference.*

Humor

RHD patients may have difficulty responding to certain aspects of jokes (Bihrle, Brownell, Powelson, & Gardner, 1986; Brownell, Michel, Powelson, & Gardner, 1983). Brownell et al. (1983) noted that jokes depend on two properties: *surprise* and *coherence.* At first the punch line is surprising, then it becomes coherent when it is replayed back onto the body of the joke. The punch line contains surprise because it would not have been predicted from the preceding narrative. Thus, the initial interpretation of the punch line must be revised and reintegrated into the body of the joke to make it coherent. This is the, "Oh, I get it!" phase of responding to jokes. Brownell et al. (1983) and Bihrle et al. (1986) found that RHD subjects were able to respond to the surprise element of jokes by picking punch lines and final cartoon frames that were surprising and funny, but their choices did not necessarily fit with the body of the joke. They appeared to recognize humor (a man slipping on a banana peel), but were not very able to manage in-

tegrating new information and revising their original interpretations.

Deficits among RHD patients in comprehending and using various forms of figurative or non-literal language are important on two levels: the functional and the theoretical. On the functional level, RHD patients may miss information because they have problems using and interpreting irony, sarcasm, joking, indirect requests and other forms of non-literal language that are sprinkled throughout standard conversational and narrative discourse. On the theoretical level, deficits in processing figurative language are of interest because of what they tell us about underlying causes of some discourse deficits. Problems in generating and maintaining alternate meanings for a lexical entry suggest a certain rigidity, deficits in using context appropriately, and possibly, a semantic level breakdown in easily applying connotative meanings.

Inference Revision

Many RHD patients have looked at picture A in Figure 6–4 and concluded that it is a picture of a man, a woman, and a cabbage. Elderly adults also sometimes think the baby in a bonnet is a cabbage, but they quickly abandon that impression and conclude that it is a family consisting of a man, a woman, and something that looks like a cabbage, but must be a baby. Resolving ambiguous stimuli requires effort because we often must revise our initial interpretations. Accurate interpretation of the ambiguous baby bonnet in Figure 6–4 occurs with the integration of it with other contextual features, such as the overall emotional tone of the picture, the facial expressions, the clothing, and the general demeanor of the man and woman which suggest that this is not a humorous or whimsical picture, but rather a serious one. Connecting these features with the "cabbage" is a type of bridging inference in which a bridge or "conceptual link," (Brownell, 1986) is made across features. In isolation, the baby may appear as a cabbage; integrated into the whole she becomes a baby in a bonnet. RHD patients have problems revising inferences and often seem satisfied with their first impressions and initial interpretations.

Inference revision has been explored in paradigms in which ideas appear at first to be incompatible or inconsistent with one another (Bloise & Tompkins, 1993; Brownell et al., 1986; Tompkins, Bloise, Timko, & Baumgaertner, 1994). Brownell et al. (1986) investigated comprehension of sentence pairs in which one sentence was misleading. For example, the sentence, "Barbara became too bored to finish the history book," leads one to conclude that Barbara is reading a textbook. However, when followed by a second sentence, "She had already spent five years writing it," the initial impression must be altered. The position of the misleading sentence was varied under the assumption that placing it first might prove more difficult because it would require an inference revision, as the previous example demonstrates. Indeed, unlike NBD controls, RHD subjects had more problems answering inferential questions when the misleading information occurred first. The authors concluded that deficits in revision may make it difficult for RHD patients to "infer the most appropriate link or conceptual bridge between individual sentences in a discourse" (p. 319). They went on to state that, "Where normal listeners are concerned to weave a coherent interpretation of an entire discourse so that each component jibes with the broader reality, RHD patients are often stuck with, or are satisfied with, a limited and piecemeal understanding" (p. 319). This description echoes previously mentioned findings in which RHD patients focus on objects or ideas in isolation rather than integrating them into the context as they interpret pictures and narratives.

Affective material also has been used to investigate inference revision ability. Tompkins et al. (1994) studied "attitudinal inferences" by exploring the capacity of RHD adults to answer factual and infer-

ential questions about short vignettes in which the final comment of one of the characters was either *congruent* or *incongruent* with the preceding context. In incongruent stimuli, a given set up might lead one to infer that the main character was unhappy, yet his or her final comment was positive and thus at odds with the story development. Such stories had to be re-evaluated to accommodate the apparent inconsistency, leading to the conclusion, for example, that a character was actually making a sarcastic comment. They found that RHD, LHD, and NBD subjects all had more problems with incongruent than with congruent attitudinal inferences. RHD subjects had no more difficulty with the incongruent stimuli than did NBD subjects. In addition, in this study and one by Bloise and Tompkins (1993), differences between NBD and RHD subjects on the type of two-sentence inferences used by Brownell et al. (1986) did not occur. However, Tompkins and her colleagues altered Brownell's original stimuli; and their RHD group was mildly impaired. Not surprisingly, subjects who fell below the range of normal performance were among those that were the most impaired on tests of neglect, again suggesting a link between neglect, attention, and cognitive performance.

Factors Contributing to Deficits in Processing Alternate Meanings

Problems in accessing figurative forms of language, resolving ambiguities, revising original interpretations, and generating alternate meanings probably are influenced by numerous variables including: (a) the complexity of the inferences to be made (i.e., the amount of distance between the alternate meaning and the supportive context), (b) the amount of effort required to link ideas together (i.e., how explicitly the ideas are stated and how redundant the supporting information), (c) the amount of competing information in the environment, (d) the speed of processing required and the time allowed for revision, and

(e) the cognitive and attentional status of the patient. The influence of general attentional and cognitive impairments and of specific mechanisms for problems in generating alternate meanings are explored in the following sections.

The Impact of Attentional and Cognitive Impairments

The finding that patients with neglect were the most impaired in inference revision in the studies by Tompkins et al. (1994) and Bloise and Tompkins (1993) suggests the now-familiar possibility that neglect is related to a decline in cognitive resources. The study by Tompkins et al. (1994) explored that possibility by measuring "working memory" in hopes of discovering associations between it and performance on inference revision tasks. *Working memory* is considered *a measure of the amount of activation allocated to support information processing and storage concurrently* (see Just & Carpenter, 1992, for a detailed explanation). That is, working memory consists of the amount of resources necessary to perform the operations for comprehension *and* for storing the information that is comprehended as one builds an interpretation (Tompkins et al., 1994). Often it is measured by having subjects answer true/false questions about sentences while concurrently remembering the last word in each sentence as they go. In normal adults, working memory capacity correlates with inference revision abilities (Daneman & Carpenter, 1983; Just & Carpenter, 1992). Tompkins et al. (1994) found that, in RHD subjects, working memory was associated with problems on difficult inference revisions. Interestingly, working memory capacity was not associated with performance on simpler inferential stimuli. The authors also found that RHD subjects with neglect performed more poorly on both working memory measures and attitudinal inferences than did RHD subjects without neglect. The authors suggested that their results were consistent with proposals that

neglect reflects reduced availability or impaired allocation of mental resources.

Reduced attention may interact with task demands for other types of alternate meaning stimuli. For example, Tompkins (1990) conducted a priming study using ambiguous words with a literal and nonliteral meaning in a lexical decision task. She found that RHD subjects had problems only under certain conditions of effortful (versus automatic) processing in which they had to develop a strategy for dealing with inconsistent or incompatible information.

According to Tompkins et al. (1994), reduced cognitive capacity or reduced or misallocated attentional resources might influence performance in two ways. First, having fewer resources available may interfere with building an initial representation such that there is an incomplete representation available for further analysis or computations. Alternatively, patients may form adequate representations, but have problems further down the line where computations such as generating bridging inferences or revising initial representations are brought to bear on already formed representations.

Thus, RHD patients, especially those with neglect, may have fewer resources available to: (a) generate and maintain alternate meanings, (b) resolve ambiguities, (c) revise initial assumptions, and (d) generate secondary meanings for figurative language in cognitively demanding situations. These deficits may occur either because RHD patients have incomplete information or because they are unable to conduct the necessary operations on that information.

Rigidity

RHD patients might be less sensitive to new information because of a certain cognitive rigidity (Brownell et al., 1986; Joanette & Goulet, 1986). Few studies have investigated reduced flexibility as it pertains to difficulty conceiving alternate meanings. However, Schneiderman and Saddy (1988) found that RHD patients demonstrated in-flexibility in a linguistic task called the "insertion test." The insertion test asks subjects to insert a word into a sentence without altering its meaning (e.g., inserting the word "white" into the sentence, "I see the snow"). RHD subjects were able to manage these simple insertions adequately. In a second condition, the insertion required a *shift* in the syntactic function and relationship a given word had to other words in the sentence. For example, inserting the word "daughter" into the sentence, "Cindy saw her take his drink," requires a reassignment of the pronoun "her" to a different grammatical category as in, "Cindy saw her daughter take his drink." In the shift condition the performance of RHD subjects fell significantly below that of NBD and subjects who had mild to moderate aphasia. Equally interesting was the nature of their responses. They either gave up entirely or expressed dissatisfaction with their incorrect insertions, but said that they could not think another way to include the insertion item, which suggested to the authors that although they understood the task, patients "were incapable of repairing a sentence which they recognized to be unacceptable" (p. 44). The authors concluded that this instance of *rigidity* in syntactic representation "might have repercussions in all cases of semantic reinterpretation whether at the sentential or at the discourse level" (p. 51). More studies investigating the nature of semantic rigidity would help to establish the conditions under which it occurs and its potential impact on discourse events that require discarding one meaning and choosing another.

Activation Deficit

Another possible source of deficits in generating alternate meanings is failure to activate multiple meanings. Chapter 5 reviewed proposals that the intact RH generates multiple, loosely connected, subordinate meanings, whereas the LH generates more familiar, tightly connected, dom-inant meanings (Beeman, 1993; Brownell et al., 1984; Burgess & Simpson, 1988; Chiarello et al., 1990). It is thought that damage to the RH may reduce the capacity to generate alternate meanings for single words and phrases under conditions of effortful processing, resulting in a specific semantic deficit. This semantic deficit also may affect discourse processing in that alternate meanings are not activated during conversational speech and discourse tasks.

Research with NBD adults has suggested that the two hemispheres may code both verbal and visual information differently. As stated in Chapter 5, the RH is thought to *coarsely code* information while the LH is thought to conduct *fine coding*. Processing in the RH is thought to be broad-based and diffuse, connecting distant concepts. Processing in the LH is thought to be more narrow and restricted. Thus, in the RH, the word "fan" and the word "baseball" might together elicit the image of someone eating a hotdog in the stands, wearing a baseball cap with a team logo on it. The RH makes a bridge between the two concepts because through coarse coding it is more adept at connecting distantly related concepts than is the LH, and is thus important to making bridging or coherence inferences.

Activation of semantic representations or meanings is considered to be a relatively automatic process that does not consume many processing resources. For example, the noun "fan" can elicit two meanings: (a) a supporter or admirer and (b) a device used for ventilation. Supporting context will determine which meaning will remain activated and be selected for further processing.

Activation often is measured in conditions of "on line" processing in which measures are taken at the time that subjects actually process material. One method of measuring "on line" decisions is a "priming" paradigm. In priming paradigms one stimulus is expected to facilitate or speed up a decision made about a subsequent stimulus. For example, a subject might be shown one word for a brief moment, followed by a second word about which they must make a decision, called a "lexical decision." The lexical decision might be to determine whether or not a word is related to the previous word or to decide whether or not a string of letters is, in fact, a word. Thus, the word "fan" might facilitate a decision about whether or not the next word "sports" is related to the word "fan." But the word "fan" would not be expected to facilitate a decision about the word "cat," for example, because "cat" would not have been activated by the word "fan." When a subject makes a faster (and presumably accurate) decision about the word "sports," compared to the word "cat," it is assumed that "fan" facilitated the decision because the word "fan" had activated the concept of "sports fan" among other meanings. Facilitation is usually measured in terms of the amount of time (reaction time) that it takes a subject to make decisions about the second stimulus.

In a study by Beeman (1993), subjects were asked to listen to stories and to periodically make decisions about whether or not strings of letters that appeared on a monitor in front of them were words. In some cases the words on the monitor were related to inferences they should have been drawing about the narratives. The author was interested in whether or not inferences drawn as subjects listened to the narratives facilitated the lexical decisions. Thus, the task was an "on line" measure of inferences made as subjects processed the stories. "Off line" measures taken at the end of the stories consisted of inferential and factual questions about the narratives. The type of inferences studied were "coherence" inferences or those that helped tie events together and resolve discrepancies, allowing new information to be smoothly mapped onto earlier representations.

Beeman found that RHD subjects performed normally when answering factual questions, but were impaired compared to elderly controls in answering inference questions. In addition, their reaction times were not facilitated by words related to the inferences in the priming section of the study. The priming results suggested that the RHD subjects, by and large, did not activate the information necessary to draw inferences from the material. That is, they did not appear to activate alternate meanings for discrepant information, and, hence, did not draw appropriate inferences. This deficit was later confirmed when subjects responded to inferential questions about the material.

Thus, the results of this study support the idea that damage to the RH interferes with *activation* of alternate, subordinate, or distantly related concepts which, in turn, interferes with arriving at coherence inferences. That is, the information necessary to generate certain types of inferences in discourse is not activated. More studies are needed to determine if decreased activation of alternate meanings is a factor in the inference generation deficits found in many RHD patients.

Suppression Deficit

An alternate hypothesis, proposed by Tompkins and her colleagues, suggests that the problem with alternate meanings does not lie in their *activation,* but in their *suppression* (Tompkins & Baumgaertner, 1998; Tompkins, Baumgaertner, Lehman, & Fossett, 1997; Tompkins, Lehman, Baumgaertner, Fossett, & Vance, 1996). In this conception of RHD discourse deficits, *ineffective suppression of multiple meanings interferes in accurate inference generation during discourse.*

Tompkins and colleagues found that RHD subjects *are* able to activate multiple meanings under conditions of relatively automatic and non-effortful processing. Like other researchers, they found that RHD subjects were able to process relatively easy inferences in certain conditions (Bloise & Tompkins, 1993; Joanette et al., 1990; McDonald & Wales, 1986; Tompkins et al., 1994). They also found that RHD subjects can generate both literal and figurative meanings for ambiguous stimuli in automatic processing conditions. For example, the performance of RHD subjects in a lexical decision task was facilitated by words that evoked *either* the figurative *or* the literal meaning of a set of target adjectives (Tompkins, 1990). That is, both meanings were activated. Yet, in a more effortful condition RHD performance fell below that of the NBD subjects. Another study demonstrated that RHD subjects could activate the figurative meaning of familiar idioms in "on line" processing, even though they had difficulty with the figurative meaning in "off line" processing. That is, they were able to access the figurative meaning in automatic processing conditions even if they later had trouble using or defining it. Thus, it appears from this body of research that the problems do not arise at the activation level, but rather at some later stage of processing.

If activation of multiple and alternative meanings is not at issue, it may be that the problem lies in mechanisms that operate on the multiple meanings that have been activated. Tompkins et al. (in press) cited work by Gernsbacher and colleagues with normal adults that suggested that there may be twin mechanisms that operate on activated representations (Gernsbacher, 1990; Gernsbacher & Faust, 1991; Gernsbacher, Varner, & Faust, 1990). They proposed that an *enhancement mechanism* increases the activation of relevant meanings whereas a *suppression mechanism* reduces activation of irrelevant meanings.

Two recent studies explored the possibility that *RHD interferes in the suppression of alternative meanings that are inappropriate or irrelevant to a given discourse.* In the first study, Tompkins et al. (1997) explored suppression of inappropriate meanings for lexical ambiguities (i.e., words with more than one meaning). RHD subjects listened to experimental sentences such as, "He was in the front row," the final word of which had two meanings. They also listened to comparison sentences such as, "He was in the front seat," in which the final word was not ambiguous. Subjects then had to decide if a given probe word, in this case "boat,"

fit with either sentence. The probe words stimulated an alternate meaning for the final word in the experimental sentences. Slowness in rejecting a probe word such as "boat" would suggest that both meanings of *"row"* had been activated and that the irrelevant meaning had not been suppressed. All subjects were expected to be, and were, accurate in judging how well the probe words fit with the sentences.

The crucial measure was reaction time. Some probe words were presented after a short (175 ms) interval and some after a longer delayed (1,000 ms) interval. At the short interval, it was expected that both meanings would have been activated and remain, interfering in the decision about the probe word. At the delayed interval, it was expected that irrelevant meanings by then would have been suppressed. Thus, although both NBD and RHD subjects were expected to have problems judging how well the probe word fit with the experimental sentences at the short interval, the authors predicted that only RHD subjects would continue to have problems at the longer interval. That is, RHD subjects would retain the inappropriate meaning longer than normal and be slower to reject a probe word.

As predicted, both subject groups demonstrated interference at the short interval in judging whether probe words fit with the sentences. That is, both meanings of the ambiguous final words were activated. As also predicted, only the RHD group continued to demonstrate interference at the delayed probe interval, suggesting that they maintained or had trouble suppressing the less relevant meaning of the ambiguous sentence-final word. In contrast, NBD subjects improved performance at the delayed interval, suggesting that they had inhibited inappropriate meanings of the final word by that time.

Another study in which the authors looked at suppression of contextually inappropriate inferences supported these results (Tompkins et al., 1996). In this study, subjects listened to two sentence stories, the first sentence of which promoted one inference, and the second of which promoted a different inference. In one condition, each sentence was followed by a probe word that was related to the meaning of the initial sentence, but was inappropriate to the sentences taken as a unit. For example, "tourist" was the probe word for the sentence pair, "Sally admired the historic farmhouse. If she sold it, her commission would be extremely high." A comparison set of sentences conveyed an interpretation consistent with the probe word as in, "Amy showed the Victorian mansion. If she sold it, her commission would be extremely high." In addition, the sentence pairs were followed by factual and inferential questions to test comprehension of both types of information. Results indicated that both NBD and RHD subjects experienced poor suppression of contextually inappropriate inferences, but that only in RHD subjects was comprehension related to suppression effectiveness.

Thus, RHD may not interfere with the activation of multiple, distantly related meanings for words or sentences in discourse. Rather, it may interfere with the ability to inhibit them when they are no longer needed. Tompkins et al. (1996) suggested a number of ways in which ineffective suppression could account for various types of RHD discourse problems. Deficits in suppression may contribute to problems in the efficiency of discourse production and to problems rejecting the literal meanings of idiomatic expressions. It may contribute to the rigidity found in some patients. That is, they may find it difficult to let go of an inappropriate tack taken in conversation or an inappropriate response to a given stimulus.

More studies are needed to determine the validity of a suppression versus activation deficit as explanations for some of these communication impairments. At this point, these two theories hold great promise as avenues of investigating problems in dealing with competing and alternate meanings and with inference and discourse deficits in general among the RHD population. Both carry strong clinical implications as well. By being either slower to *activate* or slower to *reject* inappropriate or competing meanings, RHD patients may have problems arriving at the contextually appropriate meaning of a given concept as discourse proceeds. Because conversations are dynamic, such problems may contribute not only to difficulty understanding individual inferences, but may interfere in other aspects of discourse comprehension and production as well. The extra time and effort required to arrive at a contextually appropriate meaning could interfere in adequate comprehension of subsequent information, regardless of how explicit or implicit it is. Processing roadblocks such as deficits in the activation or suppression of loosely connected semantic concepts could interfere with adequate discourse integration. Treatment strategies for problems in activation versus problems in suppression would differ considerably, an issue addressed in Chapter 9.

THEORY OF MIND DEFICITS

Overview

One of the tenets associated with RHD communicative impairments is that RHD adults have problems with the uses to which language is put and the meaning behind communicative acts (i.e., the pragmatic aspects of communication). One avenue for investigating problems in recognizing and conveying communicative intent is the study of "theory of mind."

A *theory of mind* can be considered *a theory about the internal mental state of others that helps one interpret their external behavior.* In its original definition, theory of mind was restricted to an understanding of the mental state of another person. In the literature on RHD, the definition has become more inclusive and theory of mind has come to mean not only the ability to develop a theory about what someone knows, but also about their emotional state. It is a recognition that people's beliefs may guide their behavior and that their beliefs may be different from our own. A theory of mind allows us to make predictions about other people's behavior based on our assumptions about their purposes, intentions, and knowledge. Essentially, it is a set of inferences about another person's motivations and knowledge that allows us to adjust our communication with them. It enables us to distinguish when someone is serious, joking, or sarcastic, and to determine what they mean from what they say. It enables us to negotiate the social aspects of communication. It is a set of *inferences* because the internal mental states of others are not directly observable or explicit.

The concept of "theory of mind" originated from a series of studies conducted by Premack and Woodruff with chimpanzees in the late 1970s (Premack & Woodruff, 1975, 1978). It later was used to explain some of the deficits attributed to autistic children (Baron-Cohen, 1988; Frith, 1989). More recently, in its expanded definition, it has been invoked to explain some of the pragmatic deficits found in RHD adults.

Premack and Woodruff (1978) were interested in what a chimpanzee might know about what someone else knows. It already had been established that chimps knew enough about how the physical world worked to use some tools effectively. They wanted to know if chimps also knew how people or other chimps "worked." Could they predict the behavior of other organisms by imputing mental states to them? They called this behavior a *theory* of mind; a theory because it required a system of inferences or theories about what motivated other organisms. Specifically, they investigated a chimp's ability to predict the behavior of a human based on an inference about the human's motivation and purpose. They found that a chimp could, indeed, impute wants, purposes, and knowledge states to others. A chimpanzee could predict how a human actor in a video sequence could solve a problem such as getting out of a locked cage, using a box to reach some bananas, or lighting a heater with a match to relieve the cold. In other words, the chimp, Sarah, could impute her own motivations (wanting to get out of a cage, wanting food, wanting to be warm) onto the human character. In this sense, Sarah was able to put herself in the position of humans, "empathize" with their feelings, and pick an accurate solution to their problem. It was less clear whether she could predict what a human might *know* and how that knowledge would guide his or her solutions to a given problem.

Understanding knowledge states is important to a theory of mind and to understanding the pragmatic aspects of communication. For example, it is important to distinguish between knowing and guessing. Suppose you suddenly have problems with your computer and months of work is approaching a possible meltdown. You are so frustrated that you turn to the nearest co-worker for help. Your faith in their knowledge will be an important factor in your subsequent actions. Your co-worker may say they know what to do, and sound like they do, but you must decide if they "know what they're talking about." Do you take their advice or seek further assistance? Your next step depends on your belief or theory about their knowledge, regardless of how confident they sound. Thus, a theory of mind not only informs us about someone's motivations and affective states, but about their knowledge base as well.

Knowing what someone knows is particularly important in the give and take of conversational flow. Among the maxims of conversation is that it be relevant and informative (Grice, 1975), and that this maxim is respected by both speaker and listener. Inferences about the knowledge base of others guides our interactions with them in that we try neither to talk down to them nor confuse them by talking over their heads. We also use certain conversational conventions based on the knowledge another person has of a topic. For example, if we are discussing someone else, we may base the term of reference for the third party on our listener's knowledge of that person. If they don't know the third party well, we might use first and last names (i.e., "I saw Fred Darley last night"). If they know them well, we might just use the first name (i.e., "I saw Fred last night"). If the third party is of higher status and unknown to our communicative partner, we might use a formal reference (i.e., "I saw Dr. Darley last night"). These linguistic subtleties are examples of the type of adjustments we unconsciously make to accommodate our theory of mind about the knowledge base of another person.

In the affective realm, theory of mind helps guide us in determining how much to say. If we infer that a given topic will make someone uncomfortable, we adjust by broaching it in a delicate manner. If we infer that a topic is boring to our listener, we may acknowledge it and continue or move on to another topic. We read facial expression, body language, and linguistic information to help us arrive at an understanding of the listener's perspective.

Autistic children are known for poor social interaction and impaired communicative ability. It has been suggested that many or most of their communicative deficits might be subsumed under impaired theory of mind, including deficits in: (a) using speech to communicate, (b) turn-taking, (c) using eye gaze to guide conversation, (d) starting and ending conversations appropriately, (e) giving enough background to accommodate new information, and (f) problems in determining the boundaries of shared knowledge (Baron-Cohen, 1988, 1989; Baron-Cohen, Leslie, & Frith, 1985; Frith, 1989). In a number of studies, for example, autistic children have difficulty assuming the belief structure of another person in order to predict his or her behavior. Similarly, some autistic children are deficient in providing explanations for characters' motivations based on contextual elements in stories (Happe, 1994).

Although less dramatic, similar pragmatic impairments may occur with RHD,

including: (a) poor eye contact, (b) poor turn-taking, (c) poor use of conventions for starting and ending conversations, (d) problems in determining shared knowledge, (e) tangentiality, and (f) reduced sensitivity to the impact of their messages and the implications behind others' messages. Deficits in theory of mind have great appeal in illuminating and explaining some of these pragmatic deficits and problems with social inference in the RHD population.

It has been suggested that theory of mind is a meta-representational skill by which we are able to generate representations about representations. Our beliefs about the physical world are called "primary representations" that directly represent objects or situations (Leslie, 1987). Our beliefs about other people's mental states are called second-order representations because they are beliefs about someone else's beliefs and motivations. That is, they are representations of representations or meta-representations. This meta-representational capacity has been postulated to be one source of the development of a theory of mind (Baron-Cohen, 1988). The specific mechanisms of theory of mind are not yet understood, but it is assumed that it requires a fairly sophisticated inferential capacity that aids us in filling in the gap between what is meant from what is said.

RHD Deficits in Theory of Mind

It is well known that RHD can interfere in some of the pragmatic aspects of conversational discourse, particularly when conversations move beyond the simple and straightforward to that which requires more effortful interpretations (Table 6–4). A number of studies have documented theory of mind deficits in RHD subjects including deficits in generating second-order representations, impaired sensitivity to shared knowledge, and reduced awareness of the internal motivations guiding communicative behavior. Table 6–5 lists some of the specific theory of mind deficits found in studies of RHD subjects.

TABLE 6–4. Pragmatic deficits associated with RHD patients' impaired understanding of communicative intent.

Reduced

▶ Requests for information from a conversational partner
▶ Interest in the effect of a response on a conversational partner
▶ Ability to weigh plausibility of facts
▶ Sensitivity to paralinguistic information such as facial expression, and body language
▶ Sensitivity to indirect speech acts that signal nonliteral meanings (i.e., sarcasm, irony)
▶ Sensitivity to internal motivations of communicative partner
▶ Use of conventions signaling turn-taking and topic initiation
▶ Topic maintenance
▶ Use of conventions for conversational termination and intiation
▶ Use of conversational advancers (i.e., one-word utterances such as "yes" and "uh-huh")
▶ Levels of elaborative content
▶ Eye contact during conversational speech

TABLE 6–5. Theory of mind deficits found in RHD subjects.

---

1. Reduced reliance on extra-textual (versus linguistic) information to guide interpretations (Brownell et al., 1992)
2. Impaired application of shared social knowledge (Brownell et al., 1997)
3. Reduced ability to use second-order representations in distinguishing true from false beliefs (Siegal et al., 1996; Winner et al., in press)
4. Impaired ability to adopt the mental set of another person (Siegal et al., 1996)
5. Reduced appreciation of internal versus external causes of character actions and statements in stories (Brownell et al., 1994; Kaplan et al., 1990)
6. Reduced sensitivity to the effect of conversational violations (Rehak et al., 1992)
7. Reduced sensitivity to emotional state of story characters (Bloom et al., 1997)

RHD patients may have problems in interpreting the effect of tangential comments as a violation of conversational convention (Rehak, Kaplan, & Gardner, 1992). Tangentiality is often reported in the clinical picture of RHD conversational performance, possibly because patients are not sensitive to some of the negative effects such conversational violations have on listeners. Rehak et al. (1992) investigated responses to conversational advancers that support forward movement of conversation and to conversational blockers that divert conversation away from a participant's goal. They found that RHD subjects were able to manage straightforward cooperative conversations, but were less sensitive than NBD subjects to the effect of conversational blockers. RHD subjects judged such conversations as normal more often than did NBD subjects and were less able than NBD subjects to choose an appropriate way to repair such conversations. The authors suspected that RHD affected

the ability to interpret conversational blockers because RHD subjects might not appreciate the motivations and intentions behind such conversational violations. That is, they appeared not to recognize when a conversational partner was intentionally trying to divert and control the conversation, possibly because they had difficulty assuming the mental state of the partner and understanding their intentions.

Subjects' understanding of false beliefs in which a character in a story has erroneous information that guides his actions has been investigated in several studies (Siegal, Carrington, & Radel, 1996; Winner, Brownell, Happe, Blum, & Pincus, in press). Siegal et al. (1996) found that, under some conditions, RHD subjects had more difficulty than LHD subjects in making predictions based on a character's false belief.

Several other studies have looked at the ability to understand first- and second-order beliefs by examining subjects' comprehension of sarcasm, which is a form of verbal irony (Brownell, Carroll, Rehak, & Wingfield, 1992; Kaplan, Brownell, et al., 1990; Winner et al., in press). The intended meaning of an ironic statement is usually the opposite of its literal meaning. To say, "Way to go," to someone who has just made a social gaffe is to mean the opposite. In a positive light, sarcasm is seen as a form of banter. In a negative situation its intention is hurtful (McDonald & Pearce, 1996). To understand the difference, one must be able to understand the intention behind the words. That is, to understand how a listener might interpret an ironic and/or a false statement, one needs to understand what the listener knows and what the speaker thinks the listener knows. Damage to the RH has been found to have a negative effect on subjects' ability to perceive the difference between sarcastic and literally true statements made by story characters (Kaplan et al., 1990). Kaplan et al. (1990) suggested that RHD subjects were particularly insensitive to the mutual knowledge shared between the speaker and the listener, knowledge that specified if the speaker was intending to hurt the listener or be supportive or playful in his remarks. This knowledge would be considered a second-order representation or belief. Brownell et al. (1992) found that RHD subjects relied more on linguistic information than they did on other textual devices such as the mood of a speaker in determining if what a speaker said was intended to be plausible, or if it was intended to be joking and silly or mean and nasty.

Winner et al. (in press) looked at first and second-order beliefs by examining whether RHD subjects had problems determining if intentionally false utterances spoken by story characters were intended as jokes or lies. The difference between jokes and lies in their story stimuli again depended on recognizing what a listener knows (i.e., a second-order representation or belief). That is, a false utterance may be considered a lie if a speaker doesn't think a listener knows the truth (i.e., the speaker thinks he or she can get away with lying). The same statement may be taken as an ironic joke or sarcasm if the speaker does know that the listener knows the truth. They found that RHD subjects had more problems in attrib-

uting second-order beliefs to story characters than did NBD subjects. RHD subjects' performance was, however, quite variable. Particularly problematic were stories in which a character was lying. In these cases, according to the authors, the liar holds a *false* second-order expectation in that he wrongly or inappropriately expects to be believed. They suggest that RHD subjects have more difficulty with situations like these in which someone's second-order beliefs are wrong. In addition, they found considerable variability of performance in the NBD group, suggesting that these skills may represent some of the diffuse changes associated with aging.

Another avenue for investigating theory of mind deficits in RHD subjects has been to look at the effect of shared knowledge about a third party being discussed in conversations between two partners (Brownell, Pincus, Blum, Rehak, & Winner, 1997). In two experiments, Brownell et al. (1997) investigated the terms of reference used to describe a third party. Variables that could affect the formality with which the person was referred to (i.e., "Mr. Jones," "Bob Jones," "Bob") could vary according to how familiar that person was to the speaker and to the listener, and according to that person's occupational status relative to speaker and addressee. Decisions about the relative formality of personal reference requires not only an understanding of status but also recognition of shared knowledge—what the speaker knows about what the listener knows. They found that RHD subjects were sensitive to status, but less sensitive than NBD subjects to levels of familiarity.

Finally, a study by Brownell, Blum, and Winner (1994) investigated sensitivity to internal and external factors in explaining character actions in a story. For example, a worker loses an important file upon hearing bad news. In explaining why the file is missing, subjects might invoke an "internal" explanation such as his state of mind and mood (i.e., under stress, upset). "External" explanations might include environmental factors such as blaming his secretary. They found that RHD subjects were less sensitive to internal explanations than NBD controls, suggesting that they have problems relating to other people's internal states. Similarly, Bloom et al. (1997) found that RHD subjects made fewer references to the emotional state of characters in a pictured story than did LHD subjects.

In general, studies of theory of mind deficits demonstrated that RHD adults may have problems in making inferences based on pragmatic intent. They have been found to have problems in several areas of social interaction that require an understanding of second-order representations and beliefs. These findings are not consistent. Not all RHD adults have theory-of-mind deficits, just as not all RHD subjects have discourse deficits. However, impaired ability to adopt a theory of mind appears to be a useful way of conceptualizing some of the conversational and pragmatic deficits seen in discourse impaired RHD adults.

SUMMARY

1. *RHD may leave patients linguistically proficient, but impaired in their ability to manage complex discourse situations.* Patients may be *less sensitive to shades of meaning, speaker intentions, conversational conventions, overall themes, inferences, and the beliefs and internal motivations of others.* These deficits are particularly evident in situations demanding effortful processing.

2. *RHD discourse deficits sometimes stem from attentional deficits* which create an indirect effect on discourse proficiency. They also may arise from *specific cognitive impairments that affect the capacity to integrate information, respond to alternate meanings, and to draw and revise inferences.*

3. *RHD patients may have deficits in the capacity to draw inferences, particularly from ambiguous material.* Inference gen-

eration depends o
to and integrate
into a coherent p
ity to associate t
perience and wo
or all of these capacities may
rupted by RHD.

4. Inference problems in RHD patients include *problems in generating a macrostructure or central theme.* Macrostructure deficits may be related to problems in integration of discourse features and to attentional impairments in arousal, selective attention, and attentional maintenance.

5. *RHD patients may produce reduced levels of informative content.* Some patients produce unelaborated output, but many more are verbose. Excessive output is characterized by irrelevancies, tangentiality, and intrusive comments, all of which result in inefficient verbal expression.

6. *Confabulation can occur with denial of deficit in patients with neglect and anosognosia.* Confabulations are often attempts to make sense of things the patient does not understand.

7. *The intact RH is thought to process less frequent or alternative meanings.* RHD may disrupt this capacity and affect the capacity to manage figurative and metaphoric meanings, indirect requests, and humor under effortful processing requirements.

8. *Impaired ability to manage alternate meanings also may affect the capacity of RHD patients to revise initial inferences,* a skill crucial to following discourse.

9. Factors contributing to impaired processing of alternate meanings include: (a) *reduced attentional capacity or misallocated attentional resources,* (b) *rigidity,* (c) *a deficit in activating alternate mean-*

ings, and (d) *a deficit in adequately suppressing irrelevant alternate meanings.*

10. *RHD may impair the capacity to adopt a "theory of mind" or theory about the internal mental state of other people—their motivations, emotional state, beliefs, intentions, and knowledge.* These deficits may result in impaired "social cognition" skills or "social disconnection" and, thus, interfere with the pragmatic aspects of communication and possibly with the structural components of discourse as well.

CHAPTER

Affective Deficits

Damage to the RH can alter emotional status and/or affective behavior. These changes can take a number of forms, and they can be subtle or dramatic. Most typically, patients appear indifferent, apathetic, and unmotivated. They may seem depressed, yet oddly unconcerned about their deficits. They may make jokes, but fail to smile. They may be angry, but sound sad. They may be interested, but fail to make eye contact. They may seem less responsive to the emotions of those around them and appear isolated, emotionally distant, and detached. Some patients may simply fail to observe the accepted conventions that signal an interest in social participation. For example, they may fail to greet people before they start a conversation or end it abruptly by leaving the room. They may fail to make the kind of responses (e.g., head nods, saying "um hm," smiling) that encourage the continuation of discourse.

Some patients may seem flat and disconnected across the board, failing to make the effort required of emotional connection. Some may seem inappropriately jocular at one moment and abrupt and angry at another. Still others may be agitated, restless, anxious, and confabulatory. Even patients whose outward behavior belies any obvious affective disturbance may have problems in processing emotional material. It may take more effort than it once did for them to comprehend, respond to, and express the emotional impact of situations and events. Just as they may respond to the superficial rather than the underlying meaning in complex discourse, so, too, they may fail to adequately interpret the underlying emotional content of discourse and situational events.

Emotions *are subjective mood states that involve responsivity to an evocative stimulus, certain physiologic reactions, expressive behaviors, and motivated actions* (Borod, 1992; Silberman & Weingartner, 1986). Emotional experience is an internal experience. Affect *is the outward expression of emotion that may or may not accurately reflect the subjective experience of mood and emotion.* Affect can be detected in a person's face, voice, gestures, posture, and in the content of their language. Research has confirmed the clinical observation that damage to the RH can, in some cases, alter emotional experience and/or affective behavior. Documented affective changes subsequent to RHD can include signs of apathy, indifference, denial of illness and anosognosia, problems in the nonverbal and verbal expression of emotion, and reduced sensitivity to the emotions of others. In rare cases, psychiatric disorders involving delusions, confusion and/or misidentification of place and persons with accompanying confabulatory behavior can also occur (Table 7–1).

This chapter will address emotional and affective deficits associated with RHD. It will begin with a discussion of theories that emotional sensitivity is somewhat lateralized to the RH.

TABLE 7–1. Deficits in emotional and affective behavior that can occur with RHD.

1. Deficits in Emotional Communication
   a. Comprehension and production of nonverbal emotional information as conveyed by
      (1) Facial expression
      (2) Gesture
      (3) Posture
   b. Comprehension of verbally conveyed emotions as conveyed in
      (1) Stories, pictures and films
      (2) Conversational and narrative discourse
   c. Verbal production of emotion in
      (1) Conversational and narrative discourse
      (2) Prosodic contour
      (3) Recall of emotionally evocative memories
2. Depression
3. Delusions and confusional states
   a. Agitated confusion, delirium, disorientation, psychosis
   b. Misidentification syndromes

EMOTIONAL PROCESSING IN THE RIGHT HEMISPHERE

The RH Dominance Theory

It is generally accepted that physiologic correlates of subjective emotion and mood states are linked to the limbic system. However, a large body of evidence suggests that cortical structures also play a role in the comprehension and production of emotional behavior. There also appears to be some lateralization of hemispheric control over affective behavior. Converging lines of evidence have led to the hypothesis that the RH is dominant for the perception, comprehension, and expression of emotion (see Borod, 1992; Silberman & Weingartner, 1986; and Tucker, 1981 for reviews). This theory is sometimes referred to as the *RH Dominance Theory.*

Support for this theory comes from a variety of studies, some more convincing than others. Early laterality studies in NBD adults in which visual or auditory information was presented to one hemisphere at a time suggested RH superiority for emotional material (Kimura, 1964; Landis, Assal, & Perret, 1979; Ley & Bryden, 1979; Suberi & McKeever, 1977). Certain methodological problems make the results of some laterality studies difficult to interpret. In addition, the relative RH advantage for emotional material in some of these studies could be due to RH superiority in non-emotional processes, such as auditory and visual pattern recognition and visuospatial processing, known to be under RH control. For example, as discussed in Chapter 4, the basis for the superiority of the RH in processing "emotional" prosody may be perceptual rather than emotional. "Emotional" prosody appears to be particularly dependent on pitch, a prosodic parameter for which the RH appears to have particular aptitude.

Studies of physiologic responsivity using electroencephalographic (EEG) data suggest that there is preferential RH activation during emotionally evocative experience. For example, relative RH activation has been reported when NBD subjects recall emotionally charged situations and when they report their emotional response to evocative visual stimuli (Davidson & Schwartz, 1976; Davidson, Schwartz, Saron, Bennett, & Goleman, 1979).

Studies using galvanic skin response (GSR), an electrodermal response considered to be a reflection of arousal, to measure laterality of physiologic changes in patients with affective disorders such as depression are equivocal because it is not clear whether control over GSRs is ipsilateral or contralateral and whether it is inhibitory or excitatory (Silberman & Weingartner, 1986). As discussed in Chapter 3, RHD can interfere with autonomic sensitivity and arousal which, in turn, can interfere with emotional sensitivity by reducing attention to important mood markers (Heilman et al., 1978; Morrow et al., 1981; Yokoyama et al., 1987; Zoccolotti et al., 1982).

Changes in mood states in people with seizure disorders and mental illness also

have been cited in support of the RH dominance theory. However, studies that have attempted to find lateralized EEG alterations in patients with primary affective illness (i.e., schizophrenia, bipolar disturbance) are difficult to interpret because alterations in physiologic status of either hemisphere are subtle. Investigations of patients with unilateral epileptic foci suggest that problems in affective regulation can occur with either right- or left-sided foci, albeit with some qualitative differences in the type of affective changes observed (Silberman & Weingartner, 1986). Right-sided foci have been associated with emotional changes and left-sided foci with cognitive changes (Bear & Fedio, 1977). When reviewing laterality studies of emotion, it is important to remember that there may be differences based on the type of processing required. That is, there may be a difference between measures taken during experienced or felt emotions and those that require verbal interpretation of emotion. The latter may tend to favor LH processing, for example, because language networks in the brain are activated.

Stronger support for the RH dominance theory comes from studies of patients with unilateral hemispheric damage, particularly RHD patients. In an early and often quoted study, Gainotti (1972) found that RHD and LHD patients responded differently to the psychological stress induced by failure during task performance. LHD patients had "catastrophic reactions" (tears, swearing, and other signs of extreme frustration), but RHD patients appeared inappropriately indifferent. These findings resonated with clinical experience, and spurred further investigations of affective changes that have demonstrated that RHD patients have more difficulty with emotional communication than do LHD patients. Subjects with unilateral right- or left-sided lesions have been presented with emotionally charged words, sentences, stories, pictures, and videotapes to interpret (Borod, Andelman, Obler, Tweedy, & Welkowitz, 1992; Borod et al., 1996; Buck &

Duffy, 1980; Cicone, Wapner, & Gardner, 1980; Cimino, Verfaellie, Bowers, & Heilman, 1991; Dekosky, Heilman, Bowers, & Valenstein, 1980; Mammucari et al., 1988; Ostrove et al., 1990; Rehak, Kaplan, Weylman, et al., 1992). They have been asked to discriminate and interpret emotions in facial expressions, body language, and prosodic contour (Benowitz et al., 1983; Borod, Koff, Lorch, & Nicholas, 1986; Borod et al., 1990; Dekosky et al., 1980), and their outward displays of emotion in facial expression and verbal production have been measured for intensity and accuracy of expression (Blonder et al., 1991; Blonder, Burns, Bowers, Moore, & Heilman, 1993; Bloom, Borod, Obler, & Gerstman, 1992, 1993; Borod et al., 1985, 1990; Cimino et al., 1991; Martin, Borod, Alpert, Brozgold, & Welkowitz, 1990). In the main, this research has demonstrated that RHD can have a negative impact on the production and comprehension of affective behavior, although the mechanisms (emotional, cognitive, sensory-motor) for such disorders are not entirely clear.

The Valence Hypothesis

Another hypothesis that has received a great deal of attention is the *valence hypothesis*. It holds that *the two hemispheres are differentially important in emotional behavior,* depending on the positive or negative valence of the emotion being processed. The *RH is presumed to be more adept at processing negative emotions, and the LH more adept at processing positive emotions* (Borod, 1992; Sackeim et al., 1982; Silberman & Weingartner, 1986). Damage to either hemisphere is thought to be either inhibitory or to release the emotional valence of the opposite hemisphere. RHD patients are assumed to be less responsive to negative emotion and to see things in a more positive light than patients with LHD. In some versions of the theory, the RH is thought to control overall emotional tone, possibly because of its dominance in "regulating bilateral cortical arousal levels," but with a preference for

negative affects (Silberman & Weingartner, 1986). In others, the two hemispheres are thought to share emotional control, but with differential emphasis on positive (LH) and negative (RH) emotions.

Proponents of the valence hypothesis speculate that there may be some evolutionary basis for the emotional specialization. The global scanning and arousal functions of the RH may make it ideal for quickly determining threats from the environment and organizing avoidance behaviors. The more analytic, focused, and linguistic functions of the LH may be linked to interactive and communicative behaviors associated with approach behavior (Bear, 1983; Borod, Caron, & Koff, 1981; Davidson, Ekman, Saron, Senulis, & Friesen, 1990). It can be argued, of course, that the global scanning and orienting functions of the RH are just as important in determining positive environmental signs as they are in determining threats to survival.

The importance of the valence theory relative to RHD is that damage to the RH is thought to disrupt sensitivity to negative emotions in particular; hence the "indifference" to frustration, the denial of illness, and the occasionally inappropriate jocularity associated with RHD, but not LHD. Other researchers have characterized RHD patients as "unduly cheerful" and LHD patients as generally depressed (Robinson, Starr, Kubos, & Price, 1983). The term "euphoric" has even been used to describe the indifference that can occur in some RHD patients (Gainotti, 1972). The data from studies that specifically address the valence hypothesis in subjects with RHD, however, is inconclusive. Some studies are supportive (Ostrove et al., 1990) whereas others fail to find a valence effect (Borod et al., 1992). Investigators have suggested that the primacy of negative emotions may be related to the fact that negative emotions are more intensely expressed than positive ones, that there are more negative than positive emotions in the human repertoire, and that negative emotional expression occurs earlier than positive expressions in human development (Natale, Gur, & Gur, 1983). Interference in the more strongly felt negative emotional states may be just a by-product of generally lowered levels of arousal, rather than inhibition of negative emotions per se. Interestingly, indifference and minimization are closely associated with neglect (Gainotti, 1972) which can be considered part of a larger arousal and attentional disturbance.

Clinical reality does not seem to support the valence hypothesis. RHD patients with alterations in affective behavior do not appear inappropriately cheerful, happy, or positive. Instead, they appear to be generally less responsive, indifferent, and under-aroused. In fact, they often appear depressed. They may be cavalier and seemingly unaffected by the impact of their deficits, and they may minimize their mistakes. But these behaviors typically are accompanied by a defensive attitude, lacking in insight ("This stuff makes no sense"), rather than a positive one ("I made a mistake, but, oh well, who doesn't?"). They may make what appear to be inappropriately jocular comments (i.e., "with my hands," in response to a question about how they feel that day), but their jokes often have a gallows quality, a type of humor more likely to stem from a cynical and negative outlook rather than a positive and cheerful one.

Clinical Issues

A central issue for clinicians addressing affective changes subsequent to RHD is to determine *whether reduced emotional responsivity and other affective deficits represent true alterations of the patient's internal emotional state or mood.* For example, indifference, reduced arousal, and attenuated prosody may appear as signs of clinical depression. However, they also may represent specific organic changes that interfere with cognitive and/or motor functions, not necessarily with internal emotional status. Emotionally laden stimuli, whether visual or verbal, may require higher levels of in-

ference and more cognitive effort to understand than neutral material. *Cognitive deficits* may thus leave the patient less responsive to the emotional valence of situations simply because they are more complex or require more effort to understand and interpret. *Reduced arousal* can disturb attentional functions and may interfere with environmental scanning and awareness of cues that signal emotions in facial features, conversations, situations, and narratives. *Perceptual deficits* may interfere with awareness of the emotions conveyed by prosody. *Reduced use of prosodic features* can occur without changes in internal emotions, as exemplified by those RHD patients who complain that they are unable to convey felt emotions subsequent to prosodic impairment.

Regardless of their source, changes in affective behavior need to be recognized and, when they occur, explained to patients and families. When necessary, patients should be referred for appropriate psychiatric consultation.

RHD AND POST-STROKE DEPRESSION

Depression occurs in as many as 30% to 60% of patients in the acute phase post-stroke (Andersen, Vestergaard, Riis, & Lauritzen, 1994; Cummings, 1994; Folstein, Maiberger, & McHugh, 1977; Iacoboni, Padovani, DiPiero, & Lenzi, 1995; Ng, Chan, & Straughan, 1995; Ramasubbu & Kennedy, 1994). Signs of depression include feelings of sadness, hopelessness, sleep disturbance, reduced concentration, suicidal thoughts, loss of energy, weight loss, and physical agitation or psychomotor slowing. Depression might seem to be a natural reaction to the physical and cognitive impairments that can accompany stroke, but it is not always correlated with degree of physical disability or functional impairment (Anderson, Vestergaard, Ingemann-Nielsen, & Lauritzen, 1995; Robinson & Price, 1982; Robinson et al., 1983; Sinyor et al., 1986). In a study of 1,000 patients, for example, depression was found to be independent of physical impairment (Wade, Legh-Smith, & Hewer, 1987). In some cases, however, self-reported disability levels have correlated significantly with depression (Langer, 1995).

The mechanism for post-stroke depression is not known, but it may be some combination of reactive and organic effects (Andersen et al., 1995). *Organic effects* are thought to be the consequence of neurochemical changes, particularly those involving the neurotransmitter serotonin (Bryer et al., 1992; Cummings, 1994, 1995; Folstein et al., 1977). *Reactive effects* consist of one's response and reaction to impairments and their impact on independence, mobility, and cognitive control. Reduced attention, hypoarousal, and changes in prosody that present as "flat affect" in RHD patients may convey the impression of depression. Often these symptoms are accompanied by denial of illness or minimization of deficits. In such cases, apparent depression should not be considered reactive.

A number of studies have investigated possible relationships between clinical depression and lesion location, with conflicting results. In a series of studies, Robinson and colleagues found that severe depression was more likely in patients with left anterior lesions than in any other location (Robinson, Kubos, Starr, Rao, & Price, 1984; Robinson & Price, 1982; Robinson, Starr, Lipsey, Rao, & Price, 1984). They also determined that RHD patients with anterior lesions tended to be "unduly cheerful" whereas those with posterior lesions tended to be depressed (Robinson , Kubos, et al., 1984). Similarly, Iacoboni et al. (1995) found that dorsal lesions in the RH were associated with depression, although they excluded patients with neglect or attentional disorders. Sinyor et al. (1986) attempted to replicate the findings of Robinson and colleagues, but found no significant difference in the incidence of depression based on side of lesion.

Several studies of nonacute and long-term survivors of stroke also have failed to find a relationship between side of lesion and incidence or severity of depression (House, Dennis, Warlow, Hawton, & Molyneux, 1990; Sharp et al., 1994). Of 13 studies investigating the relationship between side of lesion and incidence or severity of depression, only one found depression more prevalent in RHD than LHD (Dupont, Cullum, & Jeste, 1988). Differences in patient sampling (acute versus nonacute, mild versus severe impairment, and exclusion or inclusion of aphasic patients), as well as differing methods used to assess depression, account for some of the differences among studies of lesion location and depression. In general, however, it appears that depression can occur following either right or left hemisphere stroke. When present, depression interferes with recovery and has an adverse effect on motivation and participation in rehabilitation. Patients who are depressed also tend to have greater intellectual and functional impairments (Cummings, 1994; Iacoboni et al., 1995).

Depression can be present even in patients who minimize or deny their deficits. Anosognosia can make the diagnosis of depression difficult (Nelson, Cicchetti, Satz, Sowa, Mitrushina, 1994). It is also important to remember that "flat affect" and depression are distinct entities that can co-occur. Hypoaroused patients may or may not be depressed. Impaired concentration, apathy, and attentional deficits may, in some cases, be the result of or exacerbated by clinical depression. However, as discussed in previous chapters, these behaviors may be independent of depression in RHD patients, and may even masquerade as signs of depression.

It goes without saying that psychiatric consultation is necessary for the accurate diagnosis of suspected depression and its management. There are a number of reports of successful treatment of post-stroke depression using anti-depressent medication (Cummings, 1994; Lipsey, Robinson, Pearlson, Rao, & Price, 1984; Reding et al., 1986; Stamenkovic, Schindler, & Kasper, 1996). Finally, it should be kept in mind that post-stroke depression does not explain all of the possible alterations in affective behavior that can occur following RHD. Subsequent sections in this chapter explore other changes in emotional communication and in mental status that have been associated with RHD that are not related to depression.

NONVERBAL EMOTIONAL COMMUNICATION

Nonverbal emotional processing includes production and comprehension of emotion as conveyed in facial expression, body language, and gesture. Prosodic comprehension and production deficits, particularly in emotional prosodic processing, are among the disorders marshaled to support the RH dominance hypothesis. Prosodic deficits are covered in Chapter 5 and will not be reviewed here except to note that they may be the result of interference in processing fundamental frequency information crucial to emotional prosodic contour.

Comprehension and production of facial expression by subjects with brain damage has been studied extensively. To test comprehension, subjects typically are asked to discriminate or identify the emotions conveyed in photographs of faces with posed expressions. Production has been tested in both spontaneous and posed conditions. Subjects may be videotaped as they recall emotional experiences or view slides with emotional content. Posed expressions are elicited on command. The emotions tested usually include *happy, sad,* and *angry,* and sometimes *surprise* and/or *fear.*

Comprehension of Facial Expression

Most studies of the comprehension of emotion conveyed by facial expressions have found that RHD patients are impaired relative to both NBD and LHD subjects (Benowitz et al., 1983; Borod et al., 1986, 1990; Bowers, Bauer, Coslett, & Heilman, 1985; Cicone et al., 1980; Dekosky et al., 1980). For example, RHD patients may have

problems determining if two people have the same or different facial expressions (smiling, fearful, angry, sad), and they may have problems identifying emotions from facial expression.

Because some RHD patients seem to have problems in pattern perception and some may have specific problems in recognizing faces, the relationship between those deficits and problems in identifying emotions conveyed by faces has been investigated. Some research has found a relationship between facial recognition and comprehension of facial expression (Dekosky et al., 1980). Other research, however, has found that impaired comprehension of facial expression is independent of deficits in facial recognition (Bowers et al., 1985; Cicone et al., 1980; Dekosky et al., 1980). That is, patients who can identify famous or familiar faces still may have problems in recognizing emotions conveyed facial expressions. There also are a number of clinical reports of impaired emotional comprehension in the presence of normal facial recognition skills (Strauss & Moscovitch, 1981). Thus, the two operations can be dissociated. In addition, deficits in the comprehension of facial expression do not appear to carry over into other aspects of visual emotional comprehension. Subjects who have problems identifying facial expressions may accurately interpret the emotion conveyed by posture and body movement (Benowitz et al., 1983).

Problems in interpreting facial expression may fluctuate within a given patient. Subjects demonstrating impairments in laboratory studies typically have a variable performance and correctly identify some, but not all, expressions.

It is difficult to know how much of a problem interpreting facial expressions poses for RHD patients in real-life situations. They rarely, if ever, complain about the problem, possibly because they are unaware of it. On the other hand, patients do appear to recognize problems with facial recognition. One patient who met weekly with this author told her that he used her hair style and voice as cues to her identity.

One day she came in wearing a hat, and before she said hello he asked her where Dr. Myers was.

It is possible that reduced eye contact observed in some patients may occur because they do not derive much information from facial expression. Facial expressions are an important source of information about the emotions felt and conveyed by those around us. Patients with such problems may be deprived of this information or may have to work harder to grasp it. They may have to compensate by using other cues that signal mood, and they may be unaware of how to do so.

Production of Facial Expression

The faces of persons with RHD may seem less animated than normal, particularly if they are hypoaroused. The faces of many stroke patients are naturally altered by unilateral lower facial weakness, and this weakness affects muscles used for facial expression. With rare exception (e.g., Blonder et al., 1993), occurrence of partial facial weakness is not identified, analyzed, or compared across groups in studies of production of facial expression.

There is a fair amount of evidence that facial expressivity is reduced subsequent to RHD. Most studies have found that RHD subjects are less expressive than either NBD or LHD subjects whether producing facial expressions *on demand,* (Borod et al., 1990), *spontaneously* (Borod et al., 1986, 1990; Buck & Duffy, 1980; Martin et al., 1990), or *in natural conversation* (Blonder et al., 1993). Buck and Duffy (1980), for example, found that observers rated RHD subjects viewing emotionally evocative slides as impaired in facial animation as patients with Parkinson's disease. In contrast, the aphasic patients in their study were even more animated than the NBD controls. Although Mammucari et al. (1988) did not find differences between RHD and LHD subjects in facial expressivity, they did find that the RHD subjects performed in ways that were different from LHD and

NBD controls. When observing films with that were particularly negative or disturbing, RHD subjects, unlike the other groups, rarely averted their eyes from the screen. The authors suggested that one reason may be that they experience negative emotion with less than normal intensity, a possibility that is in accord with findings of reduced autonomic signs of arousal in RHD (see Chapter 3 for details).

Production of facial expression during spontaneous speech has been measured during conversational speech and in monologues about pleasant and unpleasant memories. Martin et al. (1990) found that RHD patients produced less intense facial expression than control subjects in recalling emotional experiences. Their performance did not differ from patients with schizophrenia who typically have "flat affect" and a blunting of emotional responsivity. Both groups of patients demonstrated less intensity in positive compared with negative emotions, a finding that does not accord with the *valence hypothesis* which holds that RHD would interfere more with positive than with negative emotions. Other studies have found that RHD does disrupt positive more than negative facial expressions (Blonder et al., 1993; Borod et al., 1986, 1988).

Blonder et al. (1993) assessed nonverbal affective behavior in naturalisitc settings. They found that, during conversations with relatives, RHD subjects smiled and laughed less than NBD controls, but cried with the same frequency as LHD subjects. The authors suggested that reduced smiling and laughing, considered a form of social attachment and a display of friendliness, may represent a loss of "metacommunicative knowledge regarding socially appropriate nonverbal signals or the loss of inner feeling of positive affect" (p. 54). Although the answer to the puzzle about underlying mechanisms remains obscure, the effects of reduced facial animation, particularly of positive expressions that act as encouragement and links to conversational partners, may interfere with natural dialogue. It may also have a negative effect on those around the patient, thus unwittingly adding to the isolation and alienation of RHD patients in the give and take of social interaction.

VERBAL EMOTIONAL COMMUNICATION

Patients may have difficulty perceiving the emotions conveyed in conversational speech and in written materials. They also may have problems conveying emotion through written and spoken language. The comprehension and expression of emotional language appear to be independent of one another, suggesting that these problems do not stem from a central emotional deficit (Borod et al., 1996).

Comprehension of Verbally Conveyed Emotion

Comprehension of verbally conveyed emotion has been assessed at the word and sentence level and in narrative discourse. It has been found that RHD may impair the capacity to identify emotions in word clusters and sentences, and to discriminate the emotions presented in word pairs (Borod et al., 1992). Blonder et al. (1991) found that RHD subjects with deficits in the perception of emotion in facial and prosodic expression also were impaired in determining emotions from lexical semantic clues. For example, they had problems identifying the mood of sentences in which emotions were conveyed by verbal descriptors such as "He shook his fist" or "Tears fell from her eyes." In addition, they were impaired in naming the emotions conveyed in sentences in which the emotions were clearly stated. Surprisingly, they were not impaired in determining the emotions conveyed in sentences in which emotional words were not used and emotion type had to be inferred from context alone (e.g., "The house seemed empty without her."). Based on their results, the authors suggested that

the RH may house certain lexical-semantic representations of emotional expression. They also proposed that RHD may interfere in the access or activation of these representations, but not of emotional content per se, because patients were able to perform inferential tasks on emotional material.

The ability of RHD patients to understand the emotions conveyed in short vignettes may depend in part on the degree of cognitive effort required by the stimuli or by the nature of the task. Wechsler (1973) found that, although RHD and LHD subjects did not differ in recalling neutral stories, RHD subjects were more impaired than LHD subjects in recalling emotionally charged stories. Rehak, Kaplan, Weylman, et al. (1992) found that RHD subjects were impaired in choosing summary statements about emotional (versus neutral) stories and in making plausible predictions about what they thought would happen next in the stories. However, they were as able as NBD controls to describe the emotions of the main characters. In another study, in which subjects were asked to add continuations to neutral and emotional vignettes, RHD subjects made more factual errors than NBD controls, regardless of whether stories were emotionally laden or neutral (Ostrove et al., 1990). RHD subjects tended to attribute positive emotions to characters in neutral, non-emotional stories, but their performance was otherwise unaffected by emotional content. Like normal controls, their performance was best on stories that had a strong interest value (i.e., suspenseful versus dull). However, interest value had a more powerful effect on their performance than it did on NBD performance, possibly, as the authors pointed out, because interest level had to be high to overcome deficits in attention and arousal.

The sensitivity of RHD subjects to humorous cartoons has been studied by Gardner, Ling, Flamm, and Silverman (1975). Their findings illustrate how impaired attention and cognitive deficits may disturb the comprehension of affective material.

Some of their RHD subjects laughed or smiled at every stimulus even when their understanding of the items was suspect. One cannot enter into their minds, but one can imagine these patients grasping the overall nature of the task, but being afraid to demonstrate problems in interpreting the stimuli, and thus programming a "mirth" response across the board to compensate. The majority of the RHD subjects in the study failed to laugh at all, even at items in which comprehension was apparent. In this case, one can imagine lowered levels of arousal reducing responsivity, animation, and energy of response.

Verbal Expression of Emotion

Production of emotional content at the discourse level has been assessed by comparing it to production of non-emotional discourse. Productions are scored along a variety of dimensions such as intensity of expression, pragmatic appropriateness, and number of emotional content units produced. Subjects have been asked to describe their feelings in response to emotionally laden pictures, to recall emotional experiences, and to tell stories about pictured events.

Borod et al. (1985) found that, compared to LHD and NBD subjects, RHD subjects had reduced prosodic contour as they talked about emotionally evocative slides. However, the amount of affective content they produced in their descriptions was not less than that of NBD subjects. This finding is at odds with two studies that investigated narrative productions by RHD subjects in response to picture story sequences (Bloom et al., 1992, 1993). Three picture story sequences depicted differing types of contents. Two were neutral and one was emotional. The first sequence, intended to stimulate procedural discourse, showed pictures of the ingredients and tools for frying an egg, the egg frying in a pan, and the cooked egg on a plate. A second sequence, intended to emphasize spatial relations, showed a boy piling books on a chair to reach a high shelf. The third sequence depicted a child walking her dog, the dog running into traffic, and then a picture of people and the girl crying as the dog lies in front of the bumper of a car. In the first study the authors found that both RHD and LHD subjects produced fewer content units on all stories relative to NBD controls. Subjects with brain damage also differed from NBD controls and from each other relative to the emotional content in each condition. RHD subjects produced significantly more content units in response to the procedural and spatial stories, but did not differ from LHD subjects in the emotional story condition. RHD subjects also were significantly less informative when describing the emotional story compared to the two neutral stories.

Further analysis of these data (Bloom et al., 1993) revealed that RHD subjects demonstrated particular discourse problems in response to emotional stories. Discourse parameters included topic maintenance, specificity, revision strategies, relevance, and quantity of informative content. RHD subjects were significantly impaired in their ability to be concise and to revise or repair ambiguities in their discourse productions about the emotional, but not the neutral, stories. LHD subjects, on the other hand, had problems in lexical selection, revisions, specificity, and quantity of information in response to the visuospatial story, and with specificity and revisions in response to the procedural story. They were not impaired relative to these parameters on the emotional story condition, however. The authors pointed to this double dissociation between the groups and between conditions for emotional and neutral material as strong support for impaired ability to process emotional material subsequent to RHD, but not LHD.

Several other aspects of the stimuli in these two studies also may account for their findings. The neutral story sequences differed from the emotional one in ways that are significant for both RHD and LHD. By their nature, the neutral sequences depicting the procedure for frying eggs and that of solving the problem of getting a book off a high shelf require more linguistic precision and allow less lexical leeway than did the events depicted in the emotional condition. That is, the nature of procedural discourse may have been a factor in the performance of the aphasic patients. Discourse situations calling for precise language are problematic for patients with language impairment. The procedural condition may not have evoked discourse deficits in RHD patients precisely because they did not have linguistic deficits and because the concepts were relatively easy to grasp. The emotional story, on the other hand, required inferential skills that may be compromised by RHD. One has to infer that the dog has been hit by the car, that the dog is dead, and that the girl and those around her are crying because of the accident. This is not a difficult inference, but it probably is more difficult than those in the procedural or neutral stories. Other studies have found that RHD patients are impaired in describing the events depicted in simple three-episode sequences containing about the same level of inference. For example, Stachowiak, Huber, Poeck, and Kerschensteiner (1977) found that RHD patients had problems determining the events in a picture sequence showing (1) a woman walking her dog past a group of men gathered around under a car hood trying to fix an engine; (2) the woman fixing the car; and (3) the same woman walking off, waving cheerfully at the dumbfounded men. One RHD patient said that it was a story of the men asking the woman to go on a picnic. These differences in cognitive complexity and in levels of linguistic precision called for may have had an impact on the findings from both aphasic and RHD subjects in the Bloom (1992, 1993) studies.

Deficits in sensitivity to emotional content also may be explained by deficits in what can be thought of as an extension of "theory of mind," the ability to generate beliefs about other people's internal motivations, beliefs, knowledge, intentions, and

emotional states (see Chapter 6 for a review of the expanded definition of theory of mind as it relates to RHD). Bloom et al. (1997), using an analysis compatible with theory of mind, found that, when re-telling a wordless picture story, RHD subjects made fewer references to emotional content than did LHD subjects, particularly in interpreting the emotion experienced by the central character. It is possible that RHD patients make fewer references to emotional states because they have problems generating theories about other's internal states and beliefs, including their emotional status.

Verbal reports of personal experience also support the possibility that RHD patients have problems conveying emotions through speech. For example, Borod et al. (1996) asked subjects to recall experiences in response to seven emotional and seven nonemotional words. Emotional words evoked less emotionally intense productions from RHD subjects compared to those for LHD and NBD subjects. There were no differences in performance in the nonemotional condition. Cimino et al. (1991) conducted a similar study in which subjects were instructed to recall an event from their own lives that related to cue words intended to be neutral (e.g., "book," "river," "milk") and ones intended to be emotionally evocative (e.g., "angry," "surprised," "lonely"). Responses were scored for emotional intensity and specificity. Regardless of type of cue word, RHD subjects were less specific than NBD controls. Similar to NBD controls, RHD subjects were more emotionally intense when responding to affective cue words. However, their productions were less emotionally intense in both conditions compared to NBD subjects, a finding that was independent of the degree of specificity in their productions. The authors suggested that deficits in arousal may interfere with the ability "to replicate the physiological state" that occurred at the time of the experience which, in turn, would affect the ability to fully recall or re-experience the emotions generated. Interestingly, when asked to rate the level of emotion in their recalled experiences, RHD subjects tended to rate their emotional intensity higher than did independent judges, suggesting that their internal experience of emotion may not match their capacity to express that experience, and that internal emotional status may be intact subsequent to RHD.

Clinically, it is difficult to know if subjective experience of emotion is or is not reflected in the emotions conveyed verbally by RHD patients. However, it does appear that patients demonstrating indifference and lack of insight tend to share little about their emotional response to their condition, at least in the acute phase of their illness. When they do refer to their deficits, altered future plans, and physical impairments, they tend to minimize rather than convey heart-felt emotion. In addition, the ability of many patients to convey the emotions depicted in narratives and pictures used in therapy seems impoverished. One picture, used often by this author, shows a man in terror, attempting to flee while a woman tries to hold him back. Fairly typical responses to that picture from patients with adequate visuospatial ability to describe the items depicted include the following:

1. "That looks like a mother and a father. And what I imagine, they live real cheerful and cooperative and probably have a family."
2. "Looks like she's trying to get him to make love to her to me. She's expecting at least a kiss. She's looking at him pretty hard. He is a good looking man."

Thus, impaired *comprehension* of affective materials, both verbal and nonverbal, may contribute to inappropriate verbal expression of emotion. These deficits may be related to: (a) specific cognitive deficits that impair effortful inferences, (b) social reasoning impairments that seem related to what has been termed "theory of mind" that disturb the ability to apprehend others' internal states, and/or (c) reduced levels of arousal that disturb the environmental scanning necessary to picking up on cues conveying emotion. In addition, there may be specific RH functions that, when damaged, inhibit the production of emotional expression. For example, patients may have problems in retrieving the lexical semantic representations for emotions (i.e., words and phrases representing emotions). Finally, in some patients, the experience of subjective emotion may also be altered. Verbal expression may be reduced in intensity because emotions are less intensely experienced, either because of reduced levels of arousal or disruptions between limbic and cortical areas crucial to emotional experience, or both.

DELUSIONS AND CONFUSIONAL STATES

Agitated Confusion

Agitated confusion, delirium, disorientation, and various psychotic states can accompany RHD (Bogousslavsky & Regli, 1988; Caplan et al., 1986; Halligan, Marshall, & Wade, 1995; Levine & Finklestein, 1982; Levine & Grek, 1984; Mesluam, Waxman, Geschwind, & Sabin, 1976; Price & Mesulam, 1985; Schmidley & Messing, 1984). It appears that psychiatric disturbances of this type are more frequent in people with RHD than LHD (Price & Mesulam, 1985). Agitated confusion is characterized by *incoherent thought patterns*, *severe reduction in attention span*, *extreme distractibility*, *restlessness*, *disruption of goal directed behavior*, *disorientation*, *and sometimes violent outbursts*. Psychotic symptoms can include *hallucinations* and *paranoid delusions*. These symptoms may pass in a few days or, in some cases, may last for months (Levine & Grek, 1984; Mesulam et al., 1976) or even years (Price & Mesulam, 1985). In some cases of agitated confusion, extreme irrationality and violent outbursts are not present (Mesulam et al., 1976). In some cases, the symptoms have been successfully treated with antidepressant medication (Weinman & Ruskin, 1994).

Persistent agitation with psychiatric disturbances accompanying RHD are considered rare, but the actual frequency of occurrence remains uncertain. Its presence may depend on degree of brain atrophy in conjunction with stroke (Levine & Grek, 1984), although it has been documented in cases without atrophy (Price & Mesulam, 1985). Delayed occurrence of psychotic behavior and agitated confusion following RHD has been associated with seizures (Levine & Finklestein, 1982), but the symptoms can occur without seizure activity (Mesulam & Price, 1985). Site of lesion may also be a determining factor. For example, Schmidley and Messing (1984) found that only 2 out of 46 patients with lesions in the distribution of the right middle cerebral artery had symptoms of agitated confusion. Caplan et al. (1986), on the other hand, found agitated confusion in 5 of 10 patients with infarcts specifically in the distribution of the inferior division of the right middle cerebral artery. Lesion sites for agitated confusion typically include the right posterior temporal or parietal cortex, but can include frontal areas as well (Caplan et al., 1986; Mesulam et al., 1976; Schmidley & Messing, 1984).

These extreme behaviors can and often do occur in the absence of or with only minimal lateralizing motor and sensory signs such as hemiplegia and hemianesthesia (Caplan et al., 1986; Mesulam et al., 1976; Schmidley & Messing, 1984). Other cognitive and behavioral signs such as neglect, visuo-perceptual impairments, and flat affect, often are present in patients who can be properly tested (Levine & Grek, 1984). Clinicians are cautioned not to rule out focal neurologic disease in cases of acute onset agitation and confusion without prior history of psychiatric problems or metabolic or toxic disturbance.

Several mechanisms have been proposed to account for the occurrence of agitated confusional states subsequent to RHD. Caplan et al. (1986) suggested that lesions in the temporal and infereior parietal lobes can disrupt cortical connections to the limbic system and that such disconnection could explain an alteration in affective behavior and tone. Price and Mesulam (1985) and Mesulam et al. (1976) concured, and suggested that lesions in tertiary association areas such as the posterior parietal lobe could disrupt cortical connections to limbic structures and result in psychotic episodes. In addition, it has been suggested that damage to crucial attentional mechanisms may be the explanation in cases dominated by extreme distractibility and inability to think coherently, but without psychosis. Damage to selective and directed attention areas in the inferior frontal gyrus, the inferior parietal lobe, the medial frontal lobe, and the inferomedial temporal lobe may create such extreme behavioral disruptions (Mesulam et al., 1976).

Specific Delusions

Although rare, several specific delusions have been associated with RHD. Together, they can be called *misidentification syndromes.* These include misidentification of place, persons, or body parts. Often these delusions are encapsulated—that is, they occur in isolation without other symptoms of confusion. Patients themselves may acknowledge the irrationality of their delusional beliefs, but cannot be persuaded to abandon them. The beliefs may be persistent or transient. Misidentification of place has been called *reduplicative paramnesia,* a term coined by Pick in 1903. More recently, the term has been used to refer to misidentification of persons, as well. Patients with this disorder think that familiar persons or places have been duplicated. For example, they may think that an imposter inhabits the body of someone familiar to them. Or they may think that their house has been duplicated and is no longer their own home, even though it looks identical to it

(Alexander, Stuss, & Benson, 1979). Delusions about the identity of body parts is sometimes referred to as "somatoparaphrenia" (Gerstman, 1942). Each of these disorders are described below.

Misidentification of Place

Patients with symptoms of misidentification of place may think that a familiar place such as their home or the hospital, is located in more than one place, or they may think they are in a duplicate of a once-familiar place. Thus, patients may recognize that they are in a hospital, but confuse it with a hospital they were in previously. They may think they are in their bedrooms at home. They may think the hospital is attached to their houses, and so on. One patient, described by Fisher (1982), accurately named the hospital he was in but thought it located variously in China, Paris, Cape Cod, Baghdad, Chicago, Africa, and California. Misidentification of place has been associated with bifrontal lesions and with frontal and/or parietal lesions restricted to the RH (Alexander et al., 1979; Benson, Gardner, & Meadows, 1976; Fisher, 1982; Hakim, Verma, & Greiffenstein, 1988; Jocic & Staton, 1993; Ruff & Volpe, 1981). It may occur with focal RH damage or be superimposed on chronic frontal damage such as that caused by alcoholism (Hakim et al., 1988). When it occurs in focal lesions, it tends to occur more often with RHD than with LHD (Cutting, 1991; Forstl, Almeida, Owen, Burns, & Howard, 1991). For example, Feinberg and Shapiro (1989) found that, out of 60 cases of misidentification of place, 29 had bilateral lesions and 36 had unilateral RHD, whereas only 5 had LHD.

Misidentification of Persons

In 1923, Capgras and Reboul-Lachaux described a case of delusional misidentification in which a patient believed that the bodies of her husband, sons, and herself had been replaced by imposters. This problem has since become known as *Capgras syndrome,* and it typically refers to the delusion that others, but not the self, have been replaced by doubles. It is most often associated with psychiatric conditions, but can occur with damage to the RH in the absence of any previous psychiatric problems. Capgras syndrome can co-occur with misidentification of place following RHD (Alexander et al., 1979; Jocic & Staton, 1993). Typically, people with Capgras syndrome consider the duplicates or doubles as dangerous or frightening (Ellis & Young, 1990).

Other forms of misidentification of persons can occur. For example, a RHD patient this author worked with was convinced that the woman in the bed next to her was her husband, and that he was flirting with the nurses. Naturally, she was angry and confused when her actual husband came to see her on his daily visits. This symptom has been referred to as the Fregoli syndrome after an actor who could change his appearance dramatically (Courbon & Fail, 1927). It can occur in patients with brain damage, but it is not usually associated with unilateral RHD.

Capgras syndrome should be distinguished from *prosopagnosia,* which is a specific form of visual agnosia for faces in which once-familiar faces are no longer recognized. Patients with prosopagnosia may not be able to visually identify their spouses, children, or famous people from pictures or in person. Usually, they rely on specific facial features (shape of the nose or eyebrows) or vocal cues for recognition. Prosopagnosia can extend to familiar objects such as cars and to animals and pets as well (Bornstein, Sroka, & Munitz, 1969; Gloning, Gloning, Hoff, & Tschabitscher, 1966). A farmer with prosopagnosia, for example, may identify his herd of cows as cows, but have trouble identifying individual cows among the herd. Although associated with unilateral RHD by some (Landis et al., 1986), prosopagnosia most typically occurs with *bilateral* posterior lesions (Benson, 1989; Damasio, Damasio, & Van Hoesen, 1982).

Some researchers have explored a possible relationship between Capgras syndrome and prosopagnosia (Bidault, Luaute, & Tzavaras, 1986; Miller, 1994; Shraberg & Weitzel, 1979). In fact, prosopagnosia is the mirror image or exact opposite of Capgras syndrome. In Capgras syndrome, facial features are readily identified ("This person looks like John"), but the feeling of familiarity is absent ("but I do not believe it *is* John"). In prosopagnosia, the patient does not recall ever having seen the face previously. The two disorders can co-occur (Miller, 1994), but they should be considered separate deficits.

Misidentification of Limbs

Patients may be confused about the identity or location of their hemiplegic limbs. In response to sensory and motor loss, they may reject the limb or may casually explain that it belongs to someone else. This response may be fairly common in patients with anosognosia for hemiplegia. It typically occurs early post-onset and is transient. It rarely occurs with LHD.

Somatoparaphrenia is a disorder in which patients construct elaborate delusions about their hemiplegic limbs while responding normally to the rest of their bodies (Bisiach, Rusconi, & Vallar, 1991; Halligan et al., 1995). For example, Halligan et al. (1995) described a RHD patient who presented with neglect and severe visual inattention. He was without psychiatric impairment, memory loss, signs of generalized mental deterioration, or denial of illness, yet he had persisting and elaborate delusions about his left limbs. For example, he suggested to the staff of the rehabilitation facility that he, "had a bag full of spare left arms," and that his left arm belonged to someone else. He reported that his foot was actually a cow's foot, but that he sold it to some physiotherapists in Ecuador (where he had been living). The following day he explained that his mother had brought a leg and a set of fingers from the left side of his body though customs in a suitcase. A

month or so later, as his sensory function improved, he explained that his hand had come back, and went on to acknowledge that his earlier thinking about his limbs had been confused but very real and even terrifying to him. As the authors pointed out, these problems adjusting to and interpreting the reduced sensory and motor function of hemiplegic limbs may have generated specific confusions in a patient who was not generally confused. His delusions were encapsulated (i.e., restricted to his limbs), and he seemed to confabulate to make sense of, and account for, his loss. The authors suggested that brain damage interferes with cognitive processes so that insight leading to a reasonable explanation eludes the patient. Interestingly, using vestibular stimulation, Bisiach et al. (1991) were able to alleviate temporarily somatoparaphrenia in a woman with a RH lesion who believed her arm had been replaced by her mother's arm. Vestibular stimulation, described in Chapter 9, also has temporarily improved neglect and anosognosia accompanying RHD. Bisiach et al. (1991) speculated, based on results of a regional blood flow study conducted during vestibular stimulation (Friberg, Olsen, Roland, Paulson, & Lassen, 1985), that vestibular stimulation increases activation in the contralateral temporal lobe.

Mechanisms of Misidentification: Familiarity and Personal Relevance

The central theme running through the misidentification symptoms just described is a *loss of the sense of familiarity*. Things do not look different to these patients. People, places, body parts look the same, but they do not seem to *be* the same as before. There is intellectual understanding and recognition, but they lack affective content.

There are several lines of thought about the nature of this disconnection between identity and familiarity. Some have speculated that posterior areas of the right hemisphere, important for visual integration and analysis, as well as damaged frontal areas, important for analysis and problem solving, have been disconnected from limbic structures that are important to affective content (Alexander et al., 1979; Levine & Finklestein, 1982). Jocic and Staton (1993), for example, pointed out that connections from the RH to areas in the right limbic system are presumed to be important for judgements of familiarity, and they suggested that loss of familiarity may be due to impaired ability to integrate present cues with past memories. Misidentifications can occur in the face of intact memory (Hakim et al., 1988), but there may be difficulty in accessing affective memories specific to the perceived object. As Crow (1991) stated, "Recognition is achieved but there is a mismatch between the emotional associations that are provoked by the perception and those that are associated in memory with the concept of the individual perceived" (p. 80).

Other investigators have suggested that facial recognition depends on more than one visual pathway leading from visual cortex to the temporal lobes. One, the ventral route, leads to overt recognition. The other, a more dorsal route that connects visual cortex and the limbic system via the inferior parietal lobe, carries the affective content of facial features (Bauer, 1984). Together, the ventral and dorsal routes are thought to play a role in establishing the identity and familiarity of objects and places. In prosopagnosia, ventral pathways may be damaged, interfering with conscious recognition. In Capgras syndrome, the ventral route may be spared, allowing recognition, but dorsal pathway may be damaged, interfering with affective familiarity and recognition of the emotional significance (Ellis & Young, 1990). Ellis and Young (1990) explained that only certain faces (i.e., those close to the patient) carry strong enough affective content to be vulnerable to disruption of the dorsal pathway. More precise lesion location in cases of misidentification will help to clarify

the role that various routes of visual identification and recognition play in these symptoms.

Some investigators have pointed to hemispheric differences in the representation of familiarity to explain the preponderance of RH lesions in cases of misidentification. Cutting (1991), for example, suggested that the RH has a particular role to play in representing the uniqueness and individuality of objects, whereas the LH is dominant for representing objects in terms of category membership. Man is a highly socialized animal and socialization is dependent on social cognition. As Crow (1991) pointed out, language is only one route to social cognition. Recognition of the uniqueness of members of the species is another. It is possible that the RH, superior to the LH in visuospatial skills and environmental scanning, may play a crucial role in identifying and recognizing the individuality, uniqueness, and affective content contained in visual percepts. Unlike the agnosias (more commonly found in LHD than in RHD), in which an object is dissociated from its meaning, objects in misidentification syndromes are separated from their familiar associations.

Support for the role of the RH in recognizing familiarity comes from studies in which sensitivity to "personally relevant" materials has been investigated. "Personal relevance" is the capacity to feel connected or united to something else through personal experience with it. Van Lanker (1991) suggested that the subjective feeling of familiarity is a conjoining of cognitive and affective associations that form a "rich context for each personally relevant item" (p. 74). She proposed that the RH has a special role in establishing and maintaining this independent affective/cognitive function. The clinical observation that severely aphasic patients often are able to respond to and comprehend familiar proper nouns is supported by studies in which aphasic patients can match familiar names to photographs of celebrities (Van Lancker & Klein, 1990) or recognize names of familiar places or people (Wapner & Gardner, 1979; Warrington & McCarthy, 1987) despite severe language impairments. In addition, it has been found that the linguistic performance of patients with severe aphasia improves when stimuli hold personal relevance for them (Collins, 1986; Wallace & Canter, 1985).

RHD subjects without apparent language deficits are even more impaired than aphasic patients on familiar-famous name recognition tasks (Van Lancker, 1991). Thus, sensitivity to personal relevance and the ability to generate and retrieve the cognitive and affective context that signals familiarity may be disrupted by RHD. Such disruption may play a significant role not only in the delusions described in this section, but also in the social/pragmatic deficits that can occur subsequent to RHD.

SUMMARY

1. *RHD may reduce the ability to comprehend and express emotional content as conveyed in facial expression, written and spoken discourse, body language, and gesture.* Not all RHD patients have these problems. Among those that do, the degree of deficit is varied and depends to some extent on how directly emotional information is presented. Patients may appear less sensitive to emotional information and may have problems conveying their own experience of emotion.

2. *The mechanisms for alterations in affective communication are not known,* but possible factors include: (a) *deficits in inferencing* that affect the ability to interpret emotional content, (b) *deficits in attention* that interfere with recognizing significant cues about emotional information, (c) *reduced prosody,* (d) *specific semantic deficits* in the representation of emotions through language, and (e) deficits in *the ability to adopt a theory of mind.*

3. Two theories, the *RH Dominance Theory* and the *Valence Theory,* have been pro-

posed to account for the apparent predominance of the RH in emotional communication and the disruption of emotional communication subsequent to RHD. As its name suggests, the *RH Dominance Theory* proposes that the RH is dominant for processing all types of emotional material. *The Valence Theory* suggests that it is dominant for negative emotional processing.

4. A central issue for clinicians is determining the *nature of emotional changes* subsequent to RHD. Alterations in the comprehension and expression of emotion in both verbal and non-verbal channels appear to be related to cognitive, attentional, and prosodic deficits rather than to changes in internal emotional status.

5. *Depression* can occur post-stroke with einther RH or LH lesions and may be a factor in reduced emotional sensitivity in RHD patients with depression. *It does not appear that depression is more prevalent with lesions in either the RH or the LH. In RHD patients, it is important not to confuse flat affect, reduced use of prosody, and hypoarousal with clinical depression.*

6. *Problems in identifying facial expression* may occur subsequent to RHD. *This deficit appears to be independent of problems in identifying and recognizing faces.* Impaired recognition of facial expression can disrupt an important avenue of feedback in conversational discourse and can contribute to the social isolation of RHD patients.

7. RHD patients may have *reduced ability to convey emotions in facial expression and gesture.* Reduced animation and problems in the ability to signal positive emotions in particular, may interfere with accepted conventions for moving conversations forward.

8. *RHD may disturb sensitivity to and understanding of the emotions conveyed verbally in conversation and in stories and films, and also may interfere with patients' ability to verbally convey emotional information.* These deficits may be related to cognitive and attentional impairments, to deficits in theory of mind, and to problems in retrieving lexical-semantic representations of emotion.

9. Although they are rare, *agitated confusion, disorientation, and various psychotic states can occur with focal RH lesions and do so more often than with focal LHD.* Mechanisms proposed to account for the occurrence of these symptoms include (a) disruption of pathways between limbic structures and tertiary cortical association areas in the RH that serve to integrate visual information and (b) attentional impairments that interfere with environmental scanning and level of arousal.

10. *Specific delusions associated with RHD include a variety of misidentification syndromes.* These delusions are typically encapsulated. Patients may misidentify persons, places, or body parts.

Disturbances in recognizing familiar places are referred to as *reduplicative paramnesia.* The delusion that people familiar to the patient have been replaced by other people is called *Capgras syndrome.* Capgras syndrome is the opposite of *prosopagnosia* in which patients no longer recognize (or have agnosia for) familiar faces.

11. Somatoparaphrenia is a disorder in which patients, particularly those with anosognosia, *confabulate in elaborate ways about their hemiplegic limbs.* It has been proposed that posterior and frontal areas in the RH that are important to visual integration and problem solving may be cut off from limbic structures, thus interfering with the ability to integrate present cues with memories that generate a sense of familiarity.

12. By disrupting areas in the RH important to visual scanning and integration and the connections between these areas and limbic structures, *RHD may impair the ability to recognize individuality, uniqueness, familiarity, and affective content of objects, places, and people.*

CHAPTER

8

Assessment

This chapter addresses the evaluation of deficits that affect communication in RHD patients, including discourse deficits, neglect, attention deficits, prosodic impairments, and problems with emotional communication. As is true in the evaluation of other types of communication problems, assessment usually is conducted using both formal and informal measures. There are very few standardized test instruments that address RHD communication impairments and few, if any, that address all of the signs and symptoms reviewed here. There are, however, a number of non-standardized, informal techniques that can also help clinicians evaluate RHD communication disorders. Much of the information contained in this chapter is also relevant to treatment.

GOALS OF ASSESSMENT

The goals for the assessment of communication disorders in RHD patients are no different than those associated with other neurologically based speech and language problems. Goals include: (a) *gathering information about the patient,* (b) *evaluating communicative strengths and weaknesses,* (c) *determining if indeed the patient has a communication disorder consistent with RHD,* (d) *making decisions about management,* and (e) *estimating prognosis for recovery.* Assessment helps clinicians decide if patients need treatment and, if so, helps to focus the goals of that treatment. Initial contact with the patient should serve as a screening for further evaluation and as an opportunity to find out about patient and family concerns. Further evaluative sessions may be conducted independently of treatment, or may be part of the initial treatment period (i.e., diagnostic therapy). The potential deficit areas that should be addressed in evaluating RHD patients are listed in Table 8–1.

The assessment techniques presented in this chapter are offered with the understanding that comprehensive and lengthy evaluation is rarely possible in the current health care environment in which the patient's stay in acute care and rehabilitation settings is short, and funds available for rehabilitation are limited. Many evaluation tasks are presented, and it is assumed that

with experience, clinicians will be able to select those that will yield the most information for a given patient. In an ideal world, clinicians would be able to spend enough time in evaluation not only to identify deficits, but also to explore in detail all the variables that may impact on patient performance. However, clinical reality impinges on our efforts, and clinicians, more than ever before, are required to be experts at making informed choices about which tasks and tests will give them the information needed to determine whether or not the patient needs treatment and to identify the type of treatment needed. Further testing should inform the clinician about underlying processes and help establish specific goals for recovery and/or compensation.

In some medical settings, all RHD patients are referred for speech and language evaluation. More typically, patients are referred only if someone on the medical team or rehabilitative service suspects a communication disorder. Because many RHD patients do not have the typical signs of either a speech or language problem and rarely demonstrate communication deficits in superficial conversation, it is up to speech-language pathologists to inform other professionals working with RHD patients of the potential impact of RHD on communication through inservice training, informal discussion, sharing reading materials, and any other means available for increasing awareness.

INITIAL SCREENING

In acute care settings, the first contact between the clinician and patient typically occurs at bedside in the form of an *initial screening.* In rehabilitation settings and outpatient clinics, time spent during the initial contact may allow for more complete testing, (see *Further Testing* in Table 8–2). Patients in acute care may not be alert enough to endure a long period of testing. The goal of assessment in these settings is usually limited to a quick determination about the

TABLE 8–1. Areas to address in a comprehensive evaluation of communication disorders in RHD patients.

Areas of Assessment	
Discourse	Neglect
Pragmatic Behavior	Attention
Prosody	Affective Processing

TABLE 8–2. Summary of initial screening and further testing options.

Initial Screening	Further Testing Options
Interview	Formal and Informal Tests of:
Scene Interpretation	Discourse deficits
Neglect: Cancellation	Neglect
Drawing	Attention
Line bisection	Prosody
	Affective communication

patient's need for and ability to benefit from treatment. Usually, the initial assessment can be conducted in 20 min or less. *Further testing* may occur over several sessions, the goals of which are to determine something about the nature of the deficits, the goals of therapy, and the prognosis for recovery. In both the initial screening and further testing, it is assumed that the clinician has reviewed the patient's chart or history for pertinent biographical and medical information such as age, education, handedness, occupation, the nature of the current illness, lesion location, and history of previous neurologic disorder, speech and language problems, chemical abuse, or psychiatric problems.

Establishing Rapport

In the initial encounter, patients may be surprised by a visit from a speech-language clinician. They may assume that they do not have a communication problem, especially because everyone around them, often including their physicians, is relieved that they can use speech to communicate. In addition, they may have poor insight into the problems of which they are aware. It often helps to explain that, even though speech might not be affected, stroke sometimes can affect communication indirectly and that the clinician's job is to check this out through a brief evaluation of the patient's comprehension and production of written and spoken language

and conversational speech. When the clinician acknowledges that the patient may *not* have communication problems, the patient usually is cooperative and participates in the testing, often with the idea that they are helping the clinician do his or her job. Patients are more cooperative if the clinician adopts a positive, non-threatening attitude and does not shrink from the task of testing someone who may be resistant and confused about what is involved in the larger picture of cognitive and communicative deficits. It helps to acknowledge the patient's good fortune in having speech spared and to use the term "screening" rather than "testing." It also helps to explain that, even though his or her speech may be fine, there are other areas of communication that may pose problems. Many RHD patients with communication deficits may have noticed that they feel a bit confused trying to follow complex conversations, for example, or events depicted on T.V. They may be frightened by their confusion and choose to cover it up in the face of their family's apparent lack of awareness. Even when insight is poor, they may be relieved to learn that they are not alone in experiencing these problems, that help is available, and that their overall confusion can be broken down into specific problem areas. Once trust is established, the author has found patients who admitted to "feeling crazy" because everyone around them was so sure that they were free of all but their physical deficits. Other patients, particularly those with very severe neglect and/or anosognosia, may have trouble recognizing and/or admitting to deficits even when they are demonstrated by the clinician in an atmosphere of trust. In any case, the clinician's job is to explore deficit areas, reassure the patient if deficits are found, and at the same time demonstrate some of the problem areas that do exist so that the patient understands and is compliant with the recommendation for therapy.

Interview

Having explained to the patient why he or she is being evaluated, the clinician can move smoothly into the interview by asking questions about what the patient sees as his or her main problems. The interview should be conducted in a natural conversational style and can be tape recorded for later analysis. Areas covered in the interview should include the following:

1. The patient's assessment of his or her deficits (*awareness of and insight into deficits*)
2. The events surrounding their hospitalization (*orientation, narrative discourse, long-term memory, awareness of illness*)
3. The focus of their current rehabilitation (*insight*)
4. Personal history—family life, work, etc. (*narrative discourse, long-term memory*)
5. Their future plans (*insight into deficit consequences*)
6. Activities that day (*orientation, narrative discourse, recent memory*)

Taken together, these content areas can provide insight into patients' *awareness of their deficits*, their *pragmatic skills in conversational speech*, their ability to *convey events in narrative form*, their *recent and long-term memory*, and their *orientation to time and place*. Although it is a good idea to cover all of the question areas, the interview should be conducted in as natural and conversational format as possible.

A portion of a patient interview between a clinician (C) and a 72-year-old male patient (P) with a right fronto-parietal lesion, neglect, and hemiplegia is presented below with comments following.

C: "So, tell me about what you see as problems you're having."
P: "Well, they tell me some of my left legs aren't working so good."
C: "What do you mean?"
P: "I can't walk so good."
C: "O.K. What other problems are you having?"
P: "I don't know—my eyes—I can't see as good as I used to even with my glasses—my vision isn't so good."
C: "Tell me more about that."
P: "I don't know—they tell me I just don't see so well over to the left."
C: "You mean when you look to the left?"
P: "Yeah, like sometimes when I have my food tray I don't eat the applesauce because—I don't know, I just don't see it over there on the tray, I guess."
C: "Do you see it when you turn your head and look to the left?"
P: "Yes, then I see it alright and I eat it."
C: "Any other problems?"
P: "No, not that I can think of."

The patient's ability to manage the pragmatic demands of this simple conversation were normal in that he followed the rules for turn-taking. His insight into and understanding of his problems was weak, however, as demonstrated by his use of the phrase, "They tell me that," to describe his problems. As stated earlier, many patients with reduced insight and denial use this term to introduce the listener to deficits they have problems recognizing (i.e., "They tell me that I had a stroke"). His use of the plural to describe his left leg can be interpreted as a *distancing from and an abnormal relationship with his own limbs which may be a sign of anosognosia.* He also seems to have little insight into his neglect, although it is a positive sign that he mentioned it.

The example that follows is from an interview a 76-year-old woman with a right middle cerebral artery infarct:

C: "What happened to you and why are you in the hospital?"

P: "Well, I was out visiting my daughter and son-in-law. Now I don't get on with my daughter the way I once did. I can't tell you why exactly, but kids grow on and you just feel out of step. Of course, they both helped me. We were just having the nicest dinner, which I cooked because they both just work so much and I just don't think they eat properly and, well, I felt kind of funny there at dinner. We were having that new fresh corn, you know? I can still eat it because I have all my teeth. And it was hot out. I think that's a change. It really wasn't so hot this time of year when I was younger. And, oh the tomatoes, and I had a nice little hot dish which I just felt they turned their noses up at, but—where was I? Oh yes, and as I was saying, I felt funny, and then my arm went, and I just . . . well, they told me I wasn't right and my arm went all funny and I fell. Well, I kinda slipped onto the floor—just like some noodles onto the floor. Well, they called the 911 to come and get me because I couldn't get up and all and they took me over to this other hospital, and, oh, the road was so bumpy. I don't know why they can't do a better job with the roads, and, of course, some of it was on dirt roads. But anyway then they shipped me off here yesterday."

C: "Why did you end up in the hospital. What do you have?"

P: "I guess it's a stroke, um hmm, a stroke."

We expect patients with major medical events to respond to the question, "What happened to you and why are you in the hospital," by beginning with the nature of the event or illness (i.e., "I had a heart attack," or, "I have to have surgery for . . . .").

RHD patients, however, often tell the events surrounding their hospitalization without ever mentioning the nature of the illness. Like this patient, they *often default to a chronological structure to organize their information.* Although the detail included by this patient in her description of those events is not unusual for the elderly, it is unusual to fail to mention the cause of the hospitalization. This failure may be attributed to *lack of a macrostructure around which to base events and/or to some level of denial of illness that can accompany RHD.*

Questions about daily activities, progress in rehabilitation, and future plans can all reveal something about patients' estimation and understanding of their deficits and the consequences of those deficits for the future. Lack of insight may signal some level of cognitive dysfunction. In addition, patients' responses can be assessed for *structure* as well as for content. Pragmatic performance, including *turn-taking, eye contact, degree of listener burden, ability to stay on topic, use of gesture, and facial expression to convey emotion* can be monitored during the interview. Later, review of the interview tape can reveal information about discourse structure. One can get a general sense of the patient's ability to generate a macrostructure and their ability to be specific, informative, and efficient in their responses. For example, were they excessively elaborative or did they produce only minimal, unelaborated responses? Did they have a good grasp of shared knowledge? Did they make good use of bridging or coherence inferences so that they were able to follow the conversation?

Because the conversation between patient and clinician is in an interview format, the exchange will be relatively straightforward and will not give much opportunity to assess the patient's command over alternate meanings, theory of mind, or complex inferences. For that reason, it also is valuable to present the patient with an opportunity to draw inferences from more subtle material. This can be done by asking the patient to describe events in a pictured scene or re-tell a brief story to be scored later for narrative expression and comprehension. A pictured scene is perhaps the better choice because it does not tax memory.

Screening Discourse Production: Scene Description

The pictured scene used during screening should be presented following the interview. It should permit assessment of the patient's ability to *distinguish between relevant and irrelevant detail*, to *integrate information across the picture,* and to *draw inferences about the events depicted.* The "Cookie Theft" picture from the *Boston Diagnostic Aphasia Examination* (Goodglass & Kaplan, 1983) (Figure 6–5) is a good choice because it meets the above criteria, is readily available to clinicians, and there are several scoring systems, described later in this chapter, that can be used to measure performance on it (Myers, 1979; Nicholas & Brookshire, 1995).

The initial instructions to the client should be "Tell me what you think is *happening* in this picture," rather than "Tell me about this picture," or, "describe this picture," so that it is clear that the patient should talk about the overall meaning of the picture rather than simply labeling or describing the items depicted in it. One then can attribute possible failure to tie significant elements into a coherent whole to faulty processing, rather than to faulty or vague instructions. One should be sure the patient sees the whole picture because this is not a test of neglect. Point to both sides of the picture and be sure the patient follows your hand as you point. Then allow the patient to complete the description. Should he or she fail to notice anything on the left, provide a cue such as, "Look over here on the left. Do you see anything there?" Note the need for a cue.

A tape recording of the patient's description can be scored later, using one of several scoring systems. Areas of interest include the generation of a macrostructure and main concepts, the capacity to process inferences, and the efficiency with which the events are described. A scoring system designed for the "Cookie Theft" picture (Myers, 1979) can be found in Appendix 1. The concepts on the list are those produced by a group of NBD subjects describing the scene in a study by Yorkston and Beukleman (1977). Myers divided that list into literal and intepretive concepts. *Literal concepts* were defined as those that had meaning in isolation (i.e., woman) whereas *interpretive concepts* were defined as those that had meaning only within the context of the picture (i.e., mother) and thus required the integration of and inferences about the pictured elements. A patient's score is the percent of the total number of concepts on the list that are "interpretive." This yields a percent interpretive score. Interjudge reliability for scoring the descriptions of NBD and RHD subjects ranged from .94 to .99, indicating that the scoring system is reliable across users (Myers, 1979). Myers and Linebaugh (1981) found that on average 49% of the concepts produced by NBD adults were interpretive concepts whereas only 27% of the concepts produced by RHD adults were interpretive concepts. This serves as a rough benchmark against which to judge a given patient's performance. Because only the concepts mentioned by NBD adults in the Yorkston and Beukleman list were used, the scoring system does not account for all of the valid concepts that the patient might mention. Only those on the list are scored. However, it does address the issue of inferences drawn from the picture.

Another "Cookie Theft" scoring system was developed by Nicholas and Brookshire (1995). It addresses main concepts, and also relies on a concept list for the scene (see Appendix 2). The four categories of measurement for main concepts include: (a) accurate and complete, (b) accurate, but incomplete, (c) inaccurate, and (d) absent. Although it was designed for aphasic patients, the scoring system can be used with RHD patients. The authors provide a detailed set of rules for determining the accuracy and completeness of concepts in their article, which clinicians should consult before using the scoring system and which can be used for constructing main concept scoring for other pictures.

Screening for Neglect

Regardless of whether there is a statement in the patient's chart regarding neglect, the clinician should test for it in the initial evaluation. Notations in the chart may be based on casual observation only. Even if there is a report of task performance, it is difficult to know how it was scored because scoring procedures for these tests are not standardized. In addition, neglect may change rapidly in the early post-onset phase. It is very important to gather information on neglect because it is likely to influence communication and cognitive performance. Patients with neglect may be hypoaroused, flat in affect, less responsive to important environmental information, less attentive to nonverbal information, and less sensitive to subtleties of verbal interaction—possibly because of the close tie between neglect and other attentional processes. Because other rehabilitation professionals may feel that neglect is restricted to their domain, it is important for clinicians to explain the potential impact of neglect on cognitive and hence on communicative skills.

Several tests of neglect should be included in the initial screening because neglect may not be apparent on all tests. Useful and quickly administered tasks include *cancellation, drawing,* and *line bisection.* The tasks should be presented in the order specified. It is best to give the drawing task in between cancellation and line bisection so that patients do not confuse the tasks. For example, if they have just completed line bisection, patients often think they have to *bisect* each line in a line cancellation task. Although this perseveration across tasks may be diagnostically significant, it takes time to redirect the patient. Suggestions for the administration of each task are presented below. If time does not permit or if drawing seems particularly taxing, one could defer the drawing task until further testing.

Cancellation

A simple cancellation task, such as the one in Figure 2–1, should be presented first. Be sure there are an equal number of lines to the left as there are to the right of the middle of the page. Randomly placed stimuli are more sensitive as a measure of neglect than are stimuli ordered into rows because rows tend to serve as an anchor and means of organizing the movement of attention across the page. Place the paper at the patient's midline and ask him or her to make a mark through each line, saying something like, "See these lines? Make a mark through each line so I know you have seen it." There are no time limits to this test. The score should be a ratio between the number of lines cancelled to the left as opposed to the right of midline. A higher percentage of lines missed on the left indicates left neglect. This is better than simply scoring for the number missed on the left because the patient may miss about the same number of lines on the right as on the left, signaling a more general visual inattention problem. Even elderly NBD adults, particularly those over 70 years of age, may make a few omissions in cancellation tasks (Stone, Halligan, Wilson, Greenwood, & Marshall, 1991), probably due to general decline in visual attention. Thus, it is important to compute a right-left ratio.

Copy Drawing

One advantage of a *copied* scene or object is that it can be scored easily because the stimulus is external, rather than being internally generated from memory by the patient. Present the patient with a simple scene like the one in Figure 8–1 which is the author's rendition of the house, tree, and fence picture described so often in the literature on neglect (see, for example, Og-

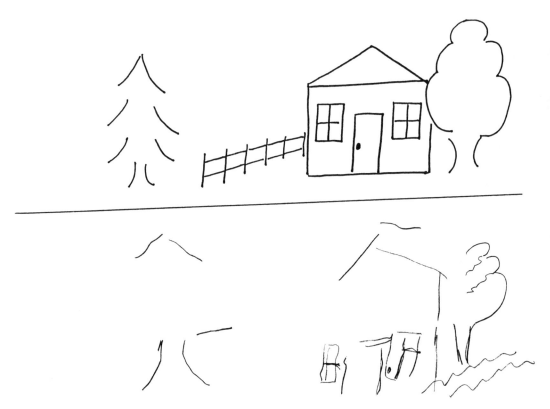

Figure 8–1. Simple scene depicting a fir tree, fence, house, and fluffy tree with a patient's copy drawing below the horizontal line. The scene was kept in the patient's view.

den, 1985a) with a copy drawing by a patient with RHD and neglect below it. The value of the scene as it is drawn in Figure 8–1 is that it has four objects across the page, a midline for the scene itself, and a midline for each object. Each object in this rendition has an equal number of lines to the left and to the right and there are an equal number of total lines to the left and right of the midline of the scene which is the left side of the house. Thus, it can be scored simply by comparing the number of left- to the number of right-sided lines included by the patient for each object and for the entire scene. It is intended to be copied so it should be kept in view as the patient copies it. It is best to present the scene on the top half of a page, with a line underneath it and space below for patients to make their copy as depicted in Figure 8–1.

A scoring system for the scene can be found in Appendix 3. Figure 8–2 shows the numbering of each line in the scene on which the scoring system is based. For example, there are four lines to the left of the fir tree and four lines to the right. The left and right of each window are assigned five lines each. The vertical line of each window is not counted since it constitutes a midline and thus would have to be counted twice. In addition to counting the ratio of left to right *lines for each object*, this system also accounts for omission of *whole objects* in that each of the two objects on the right of the midline (house and fluffy tree) and each of the two objects on the left (fence and fir tree) are given two points for their inclusion, regardless of how complete they are. The scores for the rendition in Figure 8–1 by a patient with RHD and neglect

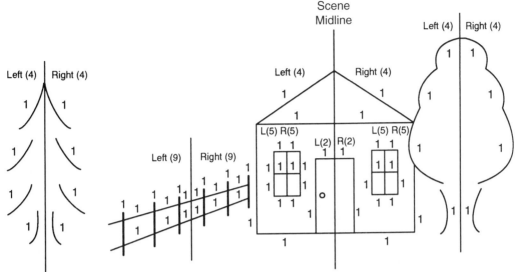

Figure 8–2. Simple scene depicted here with the point assignments that were generated for the Myers' Scoring System in Appendix 3. Each number 1 represents one point per line for the right and left sides of each object.

can be found in Appendix 4. The scoring system does not account for displacement of objects, like the door knob, nor are extra lines and marks (see Figure 8–1). It is not a perfect system, but it is useful as a means of tracking differences in the amount of right- to left-sided detail. Like other tests of neglect, this task can be presented again at a future time to probe the changes in the severity of neglect.

Freehand Drawing

A freehand drawing taps into the patient's internal imagery and does not tax the patient's visual attention and perception in the way that a copy drawing does. Thus, it serves as an additional probe into possible neglect. Ask the patient to draw a simple symmetrical object such as a man or a daisy. See Figures 2–5 and 6–6 for patients' drawings of clocks and a bicycle and Figure 8–3 for a daisy drawn by an RHD patient with neglect. One can score a daisy by comparing the number of petals on the right to the number on the left. Omission of more left-sided than right-sided detail is considered neglect. One must use this

right-left comparison because drawings by patients with either left- or right-sided damage may be quite primitive and lack detail on both sides of the object.

It is important to include a symmetrical object to test for neglect in free-hand draw-

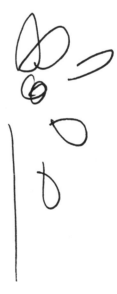

Figure 8–3. Free-hand drawing of a daisy by a patient with RHD and neglect.

ing. Clock drawing, although not essential, can provide additional information. Clock drawing is used to test the cognitive status and visuospatial skills in patients with dementia, head injury, and Parkinson's disease, as well as patients with focal brain damage. Scoring clock drawings is a complicated matter. Clocks differ from other drawing tasks because drawing a clock relies on language (number symbols) as well as on visuospatial organization skills. According to Freedman et al. (1994), clocks drawn by patients with posterior RH lesions typically are characterized by spatial disorganization. The elements may be present, but may be separated and distinct from each other. Thus the clock face may be empty and next to it a set of numbers, often trailing off down the page. The hands may be represented in yet another area of the page. Patients with right frontal lesions, on the other hand, may draw all the elements within the clock face, but have trouble attending simultaneously to the multiple dimensions of the task. For example, they may attend only to the number sequence, but fail to simultaneously maintain correct spacing between the numbers even though they include all the numbers within the clock face. Because generating the number sequence can be considered a function of the LH, RHD patients may include all of the numbers, but evidence of neglect may be seen in the drawings of both frontal and posterior RHD patients. Numbers may be crowded to the right with gaps or absence of numbers on the left. For purposes of testing for neglect, one should compare the number of right-sided to the number of left-sided numbers, the placement of hands, completeness of the circle representing the clock, and where on the page the patient has placed it (e.g., lower right-hand corner versus centered). For an extensive review of clock drawing deficits, normative data, and scoring systems see Freedman et al. (1994).

Any type of drawing can fatigue a patient, and patients often resist it, saying that they are not very good at drawing. One needs to remind patients that their drawings will not be judged on their artistic merits and to encourage them simply to do their best. Freehand drawing can be deferred until later testing if the patient seems worn out from the copy drawing task.

Line Bisection

Line bisection (see Figure 2–2) takes only a few moments. Lines used should be about 20 to 25 cm long. Shorter lines are easier to bisect and, hence, are less likely to evoke neglect. Longer lines result in considerable individual variation in NBD subjects. Instructions should be clear and explicit. Patients may not be familiar with the word "bisect," so it is best to say something like, "See this line? I'd like you to make a mark right in the middle of the line. Make a mark so that you cut the line in half." If the patient does not understand, one can demonstrate on a separate piece of paper. It is best to have the patient bisect several lines and take an average score. Deviations to the right or left of center of up to 6 mm on a 270 mm line can be considered within normal limits (Halligan, Manning, & Marshall, 1990). Sometimes, patients who have been tested on line bisection previously, will compensate in an exaggerated way. For example, one patient with documented neglect raised his pencil high over his head and, while still staring intently at the far right, then moved his arm into far left space, and came down suddenly on the far left of the page, almost missing the left end of the line. His mark in each case was only several millimeters from the far left end of the line. It pays to watch the client's performance in all of the above tests instead of just measuring the completed rendition.

Talking With Family Members

One should try to talk to family members to find out about their concerns regarding the patient. After listening to what they have to say, the clinician can list some of the deficits that can occur following RHD. Families often find it difficult to put their experience of the patient post-onset into words because they are not familiar with how to express the deficits they have noted. Like the patient, they will likely be relieved to know that some of their concerns are valid, have names, and can be addressed. In addition, families can help the clinician by describing the type of communicator the patient was prior to the neurologic event. For example, he or she may have been taciturn or garrulous by nature. Finally, the clinician can provide the family with information about the results of the initial screening.

Summary

With these simple and fairly quick tasks (interview, scene description, and several tests of neglect), one comes away from the first encounter having established rapport and gained some knowledge of the patient's ability to: (a) *manage the pragmatic demands of simple conversation;* (b) *answer open-ended questions;* (c) *acknowledge their deficits;* (d) *make inferences;* (e) *integrate information;* (f) *produce appropriate prosody, affective gesture, and facial expression;* and (g) *respond to left-sided visual input.* Thus, the Initial Screening should allow clinicians to determine if the patient does or does not need treatment. If therapy seems appropriate, the clinician has made a good beginning toward evaluation and can proceed to further testing that probes potential problem areas in more depth.

FURTHER TESTING

From information in the chart, discussion with other professionals and the patient's family, and from the Initial Screening, the clinician determines if the patient needs further testing and which areas to probe.

Most clinicians use some combination of standardized and non-standardized batteries to explore patient deficits further and to determine treatment goals.

Formal Tests of RHD Communication Impairments

There are not many published tests devoted to RHD communication disorders. Among them, the tests most frequently used include the *Mini Inventory of Right Brain Injury* (Pimental & Kinsbury, 1989), *The Rehabilitation Institute of Chicago Clinical Management of Right Hemisphere Dysfunction* (Halper, Cherney, & Burns, 1996), and *The Right Hemisphere Language Battery* (Bryan, 1995). The *Mini Inventory of Right Brain Injury* is essentially a screening and was devised to distinguish right from left hemisphere damage. The *Rehabilitation Institute of Chicago Clinical Management of Right Hemisphere Dysfunction* is the most comprehensive of the tests. Tasks in *The Right Hemisphere Language Battery* are, for the most part, based on the literature of the late 1980s. A fourth test instrument, *The Burns Brief Inventory of Communication and Cognition* (Burns, 1997), contains a section for assessing right hemisphere communication disorders as well as an inventories of left hemisphere disorders and disorders associated with complex neuropathology. All of these tests have been standardized, and they are listed with an overview of the areas tested in each in Appendix 5.

It is important to note that, unlike most tests of aphasia, none of these tests is based on a theory of the underlying processes that impair RHD communication. That is, the behaviors are tested, but without an eye toward the source of the abnormality. This is not a surprising state of affairs given that only very recently have theories begun to emerge to explain, rather than just describe, the cognitive/communicative deficits associated with RHD. As a result, the published tests give information about deficits, but do not necessarily serve as guides to the *processes* that should be addressed in therapy. To understand the impact of this problem, it is useful to consider the example of interpreting figurative language (i.e., metaphors, idioms, or proverbs), an area assessed in all of the published batteries summarized in Appendix 5. Assessment of this ability is accomplished by asking patients to match a metaphor to one of several pictures, verbally explain proverbs, or match a metaphor in a sentence to one of several printed sentences. Almost none of these tests assesses figurative language comprehension in contextually loaded discourse. In addition, asking someone to define (versus use) a proverb is both unnatural and difficult. However, assuming that there is good reason to isolate figurative language from a natural context and to ask patients to do something unnatural with it, the clinician is left without an understanding of the basis of the problem. Such an understanding, of course, would help guide therapy efforts. Without some sort of theory about the underlying disordered process, the clinician might be inclined to simply attempt to re-train comprehension and production of metaphoric speech, an ability the patient might have retained in conversational speech. Even if patients do have problems in interpreting figurative language in conversation, treatment should focus on the cause (e.g., activation/suppression of alternate meanings), not the symptoms, because it is unrealistic to expect that every figurative expression or proverb can or should be formally taught. Just as one would not attempt to rehabilitate aphasic patients by re-training word definitions from a dictionary, one would find attempting to retrain individual metaphors a useless exercise. Discovering a problem does not always translate into treating it. That is not to say that it is not valuable to have a sense of the deficits provided by these tests. It just means that clinicians must apply their *own* theories of the processes underlying impairments found on test batteries and apply those theories in the remediation of the deficits.

No test designed to assess RHD communication impairments categorizes performance by type. The *Mini Inventory of Right Brain Injury* is the only test that has a summary score representing overall severity. Given the time constraints on evaluation in most health care settings, choosing subtests based on clinical judgment can sometimes be an efficient way to look at patient performance.

Finally, no one test addresses all of the issues covered in earlier chapters, and some areas are not addressed by any of the published tests. For example, no formal battery assesses the patient's grasp of theory of mind, attentional and cognitive resources, or the capacity to suppress alternate meanings. Another point worth remembering is that, as is true of tests for aphasia and other communicative/cognitive functions, individual subtests require several cognitive and attentional functions in addition to the one noted in subtest titles. For example, tests of reading comprehension may tax the patient's visual attention, including left-sided scanning, as well as their comprehension of the overall content and the inferences contained therein.

Assessing Discourse Deficits

Discourse Comprehension

To probe narrative discourse comprehension abilities further, one can turn to several types of discourse comprehension tasks. The stimuli may be a story or paragraph read aloud by the clinician or silently by the patient. The goal should be to determine the patient's control over main events and details and their apprehension of explicit and non-explicit information. Thus, *the stimuli should require the patient to draw inferences and should be sufficiently detailed to require his or her focused attention.* Several types of tasks are outlined below, all of which use the form of yes-no or short answer questions as a means of measuring the patient's grasp of the material. These questions should be easy enough to be answered with 100% accuracy by NBD adults, but difficult enough to probe mild cognitive problems. In designing such materials, it may be useful to look at the level of the material and the norms presented in the *Discourse Comprehension Test* (Brookshire & Nicholas, 1993) described below.

Narrative Discourse Comprehension

The stories contained in *The Discourse Comprehension Test* (Brookshire & Nicholas, 1993) are very useful for probing the ability to comprehend both explicit and implied information. The test was designed for use with aphasic patients, but was also standardized on RHD subjects. Stories are followed by questions that probe the patient's ability to draw inferences from the material and to remember explicitly stated main ideas and details. The stimuli also serve as examples of the type of brief stories the clinician may want to design for use in treatment. Other stories of this type can be presented and followed by yes-no or multiple choice questions that probe comprehension of non-explicit information. Appendix 6 contains such an example.

Non-Narrative Discourse Comprehension

In addition to stories, one can present expository material such as an opinion paragraph, an editorial, a news item that is not in story form, or a conversation between two partners. Again, to check comprehension, the patient can be asked a series of yes-no questions about the main idea, the writer's opinion, the basis of that opinion, and details contained in the piece.

Discourse Production

The goal of discourse production tasks is to measure how informative, efficient, pragmatically appropriate, and inferentially astute the patient is in complex linguistic expression. Stimuli to elicit discourse production can include verbally presented sto-

ries, pictured stories, pictured scenes, and open-ended questions. The patient is asked to re-tell a story presented in verbal or written form, to tell the story contained in a picture sequence, to interpret a pictured scene, or to respond as completely as possible to an open-ended question.

Advantages and disadvantages of tasks to elicit discourse production are summarized in Table 8–3. Open-ended or divergent questions should allow the patient to explore an idea or share an opinion. They generate a more spontaneous, less controlled discourse sample than do other tasks suggested in this section. Story repetition, of course, involves memory, even if the patient is encouraged to tell the story in their own words. Picture and scene interpretation do not tax memory, but may tax visual perception. However, Myers and Brookshire (1994) found that level of visual complexity as measured by the number of objects, and, hence, the number of objects embedded, was of little or no consequence in the discourse production of RHD subjects. Subjects had significantly more trouble explaining pictures that were inferentially complex regardless of whether they were visually simple or visually complex. In general, patients were able to name pictured elements in all the pictures accurately, even when they had trouble interpreting a picture's overall meaning.

Pictured stimuli should always be placed at the patient's midline and clinicians should encourage the patient to look at the entire picture to avoid missing left-sided input. Patients should be cued to the left as necessary.

It can be difficult to measure discourse production. Areas to measure include the ability to express *main concepts, supportive (versus irrelevant) detail, inferences,* and *how efficient and informative* the patient's message is. Several methods of scoring the discourse productions of patients are described below and summarized in Table 8–4:

1. *Correct Information Unit:* One way of quantifying the concepts expressed is by

TABLE 8–3. Advantages and disadvantages of discourse production tasks.

Task	Advantage	Disadvantage
1. Story Repetition	Control over veracity of output Does not tax visual perception	Requires memory Output less spontaneous than in other tasks
2. Pictured Scene Interpretation	Control over veracity of output More spontaneous output Does not tax memory	May tax visual perception
3. Divergent Questions	Spontaneous output Does not tax memory or visual perception	Less control over output, making it more difficult to review results with the patient

TABLE 8–4. Advantages and disadvantages of sample discourse production scoring methods.

Scoring	Advantage	Disadvantage
Correct Information Unit	Quantitative Easy to score	Does not measure quality relative to irrelevancies, inferences, pragmatics
Informational Content Analysis	Measures efficiency of production	Does not measure other pragmatic and inferential features
Main Concepts	Measures ability to grasp macrostructure and supporting inferences	Does not measure efficiency Requires a list of NBD-generated concepts for each picture used

counting the number of correct information units or CIU's. For example, "The boy is on a stool" is a CIU for the "Cookie Theft" picture from the *Boston Diagnostic Aphasia Examination* (Goodglass & Kaplan, 1983) (Figure 6–5). An article by Nicholas and Brookshire (1995) contains a detailed set of rules for determining CIUs and a set of stimuli (i.e., two-picture story sequences and two pictured scenes) that are complex enough

to be useful for testing the performance of RHD patients.

2. *Informational Content Analysis:* Cherney and Canter (1993) developed a means of quantifying the efficiency of information produced by patients with either RHD or Alzheimer's disease. Their scoring system compares the amount of content-loaded information produced to the amount of information that does not convey meaningful information to ar-

rive at an *Efficiency Ratio.* An example of a content-loaded information unit for the "Cookie Theft" picture would be, "The woman is letting the water run over," whereas, "We've had such a drought this year," would not be considered relevant information. The essential features of their system are outlined in Appendix 7.

3. *Main Concepts Guidelines:* Main concepts are a good way of scoring scene interpretations. However, without norms or a list of concepts produced by NBD adults, measuring main concepts can be problematic. Appendix 8 lists the main concepts produced by a group of NBD and RHD elderly adults in a study by Myers and Brookshire (1994) for the Norman Rockwell illustrations depicted in Figures 6–1, 6–2, 6–3, 8–4, and 8–5. Next to each concept is the percentage of NBD subjects followed by the percentage of RHD subjects that mentioned these concepts. These percentages can be used as a guideline for assessing main concept performance on these particular pictures.

Stimuli for discourse production need not always be pictured, of course. One can ask *divergent* or *open-ended questions,* designed to encourage the patient to express and support an opinion. To inspire patients to respond, questions can be on a controversial topic or on a topic that the clinician suspects is of particular interest to the patient given his or her job history, hobbies, or age. Examples of age-appropriate questions that might spark the interest of middle aged and elderly adults include, "What is your opinion about the privacy rights of celebrities and politicians?" "What do you think about capital punishment?" or "Should we have dropped the atomic bomb in World War II?" There are no right or wrong answers, and brief monologues of a minute of less can reveal a great deal about verbal production skills (see Appendix 9 for sample responses to a divergent question). One can look at the *efficiency* of

production by using the informational content analysis scoring dimensions, described above. One can also rate the patient's performance on the dimension of *completeness* by checking to see if he or she provides an opinion and backs it up within reason.

Assessing Pragmatic Deficits

Although several of the tests designed to assess RHD communication impairments include observations and ratings of conversational and pragmatic behaviors, clinicians may choose to look at these behaviors in more depth. The list of Pragmatic Rating Scales in Appendix 10 contains brief overviews of some of the published methods for exploring pragmatic behaviors. These assessment tools are not tests in the formal sense of the word, and were not designed specifically for use with RHD patients, but can be adapted for them. Clinicians are encouraged to read the original sources in which these rating scales appeared to gain further insight into ways of addressing interpersonal conversational skills, nonverbal communication skills, and some aspects of discourse production such as the use of coherence structures for specificity and ease of listener burden.

Conversational analysis can be made informally by recording a conversation with the patient (e.g., the initial interview) and/or observing and recording a conversation between the patient and a person familiar to them. The most typical conversational deficits among RHD patients are: (a) *problems recognizing the limits of shared knowledge,* (b) *turn-taking,* and (c) *topic maintenance.* It is important to note that these problems may be apparent in mild form in elderly NBD adults. The clinician must judge the degree to which the problems are severe enough to warrant treatment.

Problems with *shared knowledge* can be assessed by observing the number of times the patient introduces unshared knowledge without identifying the referent or by failing to connect the new information to the original topic. Note these deficits in the

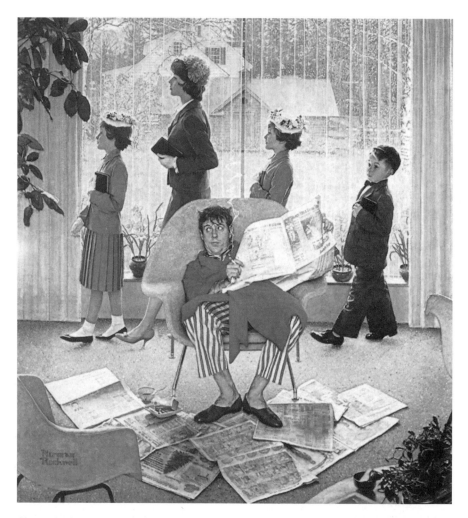

Figure 8–4. Norman Rockwell illustration depicting a Sunday morning. *Saturday Evening Post,* May 16, 1959. Reprinted with permission of the Norman Rockwell Family Trust.

following example of a conversation between a patient (P) and clinician (C) in which the clinician struggles to identify the referents:

C: "So, you are hoping to get out of the hospital on Tuesday?"

P: "It's just like with Marta. I said that to her, and she said that was all well and good to say, but did I know? So different from Dr. James."

C: "Marta? Who is Marta?"

P: "Marta always looks on the bleak side of things. Dr. James is much more um cheerful. Like he was with my other sister when we were all up north, but you wouldn't know about that."

C: "No, I wouldn't. But Dr. James? Who is he—your physician?"

P: "What? No, he isn't my physician. Of course, not. He's my brother."

C: "Oh."

In this brief interaction, the speaker makes reference to two people and one event about which the clinician has no knowledge. The patient acknowledges this lack of shared knowledge in one case (an event that occurred "up north"), but fails to do so in reference to the two people she mentions

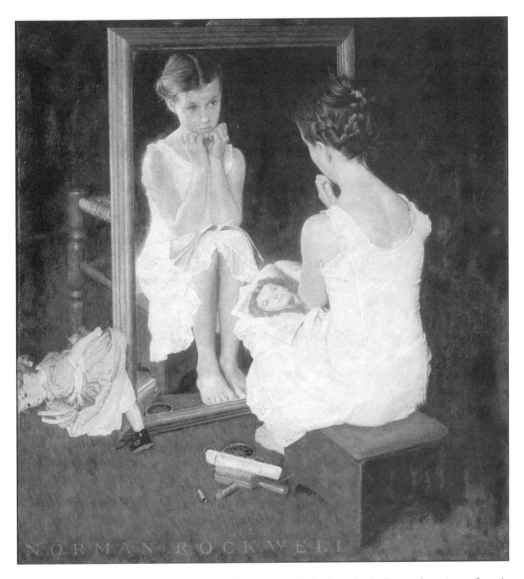

Figure 8–5. Norman Rockwell illustration depicting a girl daydreaming in front of a mirror. *Saturday Evening Post*, March 6, 1954. Reprinted with permission of the Norman Rockwell Family Trust.

by name. All of us at times are so absorbed by our own emotional state, so fatigued or so distracted that we fail to account for listener needs. The tendency to fail to acknowledge the limits of shared knowledge may occur more frequently following trauma, during illness, in the elderly, and in anyone who lacks the energy and resources to make the effort to make connections for the listener. Unfortunately, there are no absolutes or guidelines about when this behavior becomes abnormal. Clinicians must note the frequency of occurrence of reference omissions and the unwillingness or inability of patients to repair them (especially upon listener request) to judge the extent of the problem.

Patients with problems in *topic maintenance* either stay on a given topic after the conversation has moved on or switch too abruptly to a new topic. Sometimes, patients persist in discussing a topic even in the face of clear, verbal signals that their conversational partners are ready to move on. Sometimes, patients will return to a topic without the proper acknowledgement that the topic is no longer on the table or they may switch topics without the necessary new topic introduction. At other times, patients will wander off the topic in a free-form, almost stream-of-consciousness manner, as though they are unable to inhibit their internal associations. One is reminded of the patient, mentioned in Chapter 6, who said that his mind, "like a vacuum cleaner, sucked up every thought along the way and spewed them out." He seemed to be saying that the inhibition of related ideas was somewhat out of his control.

Turn-taking includes the ability to respond to cues that suggest a conversational partner wishes to have a turn to speak or has completed a turn. These cues may be signaled through facial expression, eye contact, or gesture, all of which can indicate impatience, boredom, or eagerness to speak. It is important to note whether the patient pays attention to these signals. For example, if patients do not make eye contact with their listeners, or are looking down and to the right, these visual signals will not be received. Thus, conversational interaction should be visually observed as well as read from a transcript or listened to on audiotape. Visual and vocal signals such as long pauses, a drop in pitch and volume, or resumption of eye contact can indicate that the partner has relinquished a turn. These cues may also be missed by patients who are not attending to them. After giving up a turn, the partner may have to prompt the patient to respond or take a turn, leading to a feeling of isolation on the part of the partner—a feeling that the patient is not participating, which, in fact, may be true.

The pragmatic rating scales listed in Appendix 10 are helpful in measuring the presence and degree of many of the conversational impairments listed above. Observations of conversational interaction should be about 10 to 15 min in length. For purposes of evaluation, the observed conversational interaction can be between patient and clinician, and the initial interview may give enough information for an initial pragmatic analysis. Later, during treatment, the clinician may want to analyze conversations between the patient and persons who are either familiar or unfamiliar to them in an effort to learn more about deficits detected in the initial analysis.

Assessing Neglect

Further testing of neglect can help establish a baseline performance in a variety of contexts and, most important, can help clinicians estimate the severity of the problem. The goals of testing for neglect may differ among various professionals on the rehabilitation team. For speech-language pathologists and others concerned with the impact of neglect on cognitive and communicative performance, the goal is to determine not only if it is present, but to what degree it is present, and how pervasive it is. That is, the goal is to evaluate spatial attention with an eye to its interaction with attention in general, attentional resources, arousal level in particular, and cognitive performance. Typically, for occupational and physical therapists who work directly on improving patient independence in activities of daily living, the goal of neglect testing is to determine in which activities the patient misses information on the left (e.g., grooming, eating, walking, cooking, self-care activities). Speech-language pathologists need to understand something about the severity of neglect in order to estimate the impact it may have on cognitive and hence communicative performance.

Severity can be considered in terms of the number of domains in which neglect occurs and the level of neglect in each area. Neglect may occur in one task or in several. It may show up in one frame of reference but not in another, or may occur in both the viewer-centered and the environment-centered frame of reference. Use of more than one type of task helps establish severity. Neglect also may occur across modalities, in olfaction and audition, in addition to vision and motor performance. However, although testing for olfactory and auditory neglect (beyond that established by tests of extinction) may tell us something about how pervasive neglect is, this type of testing generally is not done. Such tests are difficult to design, time consuming to perform, and are not considered necessary in most clinical settings.

On paper-and-pencil tests, if neglect occurs only on line bisection and only on long versus short lines, and if the patient is only an average of 2–3 cm off target on a 20 cm line, one could consider their neglect to be mild. If neglect also occurs on other paper-and-pencil tasks such as cancellation, and the patient misses almost all of the stimuli to the left of midline in both simple and complex cancellation tasks, his or her neglect could be considered more pervasive and more severe. Our current level of knowledge suggests that when neglect occurs in simple as well as complex tasks, and/or crosses tasks and frames of reference, it is more severe than if it occurs in a single difficult task in a single frame of reference. Occasionally, neglect that does not show up on any paper-and-pencil tasks will surface on computerized tests of visual attention. It is not known if this "subclinical" or less obvious form of neglect should be considered any more or less severe than neglect that occurs in paper and pencil testing. In such cases, severity should be considered in reference to the test protocol (i.e., number of targets missed relative to the density of the field).

Published Measures of Neglect

There are several published tests of neglect. The most well-known ones are the *Verbal and Nonverbal Cancellation Test* (Weintraub & Mesulam, 1985), the *Behavioral Inattention Test* (Wilson, Cockburn, & Halligan, 1987),

and the *Test of Visual Field Attention* (Coolspring Software) outlined in Appendix 11. The latter uses computerized presentation and scoring. The *Verbal and Nonverbal Cancellation Test* consists of a packet of standardized cancellation tests that vary in difficulty and in spatial arrangement. The *Behavioral Inattention Test* (Wilson et al., 1987) is the most complete assessment of neglect and includes functional tasks, such as reading a menu, as well as paper-and-pencil tasks. Of the paper-and-pencil subtests in this battery, star cancellation has been found to be the most sensitive measure of neglect (Halligan, Marshall, & Wade, 1989).

Informal Measures of Neglect

Line Bisection

This task was discussed in detail in the section on Initial Screening (see also Chapter 2). It is a task that can be re-administered periodically as a probe for neglect in estimating the midline according to body-centered coordinates. Another way to administer line bisection that avoids movement by the patient (i.e., avoids manual directional hypokinesia) and helps to focus on the patient's *perception* of spatial boundaries is to hold a colored pen at the far right side of the line and move it leftward along the line toward the center until the patient says "stop" to indicate that the middle of the line has been reached.

Cancellation

A simple cancellation task (Figure 2–1) was discussed previously. Further testing can be conducted by introducing various levels of difficulty that tax not only visual attention and motor exploration (eyes and hand), but also selective attention. Levels of difficulty vary with the spacing, the type of targets, and the configuration of the pattern of targets and foils across the page.

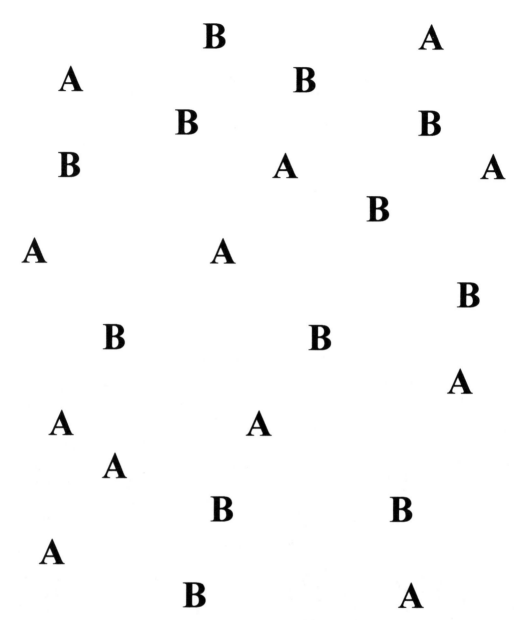

Figure 8–6. Simple cancellation task: Widely spaced, single feature, random array cancellation task in which the patient must make a mark (cancel) all instances of the letter A. Targets and foils differ only by shape.

The differences are specified below and in Table 8–5:

a. *Easy Cancellation:* widely spaced, single feature, ordered pattern

b. *Difficult Cancellation:* closely spaced, more than one feature, random pattern.

One can vary any of these features. A widely spaced, single feature, random pat-

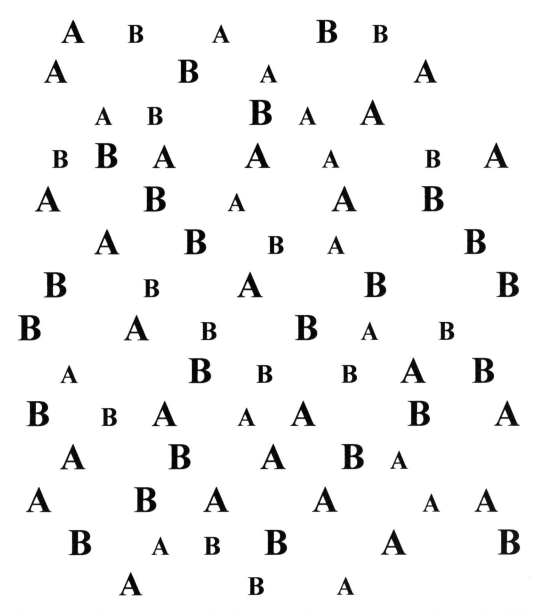

Figure 8–7. Difficult cancellation task. Closely spaced, dual feature random array cancellation task in which the patient must make a mark (cancel) all instances of the small letter A. Targets and foils differ by shape and size.

tern cancellation task can be found in Figure 8–6. The targets and foils differ only in shape. Figure 8–7 has a more crowded field with two features, size and shape, scattered in a random pattern. The patient must use selective attention to find the targets (small letter As) and screen out the foils (large let-

ter As and large and small letter Bs). Equally difficult, perhaps, is the cancellation task in Figure 8–8 because, although not crowded there is close similarity between the targets (Qs) and foils (Os). The selective attention component very likely may exacerbate the patient's neglect and

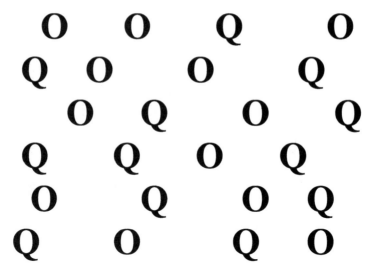

Figure 8–8. Difficult cancellation task: Targets and foils are widely spaced, but very similar in shape.

slow down performance. Level of difficulty also can be varied by selecting targets and foils from different domains (i.e., letters and numbers) which is easier than if targets and foils are all from the same domain (e.g., shapes of different sizes, or two or more numbers). Table 8–5 lists the variables that can affect cancellation task difficulty. Cancellation tasks usually are given without time limits, although one could impose a time limit. Scoring should reflect the right-left ratio of omissions. One should also note the total number of omissions. It is not unusual for elderly NBD adults to miss a target on either side of the midline. However, missing a large proportion of targets on both sides of the stimulus array suggests an overall visual attention problem. Thus, the overall score (number of targets missed) provides information about visual attention skills in general, and the right-left ratio provides information about neglect in particular.

Drawing

Drawing was described in the section on initial screening.

Reading

Reading can be assessed at the single word, sentence, and paragraph level by asking the patient to read printed material out loud. All reading material should be presented at the patient's midline.

Single Words. Single words can vary in length. Generally, the more widely spaced the letters and the longer the word, the more likely the patient will neglect the left half. Error types are listed in Table 8–6. Patients without neglect who have a visual field cut for which they are not yet compensating often omit leftward letters. The most common error for patients with neglect is a substitution (i.e., "reduction" for "induction"), probably because there is some unconscious processing of the leftward letters.

Sentences. Generally, sentences are more difficult than single words. It appears that adults with neglect do not make a sweeping left saccade to the beginning of a line of text, but instead begin at the most rightward word and make small backward

TABLE 8–5. Variables that affect task difficulty in cancellation tasks.

	Less Difficult	*More Difficult*
Field Density:	Widely spaced targets	Closely spaced targets
Target/Foil Organization:	Placement in rows	Random placement
Target/Foil type	Targets and foils from different domains	Targets and foils from the same domain
Target/foil features	Targets and foils differ in one feature (e.g., shape OR color, color OR size, etc.)	Targets and foils differ in more than one feature (e.g., shape and color or shape, color and size)

movements until what they see makes sense. Thus, patients may move their eyes to the left only until they have read enough words to constitute a meaningful phrase. When reading a random string of words, neglect is often worse because the patient becomes defeated early on. Level of difficulty can be varied by embedding a phrase within a sentence. For example, the sentence, "The boy with the dog walked our way," might be read as, "The dog walked our way," because the patient stops moving to the left as soon as a phrase becomes meaningful.

Text Reading. Again, patients with neglect do not make the long saccades from the rightward end of a line of text to the

leftward end of the next line, but instead make small backward eye movements, often stopping when they have reached a meaningful phrase, regardless of whether it makes sense within the entire context of the text. As in so many other situations, patients with neglect tend to narrow the focus of their attention to that which is immediately before them, ignoring the larger picture. An example of textual reading by a patient with neglect is provided in Chapter 2.

A sensitive test of neglect in reading was developed by Caplan (1985). He suggested varying the leftward margin so that patients do not have a physical border to use as a cue. An example of such a passage and task is given in Appendix 12. According to Caplan (1985), this task often picks up cases of mild neglect in patients who do not demonstrate neglect when reading texts with normal margins.

TABLE 8–6. Single word reading errors in left neglect.

Error Type	Examples
Substitutions: most common	barn for darn
	table for sable
Omissions: very common	tape for videotape
	dog for hotdog
Additions: least common	clock for lock
	sunglasses for glasses

Writing. The patient can be asked to copy a sentence, compose a brief paragraph or write a series of words horizontally or vertically. Response characteristics to observe are *use of margins, slant of the line, perseverative strokes, omitted strokes, omitted punctuation,* and *failure to cross t's and dot i's* as explained in Chapter 2. Patients with neglect often start in the upper right hand corner, failing to leave enough room for a complete sentence which they then write word by word vertically below the first several words. See Figure 2–6 for an example.

Baking Tray Task   (Tham & Tegner, 1996). In this task, patients are given a set of 16 cubes which they are asked to arrange on a 75 by 100 cm board with a border of 3.5 cm. Their task is to place the cubes as evenly as possible on the board as if they were "buns on a tray." There is no time limit and the score is a comparison of the number of cubes in each half field. Each cube gets a score of one point and cubes straddling the midline get a score of one-half point. According to the authors, the advantages of this task are that there is no well defined solution nor any way to memorize the outcome from an earlier effort. It taxes both global and local attention in an alternating manner. It avoids some of the perceptual problems that may be a factor in cancellation tasks, and it does not require selective attention, which can be assessed separately. It is simple to administer and score, and purportedly sensitive to neglect that may not show up in other tasks (i.e., latent or "subclinical" neglect).

Assessing Attention Deficits

Published Measures of Attention

Several formal tests, including a number of computerized tests of attention are listed in Appendix 13. They include: (a) the *Test of Everyday Attention* (Robertson, Ward, Ridgeway, & Nimmo-Smith, 1994), (b) the *Stroop Task* (Stroop, 1935), (c) the *Trail Making Test* (Reitan, 1958; Reitan & Wolfson, 1985), and (d) several computerized tasks. In addition, a number of neuropsychological test batteries designed to assess cognitive skills include tasks that tax attention.

Informal Measures of Attention

The informal measures listed below are arranged by the attentional operation that they address. It is important to remember that, even though a given task may empha-

size a particular operation, it is nearly impossible to measure attentional operations independently of one another. In addition, patients may have been tested by a neuropsychologist for attentional impairments. If that is the case, the speech-language pathologist should obtain those test results.

Arousal

It is difficult to quantify level of arousal without measuring autonomic functions such as heart rate. However, one can administer published computerized reaction time tasks that contain norms for NBD adults and can be informative about general level of arousal, attentional maintenance, and vigilance. Generally, through clinical observation, one can distinguish patients who are hypoaroused from those who are more alert by noting their inability to maintain attention for more than a few minutes, their tendency to be very slow to respond and in need of constant prompting, and by their flattened affect. Those who are not as severely hypoaroused may maintain attention longer, but still may need a great deal of prompting. As is true of all patients with brain damage, level of responsivity is worth noting during evaluation.

Vigilance and Sustained Attention

These attentional operations are best measured in tasks that require focused attention over a period of time. Reaction time tasks, as explained in Chapter 3, are a good measure of the ability to maintain vigilance. Deteriorating performance over the course of the task suggests impaired attentional maintenance. Any serial type of task such as signaling the presence of a target in a series (of numbers, letters, words) said out loud by the clinician also tests vigilance and attentional maintenance. Another test of vigilance is the Paced Auditory Serial Selection Task (Gronwall, 1977), which requires a patient to add each number to the one preceding it as the numbers are called out by the examiner. Gronwall's article provides normative data. This type of task is useful with mildly impaired patients.

Selective Attention

Cancellation tasks that conjoin two or more features such as color and size stress selective attention and can be used for that purpose as well as to test for neglect. Matching tasks in which targets (i.e., nonsense shapes) are increasingly similar to foils also can be used. In addition, the Stroop type tasks, described in Chapter 3 and mentioned in Appendix 13, are useful for measuring selective attention as well as vigilance.

Capacity (Dual Tasks)

Attentional capacity can be measured by asking patients to attend to two things at once. For example, they may be asked to list all of the animals they can think of in a verbal fluency task while sorting objects by color or shape, or to generate random numbers while canceling targets (i.e., lines on a page), or to count while sorting coins or cards by color or shape.

Alternating Attention

Alternating attention, or attentional switching, can be measured by the patient's accuracy in tasks in which targets change. For example, during a cancellation task in which the patient is searching for a target shape, letter, or number, the examiner can switch the targets and ask the patient to search for a different shape. Target switching may be better when stimuli are presented in rows, rather than in random array. That way, the patient must continue to move attention leftward (across the rows) during the attentional switching.

Assessing Prosodic Deficits

Prosodic Comprehension

Because so much of the content of the spoken word depends on its prosodic contour, poor prosodic comprehension may be a factor in impaired discourse comprehension. Because patients rarely complain of it and because it is not noticed by conversational partners, it is difficult to know if prosodic comprehension is impaired without testing. Because production and comprehension are thought to be somewhat independent of one another, it is important to test prosodic comprehension even in patients who appear to have adequate prosodic production. None of the published tests for RHD listed in Appendix 5 contain tests of prosodic comprehension; therefore, clinicians must devise their own. The tasks that follow are designed to assess prosodic discrimination independent of meaningful context. In all cases sentence stimuli should be short, about three to five words in length. Printed sentences and word choices should be placed to the right of the patient's midline to avoid the effects of neglect as much as possible. In tasks with multiple choice responses, printed choices should be arrayed vertically. Each sentence or choice should be read aloud by the patient before beginning a task to ensure his or her visual comprehension and perception of the task materials. The sentence stimuli, made up by the clinician, can be used across tasks. Scoring is based on perceptual judgments. Acoustic analysis is not considered necessary for this level of testing, although instrumentation that provides a visible display and quantifies output may be useful later in management as a means of providing feedback to the client and monitoring patient progress. Appendix 14 summarizes the tasks listed below.

1. Identify Emotional Prosody in Sentences

A simple way to test emotional prosodic comprehension is to ask patients to identify the emotional tone of a spoken sentence. The content of sentence stimuli should be emotionally neutral (e.g., "The man was tall." "The girl came home."). Sentences should be pre-recorded with one of several emotional overlays. Good choices for emotion type are *angry, happy,* and either *sad* or *indifferent.* It is best to avoid having both *indifferent* and *sad* on the list because they are often produced with a similar sounding flat intonation pattern. Similarly, *surprise* can be confused with *happy* because both are often produced with an exaggerated prosodic contour and pitch level. The emotion choices should be printed in a vertical list form and be in front of the patient as the stimuli are produced. A list of 10 sentences, each read with more than one emotion type, for a total of 30 to 40 sentences is customary. Even if the sample is smaller, each emotion should be presented more than once. It is best to pre-record the sentences and to give the task to several NBD adults, preferably in the same age range as one's patients, prior to finalizing the tape. Members of community theater groups or theater students usually are very happy to help make such a tape if the clinician feels inadequate to the task. Scoring is plus-minus.

2. Identify Emphatic Stress: Compound Nouns Versus Noun Phrases

Stimuli are distinguished on the basis of stress (e.g.,Whitehouse versus white house; hotdog versus hot dog). Patients are asked to match a spoken word or phrase to one of a set of two printed words or phrases.

3. Identify Emphatic Stress: Sentences

Patients are asked to identify the stressed word in simple printed sentences such as, "Ella loves Joe," by pointing to the stressed word (i.e., *Ella* loves Joe versus Ella *loves* Joe versus Ella loves *Joe*) as the clinician reads the sentence out loud.

4. Distinguish Sentence Types

Patients are asked to distinguish between declarative and interrogative sentences. Sentence stimuli for both choices should be identical in each set. Sentences like "Joe is in his office" are good because they can be turned into a question without changing the word order, as in "Joe is in his office?"

Prosodic Production

Clinicians can make a broad judgment about patients' control over prosodic production by listening carefully to a recorded sample of their conversational speech or oral reading. Although subjective, one should be able to judge whether the patient is using a combination of pausing, duration, pitch, and intensity changes effectively in their connected speech. One should, of course, take account of the influence of dysarthria and/or fatigue on production. The published tests in Appendix 5 contain prosodic production tasks. If a prosodic production problem is suspected, one can use those tests or some or all of the production tasks listed below to evaluate it.

1. Production of Emotional Prosody in Sentences

Patients are asked to imitate the examiner's rendition of a given emotion in a sentence. For a more spontaneous production, they can be asked to read a printed sentence with an emotion specified in advance by the examiner. One can use the set of neutral sentences from the list of comprehension tasks. The patient's productions should be tape recorded. Scoring is based on perceptual judgment by the examiner, or the collective judgment of several listeners.

2. Production of Emphatic Stress in Sentences

This task is the reverse of the one used to test comprehension of emphatic stress in sentences. The clinician must identify the stressed word from the patient's productions. Stimulus sentences should be printed and choice of the stressed word left up to the patient. Because RHD patients often rely excessively on volume for emphatic stress, the manner of stress production should be noted in scoring.

3. Distinguish Sentence Types

This task is the reverse of the one in the comprehension section in which patients are asked to identify whether sentences are declarative or interrogative. In this case, the patient is asked to produce the sentence for the examiner to judge. Stimuli can be the same as those used in the comprehension of sentence types and can include some sentences designed as questions, such as "Do you want to go?" to check the patient's control over the prosodic features of other interrogative forms.

Assessing Affective Communication

As noted in Chapter 7, RHD may have a negative impact on affective or emotional communication. Patients may not be as overtly emotionally expressive, and may have trouble comprehending facial expression, body language, and emotional content conveyed verbally. Suggestions for assessing these potential deficits are listed below.

Production of Nonverbal Emotional Expression

Measuring facial and gestural animation is problematic because (a) it is very difficult to quantify changes in nonverbal expressivity, (b) there is so much variability in NBD adults, and (c) testing can be cumbersome. Although an important component of RHD deficits, particularly in those who are hypoaroused, it is not really necessary to *measure* reduced nonverbal emotional expression. If it is observed, reduced facial and gestural expressivity can simply be noted in the overall evaluation and discussed with the patient's family without reference to numbers and scores. Should one choose to test for such deficits, one can

adapt tasks from the literature on nonverbal emotional communication (e.g., Blonder et al., 1991; Borod et al., 1990; Buck & Duffy, 1980). Typically, in experimental studies, patients view scenes with emotional content or are videotaped during conversations on emotion-laden topics. Such observations require videotape recordings and several trained judges who rate the nonverbal expressions and/or try to guess the emotional nature of the slide or conversational topic from the facial expression produced by the patients. It is important to remember the potential contribution of contralateral facial weakness when judging and/or observing facial affect.

Comprehension of Nonverbal Emotional Expression

Problems in comprehension of nonverbal emotion are more difficult to observe and, thus, more important to assess. Several published instruments, listed in Appendix 15, are available for measuring nonverbal emotional comprehension. Short of a published battery, one might consider developing tasks for discrimination and recognition. For example:

a. *Discriminate Facial Expressions*
   Goal: discriminate (same/different) emotional expressions
   Stimuli: pairs of photographs or other pictures of faces expressing an emotion (e.g., happiness, sadness, anger)
   Task: (1) state whether or not the expressions are the same or different
      (2) group photographs into sets that show the same expression
   Scoring: plus/minus

b. *Identification of Facial Expression*
   Goal: identify (name) emotional expression
   Stimuli: photographs of faces with various expressions
   Task: name the expression conveyed in the photograph

Scoring: plus/minus

A nonverbal emotional recognition task can also be conducted with pictured scenes in which emotions are depicted via contextual elements and body language, rather than facial expression. For example, a picture of a soldier crying against the shoulder of another soldier on a battle field is often described by RHD patients as a soldier who is tired, rather than as a soldier who is crying or being comforted.

Comprehension of Verbal Emotional Expression

Comprehension of verbally conveyed emotion can be tested by having patients read or listen to short paragraphs or sentences that contain emotional content. Patients can be asked to name the emotional state of the main character, to answer questions about the emotions conveyed by the story, or to infer the overall mood of a setting or plot. Questions can be yes/no or multiple choice.

There are no free-standing, standardized materials available that are specifically designed to assess emotional comprehension of verbal materials, so clinicians must devise their own. It is worth remembering that emotionally laden stimuli can be more difficult to comprehend than neutral stories because the emotions conveyed are often done so *indirectly* through context and may require difficult inferences (e.g., "He left the building, oblivious to the bright sunshine, shoulders stooped, steps slowed" is less obvious than "He felt oppressed as he left the building").

Production of Verbal Emotional Expression

Much of the verbal expression of emotion is conveyed in prosodic contour. However, emotion also is conveyed through word choice. Some RHD patients are less specific in recalling experiences in response to emotionally evocative cue words than their NBD counterparts (Cimino et al., 1991).

Few other studies have examined the spontaneous verbal expression of emotion in RHD adults. Most studies require subjects to explain or describe scenes or stories depicting neutral and emotional contents. A patient's verbal emotional expression, independent of prosody and of the ability to comprehend emotional material, is difficult to measure. One can ask patients to describe an emotional situation from their personal experience, but there are no standards for the number of emotional words, the subjective perception of emotional intensity, and the like. Verbal emotional expression perhaps is best tested by measures of prosodic production and observations of facial expression, gesture, and body language.

PROGNOSIS

Unfortunately, no test, published or not, gives guidelines about prognosis because at this point we know so little about how to measure the severity of communication impairments subsequent to RHD. The various demographic variables cited in the literature on aphasia, such as age and education, clinical history, and time post-onset also may be of predictive value in RHD patients. As in other populations with brain damage, prognosis can be considered in light of the site and size of the lesion, coexisting medical conditions, prior neurological injury, the time post-onset, and the motivation and relevant pre-morbid personality factors. With experience, clinicians should be able to make some subjective judgment about the severity of deficits and the possibility of their remediation. It is safe to say that severe attention problems are a poor prognostic sign. Experience as well as some limited data suggest that severe neglect, especially if it is accompanied by anosognosia, is also a poor prognostic sign (Pizzamiglio et al., 1992). In addition to attentional deficits, patients with neglect may have limited insight, which is also a poor prognostic sign. As more studies are done, other indicators of prognosis will be identified. For now, clinicians must rely on their best judgments, based on their experience with brain-injured patients in general and RHD patients in particular.

SUMMARY

1. Evaluation can be divided into an *Initial Screening* and *Further Testing*. The *Initial Screening should help one determine if the patient has a communication problem that warrants further testing*. It consists of *an interview, a scene description task,* and *several tests of neglect*. The interview and scene description allow observation of the patient's pragmatic and social skills, discourse ability, facial and gestural animation, prosodic expressivity, ability to draw inferences, motivation, level of alertness, and ability to maintain attention. The neglect tasks further evaluate visual attention and presence of neglect.

2. *Further Testing allows specific deficit areas to be probed in depth.* The choice of eval-

uation measures should be based on findings in the initial screening. The areas included are: (a) *discourse comprehension and production*, (b) *neglect*, (c) *attention*, (d) *prosodic production and comprehension*, and (e) *emotional expression and comprehension*. Clinicians are encouraged to choose appropriate measures from both published and informal measures at their discretion.

3. Further Testing provides additional information about individual impairments which can be: (a) *shared with patients and their families*, (b) *shared with other rehabilitation team members to help guide decisions about management*, and (c) *help set the stage for treatment*.

4. Because *none of the tests or tasks are guided by an underlying theory about the nature of the deficits, treatment based on evaluation results must be guided by the clinician's own theory about underlying cause.*

Appendix 1

MYERS' LITERAL AND INTERPRETIVE SCORING SYSTEM FOR THE "COOKIE THEFT" PICTURE

LITERAL CONCEPTS

Two	Cookies	Water
Children (kids)	High shelf	Overflowing (going over)
Little	Cupboard	Onto the Floor
Boy (kid)	With the open door	Dirty dishes left
Girl (kid)	Has finger on mouth	Reaching up
Woman	Children behind her	Lawn
Stool (footstool)	Sink	Sidewalk
Three-legged	Dishes	House next door
On the floor	Faucet on	By the boy
Puddle	Window	

INTERPRETIVE CONCEPTS

Brother	Washing (doing) dishes	Cookie jar
Sister	Feet getting wet	Asking for a cookie
Taking (stealing)	In the kitchen	Saying "shhh . . . ."
For his sister	Falling over	Trying (not trying) to help
Handing to sister	Wobbling (off balance)	Drying (wiping)
Laughing	Hurt himself	Full blast
Mother	For himself	Ignoring (daydreaming)
Disaster statement		

LITERAL AND INTERPRETIVE CONCEPT SCORING

Count each concept only once

Total Number of Concepts	_____
Number of Literal Concepts	_____
Number of Interpretative Concepts	_____
Percent Interpretive Concepts	_____

(Interpretive Concepts/Total Concepts)

Source: From "Profiles of Communication Deficits in Patients with Right Cerebral Hemisphere Lesions," by P. S. Myers, 1979, in R. H. Brookshire (Ed.), *Clinical Aphasiology: Conference Proceedings* (pp. 38–46). Minneapolis, MN: BRK Publishers. Adapted with permission.

Appendix 2

CONCEPT LIST FOR THE "COOKIE THEFT" PICTURE

1. The woman (mother) is doing dishes.
2. The sink (water) is overflowing (running over).
3. The boy is on a stool.
4. The boy (kids) is getting (stealing) cookies (getting into the cookie jar).
5. The stool is tipping (the boy is falling).
6. The girl is reaching for a cookie (the boy hands the girl a cookie) OR some mention of a plausible action by the girl or location of the girl.
7. The woman (mother) is not noticing (paying attention).

Scoring: based on the presence, accuracy and completeness of each concept

AC: Accurate and Complete

AI: Accurate but Incomplete

IN: Inaccurate

AB: Absent

Note: See article for detailed scoring rules.

Source: From "Presence, Completeness, and Accuracy of Main Concepts in the Connected Speech of Non-Brain-Damaged Adults and Adults with Aphasia," by L. E. Nicholas and R. H. Brookshire, 1995, *Journal of Speech and Hearing Research, 38,* 145–156. Copyright 1995 by the American Speech-Language-Hearing Association. Adapted with permission.

Appendix 3

MYERS COPY-SCENE SCORING SYSTEM FOR NEGLECT

LEFT SIDE OF OBJECTS

_____ Fir Tree (0–4)

_____ Fence (0–9)

_____ Right Window (0–5)

_____ Left Window (0–5)

_____ Door (0–2)

_____ House (0–4)

_____ Fluffy Tree (0–4)

_____ **TOTAL POINTS** (0–33)

RIGHT SIDE OF OBJECTS

_____ Fir Tree (0–4)

_____ Fence (0–9)

_____ Right Window (0–5)

_____ Left Window (0–5)

_____ Door (0–2)

_____ House (0–4)

_____ Fluffy Tree (0–4)

_____ **TOTAL POINTS** (0–33)

NUMBER OF LEFT OBJECTS

_____ Fir Tree (2)

_____ Fence (2)

_____ **TOTAL POINTS** (0–4)

NUMBER OF RIGHT OBJECTS

_____ Fluffy Tree (2)

_____ House (2)

_____ **TOTAL POINTS** (0–4)

COMBINED TOTAL

_____ LEFT (0–37)

_____ **RIGHT** (0–37)

RATIO: LEFT/RIGHT _____

Appendix 4

SCORES ON THE MYERS SCORING SYSTEM FOR THE COPIED SCENE IN FIGURE 8–1

LEFT SIDE OF OBJECTS

__2__ Fir Tree (0–4)

__0__ Fence (0–9)

__4__ Right Window (0–5)

__5__ Left Window (0–5)

__1__ Door (0–2)

__1__ House (0–4)

__1__ Fluffy Tree (0–4)

__14__ **TOTAL POINTS** (0–33)

RIGHT SIDE OF OBJECTS

__3__ Fir Tree (0–4)

__0__ Fence (0–9)

__4__ Right Window (0–5)

__5__ Left Window (0–5)

__2__ Door (0–2)

__2__ House (0–4)

__4__ Fluffy Tree (0–4)

__20__ **TOTAL POINTS** (0–33)

NUMBER OF LEFT OBJECTS

__2__ Fir Tree (2)

__0__ Fence (2)

__2__ **TOTAL POINTS** (0–4)

NUMBER OF RIGHT OBJECTS

__2__ Fluffy Tree (2)

__2__ House (2)

__4__ **TOTAL POINTS** (0–4)

COMBINED TOTAL

__16__ LEFT (0–37)

__24__ **RIGHT** (0–37)

RATIO: LEFT/RIGHT __16/24__

Appendix 5

PUBLISHED TESTS OF RHD COMMUNICATION IMPAIRMENTS

MINI INVENTORY OF RIGHT BRAIN INJURY (MIRBI)
Pimental, P. A., & Kinsbury, N. A. (1989)
Designed as a screening test to distinguish RHD from NBD subjects.

Tasks include:

1. *Visual scanning and tracking*
2. *Integrity of gnosis* (finger identification), *asterognosis, two-point discrimination*
3. *Oral reading*
4. *Writing:* spontaneous and copy
5. *Emotional prosodic production*
6. *Explain verbal absurdities, incongruities, figurative language, and similarities*
7. *Comprehend humor*
8. *Screen for flat affect*
9. *General behavior and "psychic integrity":* impulsivity, distractibility, and eye contact

▶ Standardized on 30 RHD and 30 NBD subjects.
▶ Available from: Pro-Ed
8700 Shoal Creek Boulevard
Austin, TX 78758-6897

REHABILITATION INSTITUTE OF CHICAGO (RICE) **CLINICAL MANAGEMENT OF RIGHT HEMISPHERE DYSFUNCTION (2nd Edition).**
Halper, A., Cherney, L. R., & Burns, M. S. (1996)

Tasks include:

1. *Behavioral Observation Profile:* observation, conversation, and interview
2. *Visual Scanning & Tracking:* cancellation of letter and word targets presented in rows
3. *Pragmatic Rating Scale:*
   ▶ Nonverbal: prosody, expression, gesture, eye contact
   ▶ Verbal : conversation initiation, turn taking, topic maintenance, referencing skills
   ▶ Narrative: completeness (based on the Story Retelling-Immediate subtest from the *Arizona Battery for Communication Disorders of Dementia* [1991], Bayles, K., & Tomoeda, C. K. Tucson, AZ: Canyonlands Publishing, Inc.)
4. *Analysis of Writing: Copy & Spontaneous*
   Scoring based on mechanics, including presence/absence of omissions, perseveration, organization of letters and lines, and neglect
5. *Metaphorical Language:* Proverb Interpretation: ability to interpret proverbs
   Scoring based on 3-point rating for accuracy and notations of responses that are literal, personal, repetitions of the proverb or lack of response

▶ Standardized on 40 RHD and 36 NBD subjects.
▶ Available from: Aspen Publications
P.O. Box 6018
Gaithersburg, MD 20877

RIGHT HEMISPHERE LANGUAGE BATTERY (RHLB) **(2nd Edition):**
Bryan, K. L. (1995)

Tasks include:

1. *Metaphor-Picture Matching:* match spoken metaphor to one of four picture depictions
2. *Written Metaphor Choice:* match a metaphor contained in a sentence to one of three sentences
3. *Comprehension of Inferred Meaning:* aspects of inferred meaning assessed in the comprehension of a written paragraph
4. *Humor Appreciation:* select a punchline for a joke from one of four printed choices
5. *Lexical Semantic Recognition:* match a target word to one of five pictures
6. *Prosody:* emphatic stress production
7. *Discourse Production:* 15 areas assessed by a 4-point rating scale

▶ Standardized on 30 NBD, 40 RHD, and 40 aphasic subjects
▶ Available from: Whurr Publishers, Ltd.
                          19b Compton Terrace
                          London N1 2UN, England

THE BURNS BRIEF INVENTORY OF COMMUNICATION AND COGNITION
Burns, M. (1997)

Tasks in the Right Hemisphere Inventory include:

1. *Scanning and Tracking*
    ▶ Functional scanning and tracking
    ▶ Scanning and tracking of single words
2. *Visuospatial Skills*
    ▶ Functional spatial distribution of attention
    ▶ Spatial distribution of attention
    ▶ Recognition of familiar faces
    ▶ Gestalt perception
    ▶ Visuospatial construction (clock)
    ▶ Visuospatial organization for writing
3. *Prosody*
    ▶ Prosody and abstract language
    ▶ Spontaneous expressive prosody
    ▶ Receptive prosody
4. *Inferences*
5. *Metaphorical language*

▶ Standardized on RHD patients
▶ Available from: Psychological Corporation
                          555 Academic Court
                          San Antonio, Texas 78204
                          1-800-211-8378

Appendix 6

EXAMPLE OF STORY COMPREHENSION TASK FOR RHD PATIENTS

STIMULUS PRESENTATION: One or more stories like the one presented below can be read to the patient or read by the patient. Questions should be printed on a separate sheet of paper.

STORY EXAMPLE:
Peter waited in eager anticipation, but with some degree of impatience and embarrassment. Like others around him, he wanted to check the time on his watch, but felt it might be inappropriate to do so. He looked to his brother, James, for support. Out of his sight, Lila adjusted her veil and smoothed her white satin dress as she stared in the mirror. Looking at her reflection, she saw she had successfully covered up her earlier tear stains with make-up. She knew time was ticking by and, yet, she felt immobilized. Through the distant strains of organ music she thought about the rumors of Peter's infidelity she'd just been privy to not an hour before. Trembling a bit, she turned from the mirror and entered the small hallway leading to the entry. With slow hesitant steps she approached her father whose face registered the same questions she kept trying to suppress in her own heart.

QUESTIONS THAT PROBE NON-EXPLICT INFORMATION

1. Who was Peter waiting for?

    a.   Lila

    b.   James

    c.   The minister

    d.   A friend

2. Was Lila about to

    a.   Go to a dance

    b.   Meet Peter at a train station

    c.   Marry Peter

    d.   Go out with her father

3. What was keeping Lila?

    a.   She was making sure her dress looked just right.

    b.   She was afraid of getting married.

    c.   She lost track of time.

    d.   She was not sure where the entry was.

Appendix 7

INFORMATIONAL CONTENT ANALYSIS

Descriptive, narrative, and procedural discourse analysis

CONTENT LOADED INFORMATION UNITS
Relevant, nonredundant, correct information

1. *Essential:*
   ▶ relevant information
   ▶ consistent with major details
   ▶ selected a priori for each task
2. *Elaborative:*
   ▶ additional relevant information
   ▶ beyond that established a priori

INFORMATION UNITS WITHOUT SIGNIFICANT CONTENT
Do not convey meaningful information

1. *Irrelevant:* Units related to the topic, but inconsistent with task requirements
   Includes:
   ▶ descriptions of items irrelevant to task
   ▶ interpretations and judgements
   ▶ personal comments and comments about task
2. *Redundant:*
   ▶ units that do not add new information
   ▶ repetitions in some fashion of previously provided information
3. *Off-Topic:*
   ▶ digressions unrelated to topic or task
4. *Incorrect:* Units intended to be accurate in the context of the stimulus or task
   Units that are:
   ▶ inconsistent with object or picture stimulus
   ▶ not included in original story
   ▶ or not part of performance of a procedure

EFFICIENCY RATIO: Number of Essential units of information, divided by total words $\times$ 100

Source: From "Informational Content in the Discourse of Patients with Alzheimer's Disease and Patients with Right Hemisphere Damage," by L. R. Cherney and G. J. Canter, 1993, in *Clinical Aphasiology, 21,* 123–134. Copyright, 1993, by Pro-Ed. Adapted with permission.

Appendix 8

CONCEPTS GENERATED BY NBD AND RHD ADULTS FOR FIGURES 6–1, 6–2, and 6–3 and FIGURES 8–4 and 8–5

Figure 6–1:

1. *Waiting room* (hospital, doctor's office) (76% vs 27%)
2. *Bandage on man's head* (59% vs 36%)
3. *The boy is scared* (worried, tense, concerned) (48% vs 14%)
4. *They are waiting* (41% vs 32%)
5. *Sitting on a bench* (couch, pew) (3% vs 23%)

Figure 6–2:

1. *Thanksgiving* (96% vs 73%)
2. *Turkey* (93% vs 68%)
3. *Mother* (grandmother) (73% vs 56%)
4. *Father* (grandfather) (48% vs 32%)
5. *Serving* (bringing in) *the turkey* (55% vs 31%)
6. *Everybody happy* (laughing, having a good time) (38% vs 14%)

Figure 6–3:

1. *Young boy* (young man, boy) (72% vs 18%)
2. *Going to college* (university, school) (76% vs 32%)
3. *Dog looks sad* (leaning on him, saying good-by; missing the boy; doesn't want him to go) (80% vs 4.5%)
4. *Dog*—without reference to position or emotion (7% vs 69%)
6. *Father* (grandfather) (55% vs 32%)
7. *Waiting for a train* (bus; at the station) (41% vs 0%)
8. *Father* (grandfather) *looks sad* (anxious; depressed) (31% vs 0%)
9. *Sitting on the running board* (24% vs 32%)

Figure 8–4:

1. *Family going to* (getting ready for) *church* (83% vs 59%)
2. *Father* (man) *reading the paper* (86% vs 73%)
3. *Family* (mother and children) (66% vs 68%)
4. *Father* (husband) (69% vs 50%)
5. *Father not dressed* (in pajamas) (41% vs 9%)
6. *Father guilty* (hiding, slouching, scrunched down) (38% vs 9%)
7. *Family ignoring him* (21% vs 0%)

Figure 8–5:

1. *Little girl* (young girl, child) (59% vs 45%)
2. *Looking at* (admiring) *herself in the mirror* (assessing her appearance) (66% vs 36%)
3. *Using make-up* (fixing herself up; fixing her hair) (62% vs 23%)
4. *Picture of a woman* (movie star) *on her lap* (55% vs 18%)

5. *Trying to emulate picture* (wondering if she'll look like the picture) (wondering what she'll look like when she grows up) (59% vs 23%)
6. *Has a doll* (has cast doll aside) (70% vs 5%)
7. *Girl trying to* (wants to be; playing at) *look grown up* (31% vs 9%)

Note: Each concept is followed by percentages in parentheses representing the percentage of NBD subjects who produced the concept followed by the percentage of RHD patients who did so (Myers & Brookshire, 1992).

Appendix 9

SAMPLE OPEN-ENDED QUESTION WITH A RESPONSE FROM AN NBD ADULT AND FROM A PATIENT WITH RHD

Question: Should we have tighter gun control laws?

NBD Response: Yes, I believe we should. You read all the time that more and more murders are being committed every day and I can't help but feel that that's because anyone can get a gun. You just have to walk into a store and take out a license. It's horrifying. They say most murders or a lot of them are due to domestic violence. And if there wasn't a gun around people wouldn't be able to use it. And what about these drug-crazed drug people and dealers? People have to have guns for protection in their homes, but only to protect themselves from people who can get guns so easily.

RHD Response: Gun laws. Yeah, all that stuff. There are a lot of guns out there. You use a gun—well, I use a gun to hunt. Now, there'd be a lot of sorry hunters if you couldn't have guns. We used to hunt in the fall, ducks mostly. Sometimes deer. We'd get one every so often but mostly we'd just sit and talk, you know. I don't know. Once we heard a prowler in our camp—turned out to be a hungry bear, looking for our food which was up in a tree because that's where you put it if you are smart. Then we thought maybe we weren't so smart because the bear might be so hungry that he'd want to eat us—but he just went off and that was the end of it right there. We had our guns, but never used them on the bear. But we were right glad we had them, you know.

Appendix 10

PRAGMATIC RATING SCALES

PRAGMATIC PROTOCOL
Prutting, C. A., & Kirchner, D. M. (1987). A Clinical Appraisal of the Pragmatic Aspects of Language. *Journal of Speech and Hearing Disorders, 52,* 105–119.

AREAS ADDRESSED INCLUDE:

1. *Verbal Aspects:*
   - Speech acts (2 areas)
   - Topic (4 areas)
   - Turn taking (9 areas)
   - Lexical selection: use across speech acts
       Specificity/accuracy
       Cohesion
   - Stylistic Variations (varying communicative style)
2. *Paralinguistic Aspects:*
   - Intelligibility and prosodics (5 areas)
   - Nonverbal aspects
   - Kinesics and proxemics (7 areas)

PROFILE OF COMMUNICATIVE APPROPRIATENESS
Penn, C. (1988). The Profiling of Syntax and Pragmatics in Aphasia. *Clinical Linguistics and Phonetics, 2,* 179–208.

AREAS ADDRESSED INCLUDE:

1. *Response to Interlocutor (6 areas)*
2. *Control of Semantic Content (7 areas)*
3. *Cohesion (8 areas)*
4. *Fluency (8 areas)*
5. *Sociolinguistic Sensitivity (10 areas)*
6. *Nonverbal Communication*
7. *Vocal Aspects (prosody—5 areas)*
8. *Nonverbal Aspects (6 areas)*

DISCOURSE ABILITIES PROFILE
Terrell, B., & Ripich, D. (1989). Discourse Competence as a Variable in Intervention. *Seminars in Speech and Language: Aphasia and Pragmatics, 10,* 282–297.

AREAS ADDRESSED INCLUDE:

1. *Narrative Discourse:* abstract; setting; episode
2. *Procedural Discourse:* (fixing toast and jelly)
   - Essential steps
   - Target step: put jelly on
   - Optional steps

3. *General Discourse Rating*
   ▶ Paralinguistic behavior (prosody)
   ▶ Nonlinguistic behavior (eye contact, gesture)
   ▶ Coherence (use of pronouns, articles, ellipses)
4. *Spontaneous Conversation*
   ▶ Turn-taking skills; topic skills; conversational repair; speech acts

Appendix 11

PUBLISHED TESTS OF NEGLECT

VERBAL AND NONVERBAL CANCELLATION TEST
Weintraub, S., & Mesulam, M-M. (1985)

▶ Packet of standardized cancellation tests
▶ Structured and unstructured verbal and nonverbal stimuli
▶ Available from: F. A. Davis, Philadelphia
                   404–420 N. 2nd Street
                   Philadelphia, PA 19123

THE BEHAVIORAL INATTENTION TEST
Wilson, B., Cockburn, J., & Halligan, P. (1987)

▶ Variety of abstract and functional tasks
▶ Standardized

▶ **Tasks include:**

Cancellation tasks   Telephone Dialing

Figure and shape copying   Reading a Menu

Line bisection   Coin Sorting

Representational drawing   Writing: copying

Picture scanning (photos of meal, toiletries, etc.)   Map Navigation

Card sorting

▶ Available from: Northern Speech Services, Inc.
                   117 North Elm Street, PO Box 1247
                   Gaylord, MI 49735

TEST OF VISUAL FIELD ATTENTION
CoolSpring Software

▶ Computerized presentation and scoring
▶ Press mouse in response to visual stimuli appearing at random locations in one of four quadrants
▶ Reaction time and error rates overall and for each quadrant
▶ Available from: CoolSpring Software
                   4 Moon Maiden Court
                   Walkersville, MD 21793

Appendix 12

EXAMPLE OF IRREGULAR MARGIN READING TASK

One of the worst storms to hit the United States was the Hurricane of 1938 which slammed into the coastline of the northeastern states on September 21st. It left a path of destruction rarely seen since. Lacking the sophisticated instruments of today, the National Weather Service failed to properly assess its strength or its course, and it hit without warning. Not only was it stronger than most hurricanes, the damp wet conditions further inland helped turn the hurricane on an inland course. It destroyed 153 of the 179 houses in West Hampton, Long Island. It crashed into Connecticut and Rhode Island. A storm wave of 100 feet broke near City Hall in Providence and left the downtown under 13 feet of water. Ocean spray left a salt residue on windows as far away as Vermont. At least 700 people died and 63,000 houses were destroyed along with trees, factories, and other property in that terrible storm.

Scoring: count number of words omitted.

Source: Passage by P. S. Myers.

Appendix 13

EXAMPLES OF PUBLISHED MEASURES OF ATTENTION

TEST OF EVERYDAY ATTENTION
Robertson, I., Ward, T., Ridgeway, V., & Nimmo-Smith, I.
Thames Valley Test Company (1994)

▶ Assesses: selective and sustained attention and alternating attention
▶ Standardized

Tasks include:

1. *Map Search*
   a. Timed—find symbols on map
   b. Selective attention
   c. Loaded on same factors as Stroop task

2. *Elevator Counting*
   d. Establish floor by counting tones
   e. Sustained attention

3. *Elevator Counting with Distraction*
   a. Count low, ignore high tones
   b. Selective and sustained attention

4. *Visual Elevator*
   a. Counting up and down following a series of visually presented floors
   b. Attention switching (flexibility)
   c. Loaded on same factors as Wisconsin Card Sort Test

5. *Auditory Elevator with Reversal*
   a. Same as subtest 4, but auditory
   b. Flexibility

6. *Telephone Search*
   a. Look for key symbols while searching entries in a simulated classified phone directory
   b. Selective

7. *Telephone Search: Dual Task*
   a. Search directory while counting strings of tones
   b. Divided attention

8. *Lottery*
   a. Listen for winning numbers ending in "55"
   b. Sustained attention
   c. Loaded on same factor as elevator counting

▶ Available from: Northern Speech Services
117 North Elm Street
P.O. Box 1247
Gaylord, MI 49735

STROOP TASK
Stroop, J. R. (1935)

▶ Tests selective attention and vigilance
▶ Original Article: Stroop, J. R. (1935). Studies of Interference in Serial Verbal Reactions. *Journal of Experimental Psychology, 18,* 643–662.
▶ Also available in published form as:

THE STROOP NEUROPSYCHOLOGICAL SCREENING TEST (SNST)
Trennerry, M. R., Crosson, B., DeBoe, J., & Leber, W. R.

Tasks: (1) Color Task—112 items
(2) Color-Word task 112 items

▶ Time: 5 minutes
▶ Standardized through age 79 years
▶ Available from: Psychological Assessment Resources, Inc.
Box 998
Odessa, FL 33556

TRAIL MAKING TEST
Reitan, R. M., 1958; Reitan, R. M., & Wolfson, D., 1985
Part of Halstead-Reitan Neuropsychological Test Battery

▶ Tests alternating attention
▶ Available from: Neuropsychology Press
Tucson, AZ

COMPUTERIZED TESTS OF ATTENTION

AUDITORY REACTION STIMULUS DISCRIMINATION
VISUAL REACTION STIMULUS DISCRIMINATION

▶ Both tests measure selective attention and inhibition of responses
▶ Available from Psychological Software Services

CALCAP COMPUTERIZED REACTION TIME
Satz, P., & Miller, E.

▶ Assesses reaction time using MS-DOS or compatible computers
▶ Assesses speed and accuracy for simple and choice RT's to visual scanning, discrimination, and divided attention
▶ Standardized on 600 subjects
▶ Available from: Norland Software
             P.O. Box 84499
             Los Angeles, CA 90073-0499

CONNERS' CONTINUOUS PERFORMANCE TEST COMPUTER PROGRAM
Connors, K.

▶ Reaction times to appearance of letters on screen
▶ Presents extensive data summary in graphic and tabular form
▶ Available from: Psychological Corporation
             555 Academic Court
             San Antonio, Texas 78204
             1-800-211-8378

PACED AUDITORY SERIAL ATTENTION TEST

▶ Computerized version of the PASAT (Gronwall, 1977)
▶ Tests RT, focused attention, and vigilance
▶ Data presented in graphic and tabular formats
▶ User can vary pacing and test duration
▶ Available from: Psychological Corporation
             555 Academic Court
             San Antonio, Texas 78204
             1-800-211-8378

REACT (Reaction Time Programs)

▶ Computerized reaction time tasks
▶ Available from Life Science Associates

VIGIL CONTINUOUS PERFORMANCE TEST (PC Software)

◗ Standardized ages 6–65
◗ Short—8 minutes
◗ PC-based version of the Continuous Performance Test
◗ Vigilance and Sustained Attention
◗ Computerized presentation and scoring
◗ User can modify timing, stimulus complexity, and clarity
◗ Standardized: ages 6–90 years
◗ Available from: Psychological Corporation
                    555 Academic Court
                    San Antonio, Texas 78204
                    1-800-211-8378

Appendix 14

INFORMAL MEASURES OF PROSODIC PERFORMANCE

COMPREHENSION

1. *Identify Emotional Prosody in Sentences*

   a. Task: determine the emotional tone of spoken sentences through prosodic contour

   b. Stimuli: 3 to 5 word sentences, neutral in content, spoken with an emotional overlay (e.g., happy, sad, angry prosodic contour)

   c. Response: point to one of three emotions with which the sentence is produced

   d. Scoring: plus-minus

2. *Identify Emphatic Stress: Compound Nouns Versus Noun Phrases*

   a. Task: discriminate between compound nouns and noun phrases through stress

   b. Stimuli: noun or noun phrase spoken by the examiner

   b. Response: point to one of two printed words representing the target

   c. Scoring: plus-minus

3. *Identify Emphatic Stress: Sentences*

   a. Task: identify stressed words in spoken sentences

   b. Stimuli: Simple 3 to 5 word sentences read aloud by the examiner

   c. Response: point to the stressed word on a printed version of the stimulus sentence

   d. Scoring: plus-minus

4. *Distinguish Sentence Types: Interrogative Versus Declarative*

   a. Task: use prosodic contour to identify sentence type

   b. Stimuli: sentence pairs of 3 to 4 words spoken by the examiner as either a question or a declarative

   c. Response: Identify sentence type by pointing to one of two printed choices Specifying either a question or a declarative

   d. Scoring: plus-minus

PRODUCTION

1. *Imitate Emotional Prosody in Sentences*

   a. Task: measure ability to imitate the emotional contour of spoken sentences

   b. Stimuli: neutral sentences spoken by the examiner with emotional prosodic overlay indicating mood: happy, sad, angry

   c.   Response: repeat sentence and imitate emotional tone (tape recorded)

   d.   Scoring 1: perceptual judgment; Rating scale of 4 points or more:

Normal	Somewhat Attenuated	Attenuated	Very Attenuated
4	3	2	1

   e.   Scoring 2: several listeners identify the emotion conveyed in the patient's production

2. *Produce Emphatic Stress in Sentences*

   a.   Task: measure control over emphatic stress production

   b.   Stimuli: simple 3 to 5 word printed sentences

   c.   Response: Patient stresses an individual word in a printed sentence
                Clinician judges which word was stressed

   d.   Scoring: plus-minus with notation about the prosodic feature(s) used to convey stress by the patient

3. *Distinguish Declaratives From Interrogatives*

   a.   Task: use prosody to convey differences in intonational contour

   b.   Stimuli: simple 3 to 5 word printed sentences

   d.   Response: Patient reads a declarative sentence as either a declarative or as a question
                Clinician judges which pattern the patient has produced

   e.   Scoring: plus-minus

Appendix 15

PUBLISHED MEASURES OF
NONVERBAL EMOTIONAL COMPREHENSION

PROFILE OF NONVERBAL SENSITIVITY (PONS)
Rosenthal, R., Hall, J. A., DiMatteo, M. R., Rogers, P. L., & Archer, D. (1979)
Sensitivity to nonverbal communication: The PONS test.

1. Stimuli: a film containing 220 2-second segments of emotional expressions which are portrayed without context
2. Variables:
   a. Views: 1) facial expressions; 2) body movements; 3) face + body
   b. Emotions: combinations of positive-negative and dominant-submissive
   c. Formats: 1) video alone; 2) audio alone (content-filtered speech); 3) video + audio combinations
4. Task: determine which of two descriptions best fits the depicted segment

   ▶ Standardized on several thousand subjects
   ▶ Available from: Johns Hopkins University Press
                      Baltimore, MD

FLORIDA AFFECT BATTERY
Blonder, L., Bowers, D., & Heilman, K. M.
The test consists of a facial expression set of subtests and a set of prosodic comprehension and discrimination subtests

FACIAL EXPRESSION

▶ Stimuli: photographs of models' faces depicting one of five emotions (happy, sad, angry, frightened, neutral)

▶ Tasks:
1. Discrimination of facial identity: same/different judgments
2. Discrimination of facial emotion: same/different judgments
3. Name the emotion on the face: select from 5 printed emotions that best characterize the facial expression
4. Point to the emotional face: pick the face best representing the emotion named by the examiner
5. Match the emotional faces: match one expression to one of five expressions

PROSODIC PROCESSING

1. Discrimination of neutral prosody: discriminate between interrogatives and declarative sentences
2. Discrimination of emotional prosody: same/different judgments of prosodic contour
3. Name the emotional prosody: match a printed emotion word to the prosodic tone of sentences
4. Match the emotional prosody to the emotional face: choose from three photographed expressions the one that best matches the prosodic contour of a stimulus sentence

5. Match the emotional face to emotional prosody: choose from three recorded sentences the one that best corresponds to a facial expression

▶ Available from: Dawn Bowers, Ph.D.
Department of Neurology
University of Florida
P.O. Box 100236
Gainsville, FL 32610-0236

Further information on this test is available in Blonder et al. (1991).

CHAPTER

Treatment

Treatment of the cognitive and communicative disorders associated with RHD is relatively new, and there are few data demonstrating the efficacy of any given therapy approach. This is an unfortunate state of affairs. Treatment studies are needed not only to help inform us about strategies that do and do not work, but also to help inform theories of the underlying deficits. The ideas and suggestions about management presented in this chapter reflect principles of accepted practices for treating acquired neurologically based communication disorders in general, and they also variously represent: (a) accumulated clinical experience with RHD patients, (b) treatment suggestions that have appeared in the literature on RHD, and (c) treatment ideas that follow logically from research describing RHD cognitive/communicative deficits, and, when possible, from theories about the mechanisms that may underlie those deficits. It should be understood that therapy approaches vary not only with the nature and severity of deficits, but also with time post-onset, presence of additional neurologic deficits and other health problems, personality, patient goals and lifestyle, and premorbid cognitive strengths and weaknesses.

TREATMENT APPROACHES

Two major treatment approaches, *task-oriented* and *process-oriented*, are used to improve the communication skills of patients with brain damage, regardless of side of lesion (Table 9–1). Both approaches are oriented toward reducing disability or handicap, but in different ways.

Task-oriented approaches are geared toward helping the patient improve performance on a

specific activity. They address specific disabilities and generally focus on symptoms, rather than on underlying processes, even though various processes are addressed in the course of training the patient to a task. Task-oriented treatments are often called "functional" because they seek to improve a specific function in the patient's daily life (e.g., calling an emergency number for help).

Process-oriented approaches address impairments rather than disabilities, and focus on the presumed underlying cause, rather than symptoms. By so doing, they attempt to reduce the impairment(s) that have led to disabilities. Process-oriented strategies typically address a number of functions indirectly and simultaneously. In theory, they have a greater potential for generalization than do task-oriented techniques.

Clinicians typically incorporate some combination of task-oriented and process-oriented strategies in treating patients with neurological speech and language impairments. The two approaches are reviewed briefly below as they apply to RHD patients.

Task-Oriented Therapy

Task-oriented treatment, designed to improve performance on a given task, is by nature highly individualized to the patient.

TABLE 9–1. Treatment approaches for acquired neurologic communication disorders.

Approach	Advantages (A); Disadvantages (D)
Task-Oriented	
▸ Teaches a specific task for immediate functional gain	A: Addresses immediate functional needs of the patient. Rationale easily understood by patients and others
	D: Addresses symptoms not cause, often with poor generalization to other skills
Process-Oriented	
▸ Uses intact processes to compensate for ones that are impaired	A: Addresses cause, not symptoms, with improved potential for generalization
▸ Stimulates recovery of impaired processes	D: May not appear to have immediate applicability to daily activities

It consists of re-training specific job skills or some aspect of self-care or social interaction, usually by teaching a new strategy for accomplishing the activity. Examples include tasks such as balancing a checkbook, reading a menu, using the phone book, preparing a document for work, and using a calculator or copy machine. These types of tasks are designed to meet some immediate need of the patient via compensation and often are "trained" through the efforts of a team of rehabilitation professionals. For example, through an analysis of the cognitive and physical demands of wheelchair transfer, the combined efforts of a physical therapist, occupational therapist, and speech-language pathologist enabled a RHD patient to use a written guide for making transfers to and from his wheelchair. Their effort succeeded in improving his independence except when he could not locate the written instructions, which was often.

When they are successful, these "functional" treatment approaches have the advantage of being of immediate benefit to the patient's quality of life, easy to explain to family members and other professionals, and easy to justify to reimbursement sources interested in functional outcomes. The disadvantage is that, because symptoms are treated rather than underlying processes, improvement, treatment rarely, if ever, generalizes to other tasks. Ultimately, this may result in limited overall improvement and inefficient use of rehabilitation resources. For example, in the case mentioned above, wheelchair transfers initially were broken down into 25 steps and later reduced to 15. It took many lengthy sessions of practice for the patient to learn to use the written guide and complete the program. It is likely that most of the patient's problems with transfers were the result of neglect. To illustrate, he would forget to put on his left-wheel brake or fail to use his left arm for balance. Because he never internalized the written instructions, he was completely dependent on them. Because he had neglect, he had trouble scanning the environment for the instructions when they were not immediately in view (i.e., in right hemispace). By addressing neglect, the underlying cause of the disability, rather than the symptom (poor transfers), treatment might have met with more success, and reduced neglect also may have led to improvement in other "functional" activities. Thus, although functional tasks have good superficial face validity, they may not always lead to optimal outcomes. *Functional tasks should play a role in treatment but they should not be the only focus of treatment for most patients.*

Process-Oriented Therapy

Process-oriented therapies address processes and mechanisms underlying observed disabilities. For that very reason, they must rely on theories or assumptions about the nature of the disturbed processes. They include techniques that help the patient *compensate* for impairments and those that help *facilitate recovery of function* (i.e., *reduce impairment*).

Compensation Techniques

Process-oriented compensation techniques provide a means of working around deficits by using intact processes to overcome impaired processes. Use of compensation techniques typically occurs because (a) the processes underlying a given disability are not known, (b) the underlying processes are identified but the patient is not likely to recover them, or (c) the underlying processes are considered too complex to address in a given patient.

Unlike the compensation techniques provided in task-oriented therapy, compensation in process-oriented therapy usually is not focused on a specific task in a specific situation, but rather on compensating for a process that may be impaired *across skills.* For example, impairments in developing a macrostructure are fundamental to many of the discourse deficits identified in Chapter 6. Problems in automatic integration might be identified as one of the processes underlying reduced macrostructure and inference generation in general. A process-oriented compensation technique might include training the use of a new strategy that takes advantage of intact verbal and sequential skills to circumvent problems in automatic integration (e.g., listing the key features in a pictured scene and verbally reviewing their possible relationships to one another). Compensation for the disordered process may then generalize to other discourse situations calling for integration and inference generation.

Facilitation Techniques

Facilitation techniques attempt to facilitate the *recovery* of processes that are impaired, as opposed to *compensating* for them. For example, to facilitate recovery of inference abilities, one might work directly on selective attention if one believes it plays a significant role in the impairment. Or one might work to improve integration in simple nonverbal patterns or puzzles.

Facilitating recovery typically is conducted in a program of systematic and controlled stimulation of the processes that are impaired, but not lost, in the hopes that repeated stimulation will engender recovery. Facilitation techniques sometimes are called "stimulation therapy" after Hildred Schuell (Schuell, Jenkins, & Jimnez-Pabn, 1964) who developed a method for stimulating recovery of disordered linguistic processes for aphasic patients (see Duffy, 1994, for a review of stimulation approaches to aphasia). General attributes of the method are familiar to most clinicians, and they are summarized in Table 9–2. *Stimulation* is the operative word in stimulation therapy, under the assumption that the more a process is stimulated, the better the chance for its recovery. However, the process must be stimulated at a level that is adequate for each stimulus to elicit a response. Patients must be given response opportunities in which they will be successful most of the time. For that reason, error rates are kept low. Responses are elicited through drills in which feedback is provided about re-

TABLE 9–2. Features of Schuell's stimulation method for facilitating recovery of function.

1. Manipulate stimulus dimensions to enable patients to make a maximal response.
2. Elicit responses through intensive and systematic stimulation.
3. Elicit responses; do not force them.
4. Error rates should not exceed 20%.
5. Feedback is given; lengthy explanations are avoided.

sponse adequacy, but explaining the nature of errors is avoided. Rather than correcting errors, clinicians provide cues to help elicit an accurate response. Cues should be consistent and organized into a hierarchy from those that provide the least amount of information to those that provide the most. Cueing hierarchies are used in task-oriented and process-oriented compensation therapies, as well as in facilitation techniques. Cues are not always used. For example, one might treat impaired vigilance using a computerized reaction-time program in which the focus is on providing opportunities for vigilant attention and in which feedback is provided only at the end of the task.

Summary

Although task-oriented and process-oriented therapy can be distinguished from one another, there are many situations in which the two approaches converge. For example, in one case, it was determined that a patient's prosodic production deficits were the result of impaired pitch perception, but his pitch perception was resistant to treatment. The patient was then trained to compensate for the underlying impaired process (e.g., pitch perception) and the impaired skill (prosody) by using words rather than prosodic contour to signal his emotional state (e.g., "I am very happy," or "That makes me sick"). Family members were counseled to use the same strategy when expressing their emotions to the patient. The treatment can be considered task-oriented in that it worked directly on and may have immediately improved the patient's functional communication. It also can be considered a process-oriented compensation approach because it identified, attempted to treat, and then circumvented an impaired process.

As the term is currently used, "functional" has come to refer to therapy tasks with immediate, direct, and readily observable applicability (i.e., task-oriented). In the face of pressure for therapy to be "functional," it is important for clinicians to remember that *all* legitimate tasks are *functional* in the sense that they are oriented toward improving the patient's ability to function in the world. Because they address underlying mechanisms, process-oriented approaches work on functional skills less directly, and may seem to have less immediate utility. However, clinicians should not forget the crucial importance of understanding the *processes* that underlie communication, ways in which those *processes* can break down, and ways in which those *processes* can be managed. At the same time, clinicians should keep in mind that the value of a given approach, either task- or process-oriented, rests on its functional merits. Ultimately, improvement in any treatment program must translate into improvement in cognitive and communicative skills that are important in the daily life of the patient.

The remainder of this chapter reviews *selected* tasks that are representative of a process-oriented approach to the management of RHD communication disorders. It is not an exhaustive review. For the most part, these representative tasks reflect theories about the impaired processes that were discussed in Chapters 2 through 7. Task-oriented approaches will not be discussed further because they are considered unique to a given patient and situation. When appropriate, the reader will be referred to tasks and scoring methods presented in Chapter 8. Additional sources of treatment tasks for RHD patients can be found in Halper et al. (1996) and Tompkins (1995) as well as in workbooks and programs for treatment of cognitive and attentional deficits (see for example Helm-Estabrooks, 1995, and Sohlberg & Mateer, 1986). It is hoped that the treatment methods presented in this chapter will inspire clinicians to develop additional tasks based on their understanding of processes underlying the communication deficits of the patients they serve.

TREATMENT OF DEFICITS IN ATTENTION

As stated in Chapter 3, attention can be considered: (a) fundamental to cognitive function, (b) somewhat lateralized to the RH, and (c) an underlying explanatory mechanism for many of the discourse deficits associated with RHD. RHD patients may have reduced arousal, vigilance, maintenance of attention, and/or selective attention. When present, these problems play a role in almost every aspect of communicative performance, from following the twists and turns of conversational speech, to drawing and revising inferences, and interpreting ambiguous material. Thus, treating disorders of attention directly can be considered one means of indirectly facilitating improvement in cognitive and communicative performance. That is, attention is the process, and communication is the skill.

Most attention tasks tap more than one attentional operation. For example, all attention tasks enlist the arousal system and require maintenance of attention. Most tasks for selective attention tax vigilance as well. Table 9–3 contains a list of selected tasks that address attention deficits. The primary targeted attentional operation is listed for each task with the understanding that each task requires a certain level of arousal, vigilance, and sustained attention.

There are a few published materials for improving attention in brain-injured adults.

TABLE 9–3. Selected tasks for treating deficits in attention.

Task	Targeted Attentional Process
Simple Reaction Time Tasks	Arousal and sustained attention
Complex Reaction Time Tasks	Arousal, vigilance, and sustained attention
Serial Tasks: Responding to targets embedded in a series of distractors	Selective attention, vigilance
Visual Matching Tasks	Selective attention
Stroop-Type Tasks	Vigilance, selective attention
Cancellation Tasks	Selective attention, vigilance
Alternating responses during cancellation or serial tasks	Selective attention, flexibility, vigilance

Dual Tasks
  (a) Performing two tasks simultaneously
  (b) Attending to more than one type of information within a task
	Sustained attention, flexibility

For example, *Attention Process Training* (APT) (Sohlberg & Mateer, 1986) is a systematic, hierarchical attention training program, often used with adults with traumatic head injury, but applicable to patients with focal RHD as well. It addresses sustained, selective, alternating, and divided attention in the visual and auditory modalities. In addition, there are a number of published computer programs that use a reaction time format for training vigilance and orienting (for example, see those listed in Chapter 8, Appendix 13).

The attention tasks reviewed here are meant to facilitate recovery of function, and they should be conducted using the principles of stimulation therapy previously described. It is important to remember that treatment of attention deficits, particularly in patients with focal versus diffuse brain damage, is in its infancy. There are no data available on the efficacy of such treatment techniques for RHD patients. A few studies have addressed treatment outcomes following attention training in head-injury patients (Ponsford & Kinsella, 1988; Sohlberg & Mateer, 1987; Wood, 1987), with conflicting results, but more needs to be learned about the gener-

alization of such training. As Whyte (1992) points out, however, "There are many treatments that have been shown to have *some* benefit for *some* patients in *some* tasks" (p. 1102). Based on individual patient evaluations, clinicians must decide which patients might benefit from attention training and which tasks seem best suited to the patient's needs.

Arousal and Vigilance Tasks

Many RHD patients, particularly those with neglect, are hypoaroused. That is, they may be less alert, less responsive, and less aroused than normal. They also may be less vigilant in that they have difficulty sustaining tonic readiness to respond. Behavioral (versus pharmacological) interventions for improving arousal (i.e., the automatic readiness to respond) and vigilance (i.e., the voluntary readiness to respond) typically take the form of reaction time (RT) tasks in which the patient must respond as fast as possible to the appearance of a target stimulus. The stimulus may be auditory or visual, and the response is usually manual (e.g., pressing the space bar on a computer keyboard). Typically, these tasks are presented in a computerized format that controls stimulus presentation and records and scores reaction times (see Chapter 8, Appendix 13). Many computerized RT programs can be adjusted for task duration and inter-stimulus interval, thus allowing adjustments of stimulus presentation to fit individual patient needs and goals. Varying the inter-stimulus interval, for example, taxes vigilance because the patient cannot be certain of the duration of time between one stimulus and the next.

RT tasks are consistent with the stimulation method in that stimuli are manipulated in such a way as to give patients maximal opportunities to respond at or just above their thresholds for adequate performance. It is assumed that continued practice stimulates arousal and vigilance, thereby facilitating their recovery. The critical assumption is that there will be concomitant improvement in cognitive and, hence, communicative, processes. An advantage of computerized RT programs is that, once trained to the nature of the task, patients can work on them independently, freeing the clinician to work with them on other aspects of communication.

Sustained Attention Tasks

RHD patients also may have problems sustaining attention which can interfere with their ability to maintain an appropriate level of cognitive effort over time and to attend to lengthy communicative events. Computerized RT programs, by their very nature, tax attentional maintenance. As stated in Chapter 3, the performance of RHD patients, unlike those with LHD, tends to deteriorate rather than improve over time. Clinicians can adjust the duration of RT tasks in light of patient performance. The inter-stimulus intervals also can be manipulated to increase or decrease task difficulty. For example, because their attention tends to drift, the performance of RHD patients with sustained attention problems may worsen as the interval between stimuli is lengthened.

Non-computerized sustained attention tasks also can be designed to encourage sustained attention in situations requiring minimal cognitive effort. Tasks may include: (a) a series of simple yes/no questions, (b) a series of simple addition problems, or (c) sorting a series of colored geometric forms by a single feature (color or shape). Reduced cognitive demands in such tasks helps to focus the treatment on the ability simply to maintain attention over periods of time.

Selective Attention Tasks

Selective attention deficits can be treated in visual or auditory tasks in which the patient must select target stimuli from among a series of targets and foils (i.e., screen out distractors when responding to targets). Auditory tasks might take the form of responding with a finger tap to the appearance of a target number in a series of verbally presented numbers, or selecting a target word in a series of words read aloud by the clinician. Visual matching tasks or cancellation tasks that require searching for targets embedded in a set of foils may also be used. Level of difficulty can be manipulated by varying the number and the similarity of the foils to the target (see Chapter 8).

It is important to remember that neglect can interfere in visual selective attention tasks. Thus, response choices should be placed in the patient's right hemispace and, when possible (e.g., in matching tasks), choices should be vertically arranged. These manipulations will not, however, completely circumvent neglect because information on the left of a single stimulus may be neglected, regardless of the hemispace location of the stimulus (see Chapter 2 and Figure 2–9). The clinician should evaluate results carefully to determine if neglect is playing a role in the patient's response patterns (e.g., all or most of the responses are rightward stimuli).

Stroop tasks (See Chapter 3 and Chapter 8, Appendix 13) are another method of addressing selective attention deficits because patients must inhibit a habitual response (e.g., reading) in favor of the target response (e.g., naming ink color). Other Stroop-type tasks include switching between reading words to indicating their size in an array of words printed in large and small type faces (Tompkins, 1995).

Alternating attention tasks in which response demands change midway through a task also may be used to improve inhibition, selective attention, and cognitive flexibility. Examples include: (a) shifting the target response from shape to color midway through a cancellation task, (b) shifting targets from shape to color or size in a pointing task, (c) shifting the target number midway through a number series task; and (d) shifting the target response midway through a Stroop-type task. Halper et al. (1996) suggested a number of alternating attention tasks in which targets in a string of letters shift from upper to lower case letters and from vowels to consonants, and targets in a string of words shift from phonemic to semantic to visual properties.

Divided Attention Tasks

Requiring patients to divide attention between two tasks is another means of treating attention. Examples of these "dual tasks" include asking the patient to: (a) count out loud while completing a cancellation task, (b) sort coins while tapping their foot whenever an auditory stimulus is presented, and (c) say the alphabet while connecting dots. Finally, patients may be required to attend to more than one type of information within a task such as finding instances of a given letter *and* a given number in a cancellation task.

TREATMENT OF NEGLECT

A central theme running through this book has been that the presence of neglect can have negative consequences for cognitive and communicative performance because it seems to represent part of a broad atten-

tional impairment (see Chapters 2 and 6). Neglect can narrow the focus of spatial *and* nonspatial attention and interfere with selective attention. It can reduce sensitivity to important verbal information during communicative interaction. As an impairment in environmental scanning, it also may reduce sensitivity to nonverbal information important to the emotional, pragmatic, and social aspects of communication. Because it may reduce attentional resources, it also may interfere in complex activities such as inference generation and revision. It appears to influence the integration of abstract verbal as well as visual material. As discussed in Chapter 6, RHD patients with severe neglect may have more difficulty than those with mild or no neglect in various discourse tasks such as generating concepts, inferences, and macrostructures for pictured scenes and stories.

The most common methods of managing neglect are compensatory strategies that reduce the effects of neglect in spatial scanning. Less commonly used, but probably more effective, are tasks that help stimulate leftward scanning independent of external cues or devices.

Compensatory Strategies for Neglect

Compensatory strategies used to circumvent neglect include verbal, visual, and tactile reminders to look to the left (Table 9–4), and restructuring the environment. The use of auditory, visual, and tactile cues for compensation may be helpful in some circumstances, but rarely improve independent performance.

Verbal Cues

Verbal reminders to look to the left can be given during any type of reading or leftward search task. For example, the clinician can say "go left" each time the patient reaches the end of a line of text as a reminder to search for the far left margin of

TABLE 9–4. Compensatory strategies for RHD patients with neglect.

Strategy	Examples
Verbal reminders to look to the left	Patients are told to look to the left during therapy tasks and daily activities
Salient visual and tactile cues used to draw attention toward the left	A red line or velcro strip at the left margin of printed texts or other materials used in the daily life of the patient
Restructuring the environment	Items important for self-care and independence are placed to the right side of the patient. Conversational partners are encouraged to stand on the right side of the patient

the next line. Verbal reminders to look to the left are usually effective only as long as they continue to be presented. Patients generally fail to internalize these reminders even though they can state with certainty that they "must remember to look to the left." That is, their intellectual understanding rarely translates into independent action that reflects that understanding.

Visual and Tactile Cues

A colored line or other salient marker such as a velcro strip can be placed on the left margin of printed text, or the left side of a dinner tray or plate, to draw attention to the left. Patients can be trained to find the cue visually or manually before and during an activity such as reading or eating. However, because patients with neglect rarely look into leftward space on their own, they may not look for or find the leftward cue independently, no matter how salient it is. That is, their attention must be drawn toward the left in the first place.

Anchors

Anchors take the form of letters or numbers printed at the right and left ends of lines of text, at the edges of a field of items to be canceled, or at the right and left ends

of a line to be bisected. The patient periodically is told to read the anchor letters or numbers before proceeding with the task in the hope that finding the anchors will help move attention to the left for the next part of the task.

Restructuring the Environment

Right-Sided Placement

This compensation strategy is used to help patients gain or maintain some independence in daily activities. Important items like the phone, water pitcher, and call button can be placed in right hemispace. Visitors are encouraged to stand on the patient's right during conversation. These measures may be helpful in the early postonset phase before the patient is ready to engage in therapy or respond to cues.

Left-Sided Placement

This is less of a compensation strategy and more of a facilitation technique. It is included here because it also involves restructuring the environment. As the patient begins a course of therapy to increase leftward attentional scanning, important objects are placed on the left and communicative partners stand to the left of the patient to encourage carry-over from therapy into daily life under the assumption that the more the patient must look to the left, the more the damaged directional attention network will be stimulated.

Facilitating Recovery From Neglect

Methods of facilitating recovery from neglect include medical and behavioral treatments. The medical treatments represent some of the non-behavioral interventions that have attempted to alleviate neglect. Behavioral techniques focus on stimulating leftward orienting of attention through search and scanning tasks *in the absence of external reminders and cues.* To date only a few reports in the literature have documented the effectiveness of behavioral interventions. The reported results of search tasks is promising but incomplete because there has been little consistency in the types of training and types of patients studied (e.g., the locus and nature of lesions; severity and type of neglect). Diller and Weinberg and their colleagues found some amelioration of neglect in some patients using a systematic program of cueing and compensation tasks (Diller & Weinberg, 1977; Weinberg et al., 1976, 1979). Robertson, Gray, Pentland, and Waite (1989), found little benefit from computerized search and scanning programs, whereas Pizzamiglio et al. (1993) found that a program using a variety of behavioral interventions, including computerized visual scanning tasks, not only increased leftward scanning and attention in functional activities, but also heightened awareness of deficit, improved patient mood, and increased willingness to participate in rehabilitation. More studies are needed on the effect of behavioral intervention on neglect and on the generalization of such training to other tasks. It is likely that some types of training benefit some patients more than others, depending on the type and severity of their neglect symptoms.

Medical Treatments

Pharmacological Treatment

Several studies have found that apomorphine, a dopamine receptor agonist, successfully reduces neglect in animals (Corwin et al., 1986; Marshall & Gotthelf, 1979). Dopamine agonist therapy also has been found to reduce, though not eliminate, neglect in humans. Fleet, Valenstien, Watson, and Heilman, (1987) reported two cases with chronic neglect whose performance on neglect tests improved during a course of bromocriptine. The authors advocated additional studies both with chronic and with more acutely ill patients to test the effectiveness of this pharmacological therapy.

Vestibular Stimulation

Sometimes called caloric stimulation, stimulation of the vestibular system by irrigating the right ear canal with warm water or, more typically, the left ear canal with cold water, has been found to induce a *temporary* reduction in various neglect symptoms, including: (a) personal neglect, (b) extrapersonal neglect (e.g., visual neglect in paper-and-pencil tasks), (c) anosognosia, (d) somatophrenic delusions, and (e) neglect masquerading as hemisensory loss (Cappa, Sterzi, Vallar, & Bisiach, 1987; Rode et al., 1992; Rubens, 1985; Vallar, Bottini, Rusconi, & Sterzi, 1993; Vallar, Sterzi, Bottini, Cappa, & Rusconi, 1990).

There is uncertainty about how vestibular stimulation works to ameliorate neglect (see Vallar et al., 1993, for a theoretical review). Because it evokes nystagmus, it may be that eye movements to the left increase awareness of left visual stimuli. However, it has been found to improve tactile neglect even when subjects were blindfolded (Vallar et al., 1993). Another possibility is that it stimulates general RH activation because the cortical projection of the vestibular system is mostly contralateral. However, neglect also has been reduced by irrigating the right ear with warm water, and irrigating the left ear with warm water can increase symptoms of neglect. Other explanations include alteration of the internal representation of egocentric and extrapersonal space by restoring balance in the bilateral neural processes, including vestibular afferent inputs, that contribute to these representations. Vestibular stimulation has been used to explore various theories about the mechanisms of neglect, and is mentioned here only because it is a known way of temporarily reducing neglect symptoms. However, it is not recommended as a treatment because its effects are so fleeting.

Behavioral Treatments

Behavioral interventions used to facilitate recovery from neglect include techniques and tasks that increase leftward orienting and, theoretically, increase RH activation. Left limb stimulation (described below) may be applied prior to other behavioral stimulation methods. The search tasks discussed encourage spontaneous leftward attentional movement. Some tasks stress voluntary control over attentional shifts to the left. Others foster more automatic leftward movements of attention. All of the tasks foster independent attentional movement without reliance on external cueing.

Left Limb Stimulation

A number of studies have found that voluntary movements or use of the *left hand in left hemispace* reduces neglect in some RHD patients (Halligan & Marshall, 1989; Joanette, Brouchon, Gauthier, & Samson, 1986; Robertson & North, 1992, 1993). The beneficial effects of left limb movements may even occur with movements of the left leg or foot. Passive movements of the left hand and movements of the left hand in right hemispace have little or no effect (Robertson & North, 1993). The effect of active left limb movements in left hemispace has been attributed variously to increased attentional activation in the RH, to a visual cueing effect, and to a motor cueing effect

in cases of motor neglect (Halligan et al., 1991; Robertson & North, 1992). Left limb movements stimulate RH sensorimotor pathways and may thus increase motor and attentional activation and prepare that hemisphere for further action. In some cases, left-sided body movements such as left finger tapping may be a visual and kinesthetic cue that increases awareness and perception of left-sided input. In other cases, use of the left limbs in left hemispace or toward the left edge of left hemispace may stimulate RH motor programs and readiness to respond motorically. In all cases, the approach is most effective if the patient moves his or her left limbs in left, not right, hemispace. However, although performance improves on tests of neglect, it is not certain how long the ameliorative effect of left-sided limb stimulation lasts or how it might translate into daily life, short of having the patient become left-handed. If the basis for improvement of neglect is RH activation, it might be valuable to use left limb movements prior to presenting the patient with neglect tasks. For example, before starting a reading or cancellation task, a patient could be encouraged to trace the left border with the left hand, move their left arm up and down, or tap their left foot during a scanning task conducted with the right hand. This technique may help not only patients with perceptual neglect, but also those with motor neglect. Obviously, it is not appropriate for patients with hemiplegia, unless it is suspected that the hemiplegia is actually neglect masquerading as hemiplegia (see Chapter 2).

Leftward Search Tasks I: Stimulating Unconscious Perception

The theory behind the following tasks is that by manipulating stimulus dimensions in such a way as to *encourage unconscious perception* of left-sided information, attention is more automatically drawn toward the left; this in turn stimulates the leftward orienting and directing of attention. Unconscious perception is the phenomenon in which patients with neglect process left-ward information without conscious awareness of having done so (see Chapter 2).

a. Meaningful Stimuli
1. **Task:** Read sentences and words; Identify objects
2. **Procedure:** Name objects and/or read words and sentences that span the area of neglected and non-neglected space relative to viewer-centered coordinates.
3. **Stimulus Dimensions and Manipulations:** Meaningfulness is a variable that can be manipulated to draw attention leftward automatically or involuntarily (Brunn & Farah, 1991; Kartsounis & Warrington, 1989; Sieroff et al., 1988). Examples of meaningful stimuli are words (versus letter strings) and real objects (versus nonsense forms). To be effective, the clues that give the stimuli unambiguous meaning in this task must be only on the left side of each stimulus so that attention is drawn leftward to disambiguate the stimulus. Figures 9–1 and 9–2 contain examples of left-cue stimuli. In Figure 9–1, objects (A) and (B) encourage leftward scanning. The ax cannot be identified by the blade alone. The handle, to the left, gives the object meaning. Similarly, one must look to the left of midline to disambiguate object (B), an anchor. However, because object C, the telephone, is symmetrical, there are enough clues to the right of midline to identify it. In Figure 9–2, leftward scanning is encouraged in the first sentence because the three words to the right of midline are not meaningful as a phrase or as a sentence. In the second sentence the words to the right of midline make a meaningful sentence, so that leftward scanning is likely to stop at the word "Tom." Similarly compound words such as "steamship," do not encourage leftward scans because the letters to the left of midline spell a word, whereas the letters in the "o o l" in the word "school" have no meaning on their own. Thus, by manipulating the

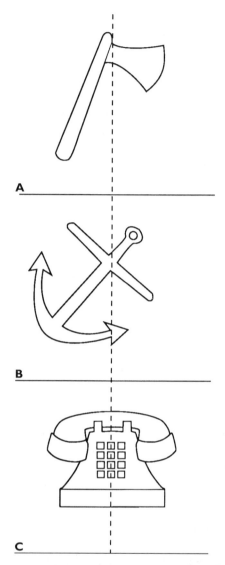

Figure 9–1. Objects A, an ax, and B, an anchor, are examples of object stimuli that encourage leftward search to disambiguate the information to the right of midline. Object C, a telephone, contains enough information to the right of midline to be identified.

placement of cues, and the overall meaningfulness of the stimuli, one may stimulate *internally generated* leftward movement of attention.

(a) Our hats were off to them

(b) She found that Tom was nice.

s c h o o l

s t e a m s h i p

Figure 9–2. Examples of verbal stimuli that encourage leftward search. The words to the right of midline in the sentence (a) and in the letters in the word "school" make no sense, thereby drawing attention further leftward. The words to the right of midline in the sentence (b) and in the word "steamship" make sense, and do not encourage further leftward search.

b. Contiguous Stimuli

1. **Task:** Identify or count printed stimuli
2. **Procedure:** Patients identify objects, presented to the left and right of midline and at varying distances from the midline.
3. **Stimulus Dimensions and Manipulations:** Contiguous stimuli seem to have a greater potential to move attention leftward than do discrete stimuli (Farah et al., 1993; Kartsounis & Warrington,

1989). The hypothesis is that, at some level, patients with neglect are sensitive to the concept of objects, independent of the type of object presented. For example, in a search task, they may attend more to leftward stimuli contained within a border than to leftward stimuli without a border because they perceive the bordered items as an object or whole (Farah et al., 1993) (Figure 9–3). They

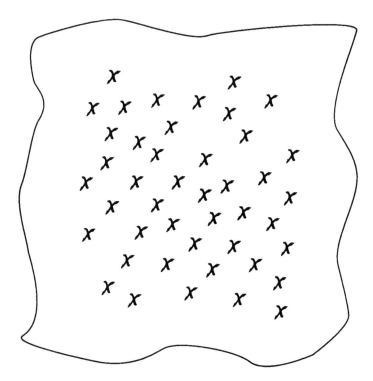

Figure 9–3. Example of a cancellation task enclosed by a border. The border may be perceived by patients as an object whole, thus drawing attention further leftward with less external cueing.

also tend to direct attention further left-ward in contiguous versus discrete stim-uli because contiguous and intersecting figures may be seen as a single object, drawing attention to their entirety. In tasks of this type, patients must point to or count the number of objects in a row. The physical connections between stim-uli can be arranged in a hierarchy of dif-ficulty, starting with sets of intersecting stimuli, moving to ones that are contig-uous, and, finally, to ones that are dis-crete and at increasing distances from one another (Figure 9–4).

c. Interactive Stimuli

1. **Task:** Describe simple scenes containing two or three objects
2. **Procedure:** Patients describe the left and right objects contained in a simple scene.

3. **Stimulus Dimensions and Manipulations:** Stimuli that interact with one another in either abstract or physical ways also may encourage leftward scans. Examples of interactive picture stimuli include situations in which: (a) a person on the right is talking to a person on the left, (b) two people, one on either side of midline, are holding hands, or (c) a person on the right is handing something to a person on the left. In other words, any simple scene in which the character on the right is interacting with the char-acter on the left constitutes interactive stimuli. For example, in a picture of a boy in a tree trying to retrieve a cat lo-cated on a leftward extending branch, the action of reaching suggests some-thing to be reached and so fosters a more or less automatic attentional shift

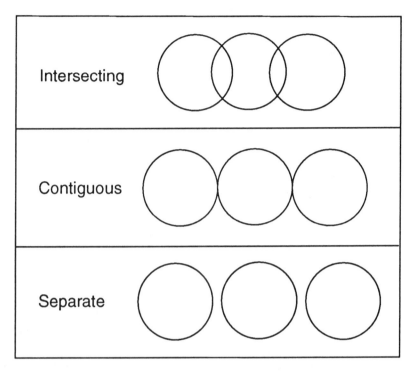

Figure 9–4. Example of stimuli used to improve leftward search. The patient must count or point to the circles in a hierarchy difficulty progressing from trials of intersecting to trials of contiguous to trials of discrete stimuli.

to the left because the boy's action raises the expectation of an event or object to the left. If the boy's hand has made contact with the cat, there is an even greater chance that attention will be drawn to the cat than if his hand is not actually touching it because the two main characters in the scene are then contiguous (i.e., considered as one).

Leftward Search Tasks II: Stimulating Automatic Leftward Movements of Attention

a. **Paper-and-Pencil Cancellation Tasks**
1. **Task:** Cancel (cross-out) instances of a target stimulus in a field of targets and foils
2. **Procedure:** As described in Chapter 8
3. **Stimulus Dimensions and Manipulations:** There are a number of ways to manipulate stimulus characteristics in cancellation tasks to foster leftward at-

tentional shifts and broadening of attentional focus. Clinicians should begin with cancellation tasks in which the patient is successful most of the time, gradually increasing task difficulty so that the processes involved in leftward orienting are stimulated again and again. As noted in Chapter 8, the less crowded the array, and the greater the difference in the physical and abstract characteristics of the stimuli, the more likely it is that patients will shift attention toward leftward targets. Other means of manipulating the stimuli include the structure within and the presence of borders outside the field. Patients tend to make fewer omissions in both right and left hemispace when stimuli are arranged in rows across the page versus in a random array (Weintraub & Mesulam, 1988). A border may increase leftward attentional movement because the border encourages patients to process the field within the frame as a single object (see Figure 9–4). Finally, removing stimuli from the right side of the page by having the patient erase, rather than cancel, targets helps to move attention leftward. In addition, one can alter the right-left balance of targets and foils by making the left hemispace array more dense than that in right hemispace.

b. Computerized Scanning Tasks

1. Task: Find targets when they appear on a computer monitor

2. Procedure: These tasks require patients to make a response (e.g., touch the space bar on the keyboard) each time a new target appears on a computer screen. Target location within and among the four quadrants can be adjusted to increase or decrease task difficulty, as can the interstimulus interval. Responses are scored for accuracy and speed. Feedback on accuracy should be immediate. Cues can be provided in the form of a warning stimulus (e.g., a sound announcing the imminent appearance of the next target) and eventually faded. A variation of this type of task, called Starry Night (Rizzo & Robin, 1990, 1996) requires a response each time a target disappears (versus appears). The number of stimuli in the field and the location of disappearing targets can be systematically controlled.

Leftward Search Tasks III: Stimulating Voluntary Shifts of Attention

The following tasks are meant to stimulate leftward scanning and broadening of attentional focus by encouraging *voluntary* control over areas to be searched. Search tasks are presented in which patients (a) enlist voluntary attention for leftward scans and (b) can easily monitor their performance without external feedback.

a. The Mackisack-Myers Edgeness Task

(Myers, 1997; and Myers & Mackisack,

1990; see also, Halper et al., 1996 for a step-by-step outline of the program).

1. Task: Find specified number of cubes on a four quadrant board

2. Procedure:

(a) *Materials:* A flat board, approximately 8 × 13 inches, divided into quadrants by grooved borders is used as the surface on which colored cubes are placed. Cubes should be approximately 1 inch in size.

(b) *Task:* While the patient is not looking at the board, the clinician places a specific number of cubes in various locations for the patient to find. The patient is then told how many cubes need to be located. Starting with a single cube in the upper right hand grid, a location that should be easy for the patient to find, the task becomes increasingly difficult as more cubes in varying locations are placed on the board. The goal is simply to find the specified number of cubes. The location of the cubes is systematically varied across the four quadrants, with the lower left being the most difficult location. The further to the left, the harder the cubes are to find. A selective attention component can be introduced by adding cubes of different colors as foils (e.g., find 5 target blue cubes in an field of 5 blue and 5 orange cubes), making the task more difficult.

The advantage of this type of task is that patients can monitor their own performance. If three cubes are to be found and only two have been found, the patient knows without being told that he or she must continue to search. If the missing cube is to the left, patients will make *voluntary* movements of attention to the left, thereby stimulating leftward scanning without external cueing. The tactile component helps the patient keep track of the number of cubes. Anecdotally, this task can be a good warm-up task before discourse tasks that require leftward attentional shifts, such as scene interpretation. Possibly by providing opportunities for stimulating internally generated, voluntary shifts of attention not only from left to right, but from narrow to broad, this task and others like it may help facilitate recovery of automatic leftward attentional shifts. Like other search tasks, the assumption is that the more attention is directed toward the left, the more the damaged directed attention network will be stimulated, regardless of whether attentional shifts are voluntary and conscious, or automatic.

b. Right-Left Alternating Tasks

1. **Task:** Find (point to, read) one leftward target for every rightward one
2. **Procedure:** Stimulus arrays are arranged with targets on the left and right in random or structured order. For example, two columns of words to be read aloud can be arranged on the page, one column on the right and one on the left. Each time a word is read from the right column, it must be followed by reading a word from the left column. Other types of tasks include pointing to or canceling objects, numbers, letters, and so on, on the right and left of a central blank area on a page, or picking up objects from the left and right side of a stimulus array. This preprogrammed shift of attention from right to left encourages voluntary control over leftward attentional shifts so as to stimulate the leftward movement of attention.
3. **Stimulus Manipulations:** Stimuli should be consistent with one another (i.e., all numbers, words, letters, objects, etc.) to avoid taxing selective attention.

Reading and Writing

It is assumed that many of the tasks to increase leftward search will indirectly help

patients scan a page when reading and use margins appropriately when writing. In addition, one might use variations of the irregular left margin reading task described in Chapter 8 (see Chapter 8, Appendix 12) for patients with mild neglect in reading as a means of increasing vigilant attention to the left border.

To improve writing, patients can practice with graph paper in which each letter must be printed in a single block on the grid to help them control spacing, reduce upward slant, and make appropriate use of margins.

TREATMENT OF PROSODIC DEFICITS

If a patient has prosodic production or comprehension impairments that are not due to dysarthria, the most effective and immediate intervention is counseling the patient and the family. This compensatory method is recommended, regardless of whether more direct treatments are applied. As noted in Chapter 5, the nature of prosodic impairments secondary to RHD is not well understood and there currently are no data available on the effectiveness of methods to foster recovery of prosodic function or when and for whom these methods might be most facilitatory. The following tasks are based on our understanding of the deficits as presented in Chapter 5 and on the tasks for assessment presented in Chapter 8.

Compensation Strategies

Compensation strategies include: (a) explaining the nature of prosody and its breakdown and (b) providing practice opportunities for compensatory techniques.

Explaining Prosody to Patients and Families

Without resorting to technical terms, clinicians can define prosody as the overall tone of voice one uses to express emotions and attitudes. One can demonstrate the changes in tone using examples that clearly distinguish emotions or attitudes. If the patient has prosodic production problems and a generally flat affect, families usually are already aware of the problem and often say that the patient's voice sounds "tired" or "flat." It helps to have the reasons clarified, particularly to understand that the patient's tone of voice may not reflect their feelings, interest, or attitudes in conversations accurately.

Helping Patients Compensate

RHD patients themselves may or may not be aware that they sound different. Mildly impaired patients often are responsive to the problem once it is defined because they have had a vague sense that they do not sound like themselves. Aside from explanations and demonstrations, the main compensatory technique for production deficits is to encourage patients to label their emotional states for their communicative partners. This is particularly useful with patients whose other cognitive and communicative impairments are mild because its effectiveness rests on (a) awareness of one's emotional state and (b) sensitivity to the needs of a communicative partner. In other words, if a patient is generally hypoaroused, chances are good that he or she will not be sensitive to the communicative situation nor muster the energy to identify or explain how they feel at a given time.

To compensate for a patient's prosodic comprehension deficits, families can be counseled to identify their own moods and attitudes explicitly in conversation. Patients can be counseled to attend to these cues and to use other cues such as facial expression to understand communicative partner's intentions and attitudes. Practice could include recognizing emotions conveyed by pictured facial expressions, although it is important first to determine if patients have reduced eye contact. Recognizing nonverbal emotional expressions is

of little value if patients do not attend to them in daily life.

Another method to help circumvent prosodic comprehension problems is to increase sensitivity to the emotional content of words themselves. For example, ascertain if the patient can identify the emotional state of main characters in simple sentences such as "Sally's favorite dog was suddenly very sick" or "I have way too much to do today and don't know how I'll get it all done." Again, using verbal, gestural, or facial expression cues to compensate for prosodic comprehension deficits assumes attentional and cognitive integrity, as well as adequate social reasoning skills, to be able to make use of these cues. It is certainly an appropriate approach with patients who either have an isolated prosodic deficit or very mild cognitive problems.

Facilitating Recovery of Function

To stimulate recovery of function, clinicians can modify and expand many of the techniques used to assess prosodic production and comprehension deficits. Specific aspects of prosody, particularly variation in pitch, may cause problems in both comprehension and expression. Low-level tasks for pitch perception can include drills in which the patient must discriminate between musical notes or vowel sounds played on a tape recorder. Pitch production drills require patients to imitate the pitch level of a vowel sound produced by the clinician. Similar drills can be set up for loudness and duration. For some patients, it may be more difficult to imitate isolated prosodic features in single vowel sounds. If so, words can be a better and more familiar stimulus option. These drills may be done in conjunction with tasks chosen from the list in Table 9–5. Each of these tasks was described in Chapter 8. They can be modified by adding systematic cues and by increasing or decreasing task difficulty.

One way to modify tasks is to add supportive context for prosodic contour. The

TABLE 9–5. Prosodic comprehension and production tasks (see Chapter 8 for details).

Comprehension Tasks
1. Identify Emotional Prosody in Sentences
2. Identify Emphatic Stress: Compound words vs. Noun Phrases
3. Identify Emphatic Stress: Sentences
4. Discriminate Sentence Types: Declaratives vs. Interrogatives

Production Tasks
1. Production of Emotional Prosody in Sentences
2. Production of Emphatic Stress: Compound words vs. Noun Phrases
3. Production of Emphatic Stress: Sentences

Initial Sentence:
Kevin was surprised by a visitor.

Second Sentence Options:
It was (a) his mother,
　　　　(b) a long lost girlfriend,
　　　　(c) a police woman.

Third Sentence Options:
She said (a) "Why haven't you called me?"
　　　　　(b) "I've missed you."
　　　　　(c) "You are under arrest."

Final Quote:
Kevin replied, "How did you find me?"
(to be read with prosody and emotional tone consistent with the first three sentences, e.g., [a] irritation; [b] excitement; [c] fear).

addition of context (a) allows more spontaneous productions, (b) makes prosodic productions less artificial because they flow from a contextual situation, and (c) may tax inferential skills. Prosodic productions that are matched to situational context may be easier than those requiring production of prosody on command in a neutral sentence. On the other hand, if the patient has inference deficits, the additional element of contextual interpretation may make the task more difficult. Two examples of modifications that increase difficulty and add spontaneity to prosodic production tasks are reviewed in the tasks that follow.

Production of Emotional Prosody

One can use a modified version of a task devised by Tompkins and Flowers (1985) to assess the influence of context on prosodic production. Rather than specifying the emotion to be used, the patient must spontaneously generate prosody appropriate to the story context. The clinician reads a three-sentence printed story ending in a quote by one of the characters which the patient reads out loud. The task allows the clinician to set up several alternative story lines using a single set of stimuli, for example:

Production of Emphatic Stress

Target sentences can be embedded in a brief printed paragraph placed in front of the patient. The clinician reads the paragraph aloud and asks questions about the key sentences or phrases in such a way as to stimulate emphatic stress. For example,

> Joe was late for the meeting so Jackie looked everywhere for him. She looked in the library, in Arnie's office, and at the vending machines. She finally realized that, of course, *Joe was in his office.*

For the target phrase, "Joe was in his office," the clinician can ask: (a) "Was Arnie in Joe's office?" to which the answer should be, "No, *Joe* was in his office"; (b) "Was Joe in the library?" to which the response should be, "No, Joe was in his *office*"; or (c) "Was Joe in Arnie's office?" to which the response should be, "No, Joe was in *his* office," and so on.

Cues: if patients are unable to produce adequate stress, clinicians can model the stress pattern for them to imitate. If imitation does not work, further instructions can be offered about how to prolong syllables and raise pitch and loudness. Drills in which the patient imitates alterations in the pitch, loudness, or duration of single vowels also may be introduced.

TREATMENT OF AFFECTIVE COMMUNICATION DEFICITS

Nonverbal Affective Communication

Comprehension of Nonverbal Emotional Expression

The types of tasks presented in Chapter 8 for identifying and discriminating emotional expressions in pictured scenes and photographs of faces may be modified to vary difficulty in treatment tasks. For example, scenes depicting emotional situations can be more or less difficult to interpret depending on how familiar the context is and how explicit the facial expressions are. The emotions depicted in Figure 6–2 are easy to interpret because Thanksgiving triggers familiar emotions and the people depicted are smiling. Even if the concept of Thanksgiving is missed, the concept of happy people gathered around a table is not difficult to grasp. On the other hand, the emotions depicted in Figure 8–4 are more difficult because the scene is novel and the expression on the girl's face is more subtle. One must use the surrounding context to accurately interpret her expression.

Production of Nonverbal Emotional Expression

As pointed out in Chapter 8, reduced facial and gestural expressivity is easily observed, but not so easily measured. Patients and their families can be alerted to the problem through counseling, but treatment aimed at recovery is difficult at best. The best management strategy may be to monitor these deficits over time. Treatment tasks that train patients to display emotions and attitudes (i.e., interest, disbelief, etc.) on command address symptoms, but not the underlying causes. Treatment is not advised for hypoaroused patients who are the most likely to have severely reduced animation, and the least likely to be aware of it. Their lack of animation is very likely linked to a lowered level of arousal and a general reduction in responsivity.

Patients with mild cognitive impairments may be more aware of and interested in improving their ability to convey emotions nonverbally. For these patients, reduced animation may be accompanied by reduced vocal variation. Improvements in prosodic production may help them compensate for reduced nonverbal emotional expressivity.

Reduced use of gesture and facial expression to signal mood and attitude may also be accompanied by theory of mind deficits. In this case, it is recommended that treatment focus on discourse tasks meant to improve the patient's capacity to identify the beliefs, attitudes, motivations, expectations, and emotional conditions of story characters.

Verbal Affective Communication

Many problems in the comprehension and production of verbally conveyed emotion are related either to prosodic impairments, covered earlier, or to discourse deficits which are covered in the following section.

TREATMENT OF DISCOURSE DEFICITS

Treatment of discourse deficits focuses on two areas, each important to discourse. The first is management of problems in narrative and conversational discourse. The second, and perhaps less obvious, is management of what might be called social disconnection. The term *social disconnection refers to reduced awareness of the social purposes served by communication and of the bonds that tie the self to people, events, and objects in the environment.* As stated previously, RHD patients may appear distant, remote, and bound up in themselves. They may be less than actively engaged in communicative interactions, make less use of conventions for conversation, seem less responsive to the communicative context, and have difficulty assessing listener needs. Chapter 6 also described theory of mind deficits in which there is an impoverished ability to develop a theory about the beliefs, knowledge, motivations, and intentions of others. Chapter 7 reviewed the extreme case of misidentification syndrome in which patients can be so isolated that they loose the sense of their own connections with once familiar objects, places and persons. They may have problems accessing affective memories that represent the bonds between themselves and the world around them. To a lesser degree, social disconnection represents interference in the mechanisms that help us establish and reinforce our connections with one another through human discourse and other communicative acts.

There is obvious interplay between narrative level discourse deficits and those representing social disconnection. There are cognitive and affective forces at work in both deficit areas, and reduced attentional resources course along as undercurrents in both discourse deficits and social disconnection. However, the two can be distinguished in a framework for treatment goals and objectives. Treatment of narrative and conversational discourse deficits specifically addresses: (a) reduced performance in inference generation, (b) reduced level of informative content, and (c) reduced ability to manage alternate mean-

ings and revisions. Treatment of social disconnection deficits focuses on: (a) reduced awareness of listener needs, (b) reduced use of the social conventions for communicative interactions, and (c) theory of mind deficits.

Narrative and Conversational Discourse

Inference Generation Tasks

As discussed in Chapter 6, inference generation deficits can have a broad impact on the comprehension and production of discourse. Inference problems include difficulty generating macrostructures or thematic inferences, problems bridging gaps through coherence references, and difficulty making individual inferences. In addition to treating inference generation directly, tasks that stimulate proposed underlying processes such as integration and selective attention may be appropriate. See Table 9–6 for a list of tasks.

Macrostructure and Other Inferences Tasks

1. **Picture/Story Interpretation**

   a. *Goal:* Strengthen macrostructure generation (i.e., central, thematic inferences) though stimulation

   b. *Procedure:* Present stories or pictured scenes for the patient to interpret

TABLE 9–6. Macrostructure and other inference generation tasks.

Task	Goal
Picture/Story Interpretation	Strengthen accurate inference production
Guided Inference Generation	Train compensatory strategy for inference production
Picture Titles/Story Headlines	Strengthen integration and macrostructure skills
Story Continuations	Strengthen integration and macrostructure skills
Individual Inferences	Strengthen comprehension of individual inferences

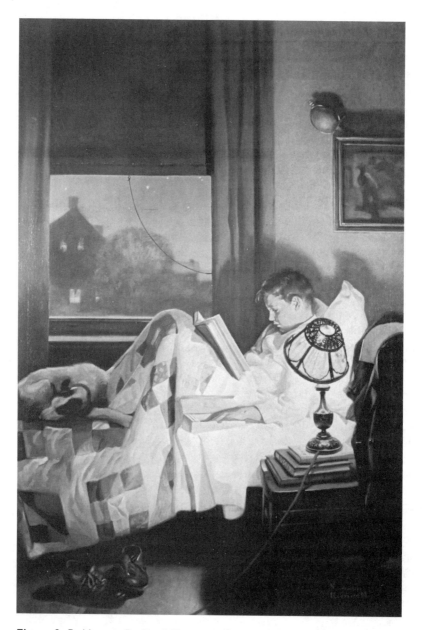

Figure 9–5. Norman Rockwell illustration depicting a boy reading in bed. Edison Mazda: Lamp Advertisement, 1920. Courtesy of the Norman Rockwell Family Trust.

and/or summarize. Stimuli should be at or just above the patient's level of adequate performance.

c. *Pictured Stimulus Manipulations:*

(1) *Visual Considerations:* It may be best to avoid black and white photographs, and instead use black and white or colored line drawings or colored photographs. There is evidence that the RH is more adept at processing the low spatial frequency information contained in the shading and shadows of black and white photographs wheras the LH may be more adept with high spectral frequencies such as those contained in the sharp contrasts of line drawings (Sargent, 1987). RHD can impair processing low spatial frequencies (Spinnler, Guariglia, Massironi, Pizzamiglion, & Zoccolotti, 1990). Thus, line drawings and colored photographs may help avoid problems at the initial level of visual processing. (Note that the original color prints of the Norman Rockwell scenes used in this book are presented as black and white figures for publication purposes only.)

(2) *Levels of Difficulty:* As reviewed in Chapter 6, inference level is the most important consideration in ordering stimuli into a hierarchy. Visually simple pictures can be as difficult to interpret as visually complex ones. Similarly, visually complex scenes that contain familiar content and easy inferences can be easy to interpret, despite the number of visual elements. More visual information can even be helpfully redundant. The picture of the boy reading in bed in Figure 9–5 is crowded, but the theme is simple to interpret. Examples of small increments in inference are depicted in Figure 9–6. The simple and familiar action of saddling up a horse in picture (A) is somewhat easier to interpret than the event depicted in picture (B). For example, to understand that the horse is not merely sleeping in picture (B), one must associate the cowboy's body language (i.e., kneeling, the way he is holding his hat) with previous experience and emotional knowledge. Another slightly more difficult inference is depicted in Figure 9–7 in which there is a greater physical distance between the events depicted. Examples of more subtle emotional content can be found in Figure 6–3 in which even the dog's emotions play a role and must be gleaned purely from his body language. By varying the level of stimulus difficulty in both stories and pictured scenes, it is presumed that the operations involved in inference will be stimulated which in turn may foster recovery.

(3) *Cues:* Cues can range from asking "wh" questions to prompts and modeling (e.g., picture (B), Figure 9–6: What is the cowboy doing? Why is he kneeling? What is he holding? Why is the horse lying on the ground?)

d. *Scoring:* Responses can be scored along various dimensions such as plausibility, accuracy, completeness.

2. Guided Inference Generation: Compensatory Strategy for Inference Deficits

a. *Goal:* Retrain inference generation by enlisting an analytic approach for that which was once automatic

b. *Procedure:* Patients are presented with a step by-step-guide for difficult inferences

c. *Stimuli:* Picture Scenes/Stories

Example 1: Figure 9–6, picture (B).

(1) *Label* elements in the picture (cowboy, horse, stall, hat, rope)

(2) Specify *key elements* (cowboy, horse, hat)

(3) Point to *elements that are related to one another* (cowboy, horse, hat)

(4) *Explain relationships* (e.g., "the cowboy is concerned about the horse," "the horse belongs to the cowboy," "the cowboy wants to

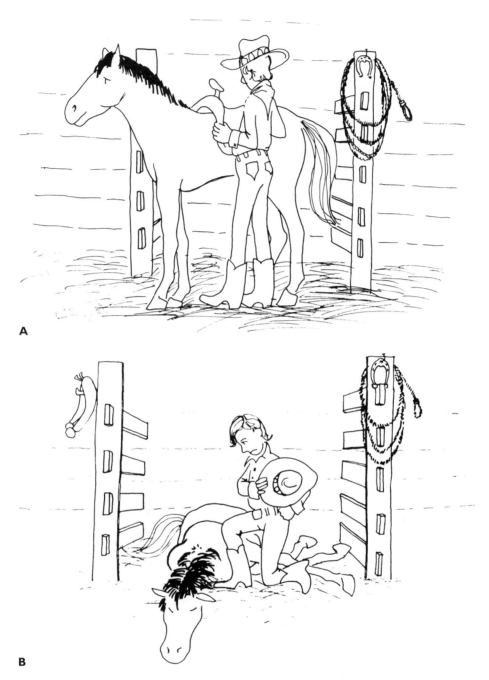

Figure 9–6. Scenes requiring a simple inference in picture (**A**), saddling up Blackie, the horse, and a slightly more difficult inference in picture (**B**), Blackie's demise.

get the horse up," "the cowboy is sad because the horse is dead," etc.)

In this example, almost all the pictured items are significant. Adding other less significant and irrelevant

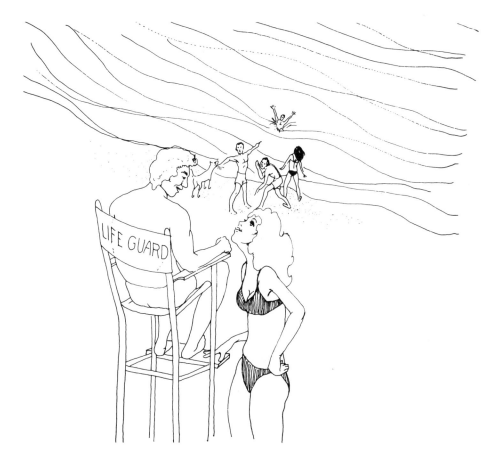

Figure 9–7. Scene requiring interpretation of emotional content.

information increases selective attention demands as in Example 2 below.

Example 2: "Cookie Theft" Picture, Figure 6–5.

(1) *Pictured elements* (mother, sink, water, curtains, cupboards, etc.)
(2) *Key elements* (mother, water, boy, girl, stool, cookie jar)
(3) *Elements related to one another* (mother, water, boy, girl, stool, cookie jar)
(4) *Relationships* (e.g., the woman is connected to the children because she is their mother; the woman is connected to the water because she is standing in it and

not paying attention; the children are connected to the water because they can tell from it that the mother is not paying attention, etc.)

d. *Scoring:* Responses for each step can be scored plus/minus for accuracy and completeness.

3. Picture Titles/Story Headlines

a. *Goal:* Strengthen macrostructure generation and information integration
b. *Task:* Patients must generate titles for short news items or titles for pictured scenes. Stimulus manipulations, cueing strategies, clinician prompts, scoring and methods of compensation

TABLE 9–7. Integration tasks.

Task	Main Goal
Sentence/Picture Arrangement	Strengthen integration and macrostructure skills
Puzzle/object Arrangement	Strengthen integration skills
Fragmented Object Identification	Strengthen integration skills and improve recognition of key features
Recognizing Commonalities	Strengthen recognition of relationships and integration skills

used in Tasks 1 and 2 may be used in these tasks.

  c. *Stimulus manipulations:* News stories and pictures can vary according to how explicit, obvious, and/or familiar their content.

4. **Story Continuations**

  a. *Goal:* Strengthen macrostructure generation

  b. *Task:* Based on story context, patients can be asked to provide their own story endings or pick an ending in a multiple choice format. In designing multiple choice questions, the appropriateness, plausibility, and relatedness of the choices can be varied. Spontaneous continuations can be scored along these same dimensions.

Example:

> Justine was racing through the hospital to the emergency room. Her son, Rob, had had an accident, and she didn't know what his condition was. When she got there, she was met by her husband, and she immediately asked him_____?

Multiple Choice Responses:

"How is Rob?"   Appropriate, related, plausible

"How are you?"   Related, plausible

"How was your day?"   Related, inappropriate

"Where's the cafeteria?"   Unrelated, inappropriate, implausible

5. **Comprehension of individual inferences:**

  a. *Goal:* Improve comprehension of individual inferences that lead to a macrostructure

  b. *Task:* The patient reads simple stories followed by questions about the explicit and implicit information in the story

  c. *Stimulus example:* see Chapter 8, Appendix 6. Level of difficulty can be manipulated using the variables that are applied in previously described macrostructure tasks.

  d. *Scoring:* Plus-minus on questions

Integration Tasks

Integration is one of the operations thought to be involved in generating inferences (see Chapter 6). The following tasks address that process directly as a means of working indirectly on inference abilities. See Table 9–7 for a list of integration tasks.

1. **Sentence/Picture Arrangement**

  a. *Goal:* Improve integration skills and strengthen inference generation indirectly

  b. *Task:* Sets of sentences or pictures must be ordered into a meaningful arrangement to tell a story or represent expository information in a paragraph. Performance rests on accurate understanding of each component and its relationship to the others in the set.

c. *Stimulus Manipulations:* The greater the number of pictured or sentence stimuli the more difficult the task. Pictured or verbal story lines can follow a chronological sequence (baby grows up) or an action-climax-resolution sequence, which may be more difficult.

d. *Scoring:* Inaccurate arrangements can vary in degree of inaccuracy. One way to measure level of accuracy is to score items according to the sequential distance they are from their target position. The scoring system in Appendix 1 accounts for degree of accuracy in this one dimension, and it helps account for completely random arrangements.

2. Puzzle and Object Arrangements

a. *Goal:* Improve integration skills and strengthen inference generation indirectly

b. *Task:* Simple puzzle pieces must be arranged into a pattern according to an abstract model or object.

c. *Stimulus manipulations:* Puzzles can range in difficulty, depending on the number of pieces and the complexity of the pattern.

Note: Occupational therapists may already be conducting such tasks, in which case it is not necessary to duplicate their efforts.

3. Fragmented Object Identification

a. *Goal:* Improve integration skills and strengthen inference generation indirectly

b. *Procedure:* Ask patients to identify pictures of objects that have been cut into pieces (adapted from The Hooper Visual Organization Test, 1983).

c. *Stimuli:* Line drawings of simple objects that have been cut into pieces, like a puzzle, and pasted on a sheet of paper in a random configuration (see Figure 9–8).

d. *Scoring:* plus-minus

4. Recognizing Commonalities

a. *Goal:* Improve integration skills and strengthen inference generation indirectly

b. *Task:* Arrange stimuli by theme. See discussion of Myers & Brookshire, (1995) and Myers et al. (1985) in Chapter 6.

(**1**) Generating categories: Sets of stimuli such as objects, action pictures, words, or pictured scenes, which must be grouped by category. Categories can range from color to function to theme. Patients must devise their own categories.

(**2**) Recognizing commonalities: Patients demonstrate their recognition of commonalities by grouping sets of stimuli and by supplying the category or collective name for sets of stimuli.

c. *Stimulus manipulations:* Task difficulty can be increased by manipulating how explicit and common the category is. The more oblique, abstract, and less familiar the category, the more difficult it will be to recognize or to group objects under it. Objects are generally easier to group than action pictures or more complex scenes because actions and scenes require more inferences. Inferential difficulty may be increased by adding emotional content. The number of stimuli may vary according to the patient's level of performance (e.g., 4 items to be grouped into 2 sets of 2 items each to 9 items to be grouped into 3 sets of three).

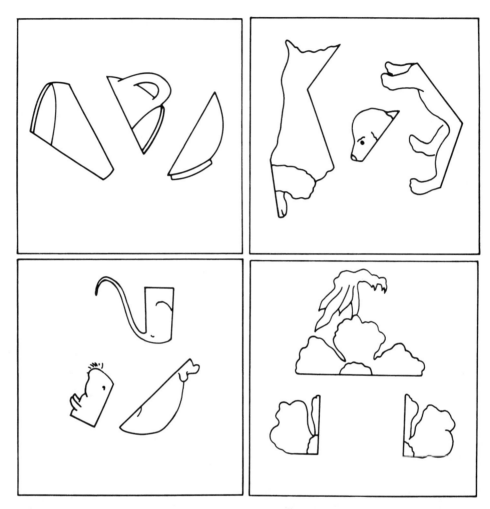

Figure 9–8. Fragmented objects. Selected items from the Hooper Visual Organization Test, copyright © 1957 by H. Elston Hooper. Reprinted by permission of the publisher, Western Psychological Services, 12031 Wilshire Boulevard, Los Angeles, California 90025, USA. Not to be reprinted in whole or in part for any additional purpose without the expressed, written permission of the publisher. All rights reserved.

Increasing Informative Content

Improving macrostructure generation and integration skills can promote improvement in the informative content of discourse. Other ways of increasing the level of informative content include tasks that address the number, relevance, and specificity of concepts produced. Representative tasks are presented below, most of which involve didactic methods of instruction in which patients are taught to recognize their errors. Educational level and estimated premorbid abilities should be considered in designing these tasks.

Typed transcripts are better than video or audio recordings for review with the patient for several reasons: (a) transcripts do not tax memory, (b) transcripts invite less chance of dispute over the what the patient said, and (c) transcripts can be physically scored by circling or otherwise marking errors in the presence of the patient. See Table 9–8 for a list of tasks for increasing informative content.

TABLE 9–8. Tasks for increasing informative content.

Task	Goal
Divergent Questions I	Increase informative content through didactic training
Divergent Questions II	Increase efficiency of production
Dimensions of Informative Content	Increase awareness of the dimensions of informative content
Concept Generation	Increase number and accuracy of concepts produced in a monologue
Pronoun Reference Task	Increase specificity by reducing the number of unreferenced pronouns

1. Divergent Questions I: Increasing Informative Content

a. *Goal:* Increase informative content through didactic training

b. *Task:* Elicit a brief monologue (less than a minute long) by asking a divergent question requiring the patient to state and support an opinion (see Chapter 8). Transcripts of taped responses are reviewed with the patient to increase awareness of the dimensions by which it will be judged including its structure, completeness, efficiency, and relevance (see Chapter 8).
Steps:
(1) Clinician selects a single dimension on which to focus (e.g., completeness).
(2) Clinician and patient review and score the transcript on the chosen dimension.
(3) Clinician and patient discuss ways in which the response could be improved.
(4) Patient is given another opportunity to respond to the same or to another question while focusing on the chosen scoring dimension.
This is a didactic method that may increase awareness. Later, the patient can score his or her own transcripts, and other scoring dimensions can be introduced as the patient improves.

c. *Stimulus manipulations:* Questions should be of sufficient interest to the patient to inspire a response.

d. *Scoring:* (1) number of errors; (2) percent of errors recognized by the patient

2. Divergent Questions II: Increasing Efficiency

a. *Goal:* Improve efficiency of discourse.

b. *Task:* A short monologue (1 min or less) is elicited and scored for efficiency. This is essentially the same task as that presented in Task 1, but uses a scoring system that places particular importance on efficiency (see Chapter 8, Appendix 7).

c. *Stimulus manipulations:* Questions that are of sufficient interest to elicit a response.

d. *Scoring:* Responses can be scored for essential, elaborative, irrelevant, redundant and off-topic information (see Chapter 8, Appendix 7).

3. Recognizing the Dimensions of Informative Content

a. *Goal:* Increase awareness of the dimensions that affect level of informative content.

b. *Task:* The patient reads paragraph length opinions on a given topic that contain errors in the dimensions of relevance, completeness, efficiency, and/or relatedness. The patient's task is to find instances of a given error type. Error types should be consistent with the types of errors the patient makes. This is a good practice task for patients who have problems with insight and reduced ability to recognize their own errors and/or problems understanding the nature of the scoring dimensions.

   c. *Scoring:* Percent of instances found.

4. Concept Generation

   a. *Goal:* Increase the amount of informative content by focusing on number and accuracy of content units.

   b. *Task:* Present stories and pictures similar to those used for macrostructure tasks for the patient to interpret in which level of difficulty is controlled by the dimensions of the stimulus.

   c. *Stimulus manipulations:* Stimuli should be at or just above the patient's level of performance (for stimulus level, see Stimulus Manipulations for Task 1 in the section on Macrostructure and Other Inference tasks). The number of concepts for each stimulus should be determined by the clinician and other judges prior to presentation.

   d. *Scoring:* Count number of accurate concepts (see Nicholas & Brookshire (1995) for method of counting concepts).

   e. *Cues:* A hierarchy of cues can be presented that range from asking "Wh" questions to modeling.

5. Increasing Specificity: Pronoun Reference Task

   a. *Goal:* Increase specificity by decreasing the number of unreferenced pronouns

   b. *Task:* Elicit personal stories about past events from the patient and review transcripts for instances of unreferenced pronouns. Training should

proceed in the manner suggested in Task 1, under Divergent Questions 1: Increasing Informative Content.

   c. *Scoring:*
     (1) instances of unreferenced pronouns produced in transcript; and/or
     (2) instances of unreferenced pronouns found by the patient in transcript review

Managing Alternate Meanings

Initial interpretations often must be adjusted and alternative meanings generated to accommodate the constant flow of new information during discourse. As discussed in Chapter 6, RHD patients may have difficulty revising inferences and managing alternate meanings in response to indirect requests, metaphoric and figurative language, and/or ambiguous information under certain conditions. One source of their deficits in this area may be reduced sensitivity to the situational context. Adequate processing of contextual features that help determine intended meaning has been addressed in tasks designed to improve arousal, selective attention, and inference generation. Damage to certain cognitive and linguistic mechanisms in the RH also has been proposed to account for alternate meaning deficits (see Chapters 5 and 6). Chapter 6 explored two alternative hypotheses that suggest RHD interferes with either the *activation* or the *suppression* of alternate meanings (see Beeman, 1993; Tompkins & Baumgaertner, 1998; and Tompkins et al., 1996, 1997).

At first glance, it may seem appropriate to treat alternate meanings impairments in tasks requiring that patients use and interpret figurative language. However, clinical experience suggests that patients rarely have problems with figurative language in conversational speech. A person who points to the picture with a lion in it in the experimental task pictured in Figure 6–7 may be perfectly capable of understanding the idiom "lion's share," in an event that has personal relevance. Most indirect requests also do not pose problems in everyday discourse for most patients. The exception may be indirect requests that are extremely oblique such as "hints" (e.g., interpreting the statement, "I'm so hot and dry," as a request for water). As explained in Chapter 6, hints require greater levels of inference about the intentions of the speaker, greater knowledge of the speaker, and greater awareness of the contextual situation than do familiar and standard indirect request forms (e.g., "Can you open the window?"). In this sense, understanding hints depends as much on the ability to adopt a theory of mind as it does on adopting an alternate meaning for a set of words. Targeting standard indirect requests and comprehension and expression of figurative language directly in therapy may be of little benefit to functional communication.

Resolving ambiguities and in revising old information to accommodate the new information are more clinically relevant tasks. The unique RH capacity to manage alternate meanings suggests that damage to the RH can interfere in this cognitive process. Because the proposals for a suppression versus an activation deficit are relatively new, there is scant evidence to guide clinical decisions. Tasks for deficits in both activation and suppression are presented below. Table 9–9 summarizes the tasks discussed in this section. Other tasks that encourage inhibition of habitual responses (e.g., Stroop type tasks) may stimulate mechanisms for the suppression of alternate responses and thus indirectly improve inhibition of unwanted or irrelevant responses in discourse.

Activation Tasks

1. Word Associations

  a. *Goal:* Stimulate activation of alternate meanings.
  b. *Task:* Ask patients to find two out of three words that can be grouped together.

TABLE 9–9. Tasks to improve management of alternate meanings.

Activation Tasks
Goal: Stimulate activation of alternate meanings
1. Word Associations
2. Homographs
3. Resovling Ambiguities
4. Inference Revision

Suppression Tasks
Goal: Improve awareness and conscious control over the suppression of inappropriate alternate meanings
1. Homographs
2. Semantic Relations
3. Sentence Interpretation I
4. Sentence Interpretation II: Providing Context
5. Sentence Interpretation III: Explaining Alternatives
6. Sentence Interpretation IV: Promoting Alternative Interpretations
4. Guided Sentence Interpretation

Example: Find two words that go together from a set of three:

　　　　salmon　　shark　　card

The two possible groupings are "salmon/shark" (superordinate category association) and "card/shark" (metaphoric association). The set "salmon/card" is inaccurate.

  c. *Stimulus manipulations:* Stimuli can be manipulated according to the familiarity and explicitness of the association. Associations can include:
  Superordinate category (cod/ halibut)
  Antonymic contrast (open/shut)
  Common association (bank/money)
  Uncommon association (bank/river)
  Metaphoric association (warm/ loving)

2. Homographs

  a. *Goal:* Stimulate the activation of alternate meanings.
  b. *Task:* Ask patient to provide two meanings for common homographs.

c. *Stimulus examples:* bank, spade, watch, club, bat, fan

3. Resolving Lexical Ambiguities

a. *Goal:* Stimulate activation of alternate meanings.

b. *Task:* Ask patients to provide two meanings for ambiguous lexical entities.

c. *Stimulus examples:* headlines, book titles with double meanings;
Note: One also could use visual ambiguities as stimuli (e.g., picture [a] in Figure 6–4).

4. Inference Revision (see Brownell et al., 1986).

a. *Goal:* Stimulate generation of alternate meanings.

b. *Task:* Patients must state the outcome or answer multiple choice questions about two sentence stories in which the premise in the first sentence is misleading. A brief delay between the first and second sentence may increase task difficulty.

c. *Stimulus example:*
Ella grabbed her bag and rushed to the gate.
Once there, she pulled out her key and unlocked it.

d. *Scoring:* Accuracy of story interpretation or plus/minus on multiple choice questions (factual and inferential)

Suppression Tasks

I. Homographs

a. *Goal:* Stimulate inhibition of alternate word meanings by requiring a rapid response.

b. *Task:* Ask patients to provide a single meaning as rapidly as possible for homographs. The task can be made more difficult by asking for the less common meaning. Speed of response may indicate something about the patient's capacity to suppress additional meanings under the assumption that

rapid responses indicate automatic suppression while slower responses indicate effortful suppression of the second meaning. The patient must serve as his or her own control.

c. *Stimuli:* See Homographs in Activation Task 1.

d. *Scoring:* Reaction time (measured by a stop watch)

2. Semantic Relations

a. *Goal:* Stimulate suppression of alternate semantic concepts for single words in a sentence context and increase awareness of and control over alternate meanings.

b. *Task:* Patients are presented with a printed sentence, the final word of which has more than one meaning. The sentence is followed by several words which vary in the degree to which they are related to the meaning of the final word. The patient must select the most closely related word as rapidly as possible. Discussion can ensue about the inappropriateness of other less related words.

c. *Stimuli:* Example:
Marilyn was about to swing her club.
Word choices: Golf (closely related)
Bat (related)
Cards (very distantly related)
Oar (unrelated)
Note: The order of related and unrelated words should be varied.

3. Sentence Interpretation I

a. *Goal:* Stimulate inhibition of alternate sentence meanings.

b. *Task:* The clinician reads aloud a printed sentence, for which there two or more interpretations. The two interpretations are printed below the sentence as story continuations and patients are asked to respond to one of the meanings as rapidly as possible (see Suppression Tasks 1 and 2).

c. *Stimuli:* Sentence example:
Brenda walked over to the bank.
Question: Where was she going?

Interpretations:
(a) Familiar: She was going to make a cash deposit.
(b) Less Familiar: She was walking by the river.

Note: The order of familiar and less familiar interpretations should be varied.

d. *Scoring:* Reaction Time (measured by stop watch)

4. Sentence Interpretation II: Providing Context

a. *Goal:* Increase awareness of and conscious control over alternate meanings to help compensate for problems with suppressing alternate meanings.

b. *Task:* This is an extension of the task in Sentence Interpretation I above with the following addition: After the patient has made his or her choice, the patient and clinician discuss the alternative choices and the patient provides appropriate context. An example of such phrases for the two alternatives in Sentence Interpretation I would be: (a) Familiar: *Brenda was worried about carrying all of the cash, so she walked over to the bank;* (b) Less Familiar: *Brenda wanted to cool off after walking by the river so* she walked over to the bank.

5. Sentence Interpretation III: Explaining Alternatives

a. *Goal:* Stimulate conscious inhibition of alternate sentence meanings.

b. *Task:*

Step 1: The clinician reads a pair of printed sentences aloud and asks the patient to select the appropriate interpretation in a multiple choice paradigm from a list of alternatives. Corrective feedback is offered, if necessary.

Step 2: The patient explains the inappropriateness of other choices. This step is meant to encour-

age conscious awareness and control over inappropriate alternatives that may be activated.

c. *Stimuli:*

Example: Elli was ready to go fishing. She got out her gear and walked over to the bank.

Alternatives: Elli decided to cash her check (related, but inappropriate).
Elli walked to the river (related and appropriate).
Elli was going to the movies (unrelated).

d. *Scoring:* accuracy of responses to Step 1 and to Step 2

6. Guided Sentence Interpretation IV (adapted from Tompkins & Baumgaertner, 1998)

a. *Goal:* Stimulate conscious inhibition of alternate meanings for sentences.

b. *Task:*

Step 1: The clinician reads aloud a printed sentence for which there is more than one meaning.

Step 2: The patient is asked to interpret the action in the sentence.

Step 3: The clinician suggests other, alternate interpretations.

Step 4: The clinician again presents the sentence, but with other contextual clues that promote a different interpretation from the one mentioned by the patient.

Step 5: The patient is asked to determine whether his/her original interpretation is inappropriate in light of the context provided in Step 4. The ensuing discussion of appropriateness of other choices is meant to encourage awareness and conscious control

TABLE 9–10. Social disconnection tasks.

Task	Goal
Conversational Conventions I	Increase use of conversational promoters (e.g., head nods, eye contact, verbal promoters)
Conversational Conventions II	Decrease of conversational blockers (e.g., interruptions, abrupt opening and closing)
Theory of Mind Tasks	Improve awareness of others' knowledge beliefs, motivations, and emotional states

over the inappropriate alternate meanings.

c. *Stimuli:*

Example: Louise stared with disbelief at the rubble that had once been her home.

Some possible interpretations:

Her home had been destroyed by fire.

Her home had been destroyed by a tornado.

She lived in a war zone.

Her nephews had had a party.

Examples of context provided by clinician to promote a given interpretation

(a) Louise had been lucky to escape the smoke and flames.

(b) Louise came up out of the basement after the howling winds had stopped.

(c) Louise had been lucky to be in a neighboring town when the troops came through.

(d) Louise could not believe she had allowed her nephew's college friends to celebrate their team's victory at her house.

Treatment of Social Disconnection Deficits

Reduced awareness of listener needs, reduced use of the social conventions for communicative interactions, and deficits in theory of mind are among the symptoms of social disconnection that can impact on discourse abilities in RHD patients. The underlying cognitive and emotional mechanisms for these symptoms are not known, although it is possible that they have an affective basis resulting from a cortical/limbic disconnection. Because treatment is cognitively based, it may not address the underlying cause.

In some cases, social disconnection deficits may not be treatable, at least with conventional therapy techniques. For example, one may be able to train patients to use eye contact or head nods at appropriate times, but these superficial changes may not alter their actual communicative behavior and nor increase their participation in communicative exchange, if the cause of the problem is a decrease in the affective motivation to be an involved and active communicator. On the other hand, if these deficits are due to reduced arousal or some purely cognitive mechanism, it may be possible to ameliorate them using compensatory strategies. Clinicians need to be aware of this issue before attempting to treat behaviors that signal social disconnection.

Most of the following tasks address the symptoms, not the cause of social disconnection. Theory of mind deficits, as defined in Chapter 6, are approached as cognitive impairments, although they very likely also have an affective basis. Table 9–10 lists several social disconnection tasks.

1. Conversational Conventions I

a. *Goal:* Increase use of conversational conventions (e.g., head nods, eye contact)

b. *Task:*

(1) Video tape brief conversations between patient and a second person.

(2) Didactic Phase: Review tapes with patient and discuss the target behaviors.

(3) Recognition Phase: Patient reviews tapes for instances of target behavior.

(4) Training Phase: Patient is given cues (e.g., verbal reminders, hand signals) at each instance of failure to use the target behavior during a taped conversation.

(5) Transition Phase: Conversations move to situations outside the confines of therapy.

2. Conversational Conventions II

a. *Goal:* Decrease use of barriers to conversational interaction (e.g., poor turn taking, abrupt beginnings and endings).

b. *Task:* See Conversational Conventions I.

3. Theory of Mind Tasks:

a. *Goal:* Improve ability to adopt a theory of mind.

b. *Task:* Present paragraph-length stories followed by questions that test the patient's capacity to adopt the perspective (knowledge, assumptions, motivations, attitudes, emotional state) of a story character.

c. *Stimulus Examples:*

(1) Audrey was on the phone discussing plans for Mick's surprise party when Mick walked in. Just as he did so, he heard Audrey saying, "I'll just invite Mick over for dinner on Saturday, and he'll never suspect a thing about the party." Audrey turned and saw Mick as she hung up the phone, and she knew he'd probably overheard her. She said, "Well, well, would you like to come over for a quiet little dinner on Saturday night?"

Sample Questions:

Fact question: Did Mick overhear plans about his party?

Belief question: Did Audrey realize that Mick had overheard her making plans for his surprise party?

Belief question: Did Mick realize Audrey knew he had overheard her?

Belief question: Was Audrey making a joke at the end of the story?

(2) Terry and Rich were on the same softball team in the town league. Rich knew that Terry had never gotten over the fact that he had once dated Terry's girlfriend. During the second inning, Rich made an error at third base and the other team scored a run. Back in the dugout Terry said to Rich, "Nice play at third, Rich."

Sample Questions:

Fact question: Did Rich miss a play at third base?

Belief question: Was Terry giving Rich a compliment?

Belief question: Did Rich believe what Terry said about the play at third?

SUMMARY

1. Two major treatment approaches are *task-oriented* and *process-oriented* therapy.

2. *Task-oriented approaches* (a) focus on improving a specific activity, (b) focus on symptoms versus cause, (c) are highly individualized to the patient, (d) are often of immediate functional utility, and (e) rarely generalize to other tasks.

3. *Process-oriented approaches* (a) address mechanisms underlying disabilities, (b) focus on cause versus symptoms, (c) address several functions indirectly and simultaneously, and (d) have greater potential for generalization.

4. *Compensation techniques are used in both process-oriented and task-oriented therapy.* Process-oriented compensation techniques use intact processes to overcome impaired processes. Task-oriented compensation techniques use intact processes to work around an impaired skill in a given task.

5. *Facilitation techniques are accomplished through a program of systematic stimulation of an underlying process to improve recovery of function.* These techniques sometimes are called "stimulation therapy."

6. *Treatment of attentional deficits is consistent with theories that suggest that attentional disorders are among the fundamental causes of RHD cognitive and communicative disorders.* Most attentional tasks tap more than one attentional operation. Although in line with theories about RHD impairments, treatment of attention as a means of improving communicative disorders is relatively new and little is known about its utility and effectiveness.

7. *Treatment of neglect is considered part of an attentional program aimed at improving cognitive and communicative functions.* Therapy for neglect can be compensatory to help patients manipulate their environment. *It also can be focused on stimulating recovery of function in an effort to improve cognitive and communicative performance.*

8. *Compensation for neglect* is accomplished through verbal and visual cues and alterations of the spatial location of objects.

9. *Facilitation strategies for neglect* include providing the patient with situations that inspire the motivation to expand the focus of attention and move attention in a leftward direction automatically.

10. *Treatment for prosodic deficits* includes counseling and compensation techniques as well as stimulation tasks to improve specific prosodic features.

11. *Treatment of deficits in the comprehension of nonverbal emotional expression* includes tasks to stimulate comprehension of emotional expressions.

12. *Treatment of deficits in the production of nonverbal emotional expression* is focused on counseling patients and families in an effort to heighten awareness. Direct manipulations of emotional expressivity rarely are recommended, particularly for patients who are hypoaroused.

13. *Deficits in the verbal expression of emotion and in the comprehension of verbally conveyed emotion are addressed in treatment of discourse deficits.*

14. Discourse treatment includes tasks that improve *inference generation, integration abilities, and informative content.* In addition, treatment of discourse includes tasks that focus on *management of alternate meanings to improve the capacity for inference revision* and *tasks to improve the ability to accommodate and disambiguate new information.*

15. *"Pragmatic" deficits are addressed under social disconnection deficits which includes management of reduced sensitivity to listener needs, reduced use of social conventions for conversational interactions, and reduced ability to adopt a theory of mind.*

16. *There are as yet no treatments to address the affective components of social disconnection deficits, and some deficits cannot be treated by available methods. Existing* treatment for theory of mind impairments approaches this disorder as a cognitive impairment, although it may have an affective basis as well.

Appendix I

SENTENCE/PICTURE ARRANGEMENT
TASKS SCORING GUIDELINE

Method: find the difference between the correct and the patient's sentence/picture place-
ments. Add the differences. A perfect score is zero. The greater the total, the more random
and less accurate the arrangement.

Example 1:

Correct arrangement	1	2	3	4	5	6
Patient's arrangement	2	1	3	4	5	6

Difference $1 + 1 + 0 + 0 + 0 + 0 = 2$ Total

Example 2

Correct arrangement	1	2	3	4	5	6
Patient's arrangement	6	4	3	2	1	5

Difference $5 + 2 + 0 + 2 + 4 + 1 = 14$ Total

CHAPTER

Conclusion

One of my primary goals in writing this book was to explore further possible relationships among the cognitive and communicative deficits associated with RHD. Writing a textbook, however, is an analytic exercise in which information is broken down into component parts; each part analyzed separately. As a result, the reality of the whole, the theme of the story, can become hidden in the systematic and sequential presentation of information. To discover the truth of the RHD story, or of any story for that matter, we must see how the pieces fit into the larger reality. What follows are some speculations about the shared features among RHD cognitive and communicative deficits as well as some suggestions for future work that may improve our understanding of the consequences of RHD for communication.

RHD SYNDROME?

As the behavioral consequences of RHD have become more widely recognized dur-

ing the past several decades, a concept of a "RHD syndrome" has begun to emerge. For example, certain patients are viewed as having "classic RHD signs," a testament to some shared impression among clinicians about these deficits. What generates this shared impression? More importantly, how might this impression inform us about the nature of the deficits?

The notion of "classic" RHD signs rests on characteristics that are independent of severity of impairment. Perhaps the most prominent characteristic shared by mildly impaired and severely impaired patients is that they seem somewhat disconnected from the world around them. Insensitivity to communicative context, listener needs, the subtleties and nuances of verbal and nonverbal communication, and the meaning behind the words helps foster this impression. The reduced animation and responsivity of hypoaroused patients, for example, may be just one end of a continuum of social disconnection. At the other end, it may be manifest in occasional lapses in the social conventions for initiating, encouraging, and terminating conversational interaction, in slightly reduced sensitivity to situational context, or in a certain rigidity of interpretation. Misidentification syndromes and anosognosia may be but extreme examples of a more pervasive deficit in appreciating the uniqueness and familiarity of objects and events. These deficits may leave even mildly impaired patients less clearly bonded to the environment, as well as less able, and perhaps less motivated, to enlist a theory of mind to help them interpret the motivations, intentions, knowledge base, and emotional condition of the people in it.

Specific cognitive and semantic impairments also may play a role in fostering the impression of social disconnection. For example, RHD can disrupt the ability to make connections among loosely related meanings, appreciate connotative meanings, manage alternate meanings at the word level. These deficits may be an important source of problems at the sentential and textual level in resolving ambiguities, revising original interpretations, and interpreting extralinguistic information.

The constellation of symptoms that contribute to an impression of a RHD syndrome is painted on a backdrop of attentional impairments that can range from extreme hypoarousal to mild problems in selective attention. There is strong evidence that the RH is particularly important to arousal, vigilance, and broad-based environmental scanning, all of which play a role in evaluating extralinguistic input. The narrowed attentional focus of patients with neglect appears to have negative consequences for recognizing the broader context in which abstract as well as physical information occurs. Neglect has also been correlated with reduced ability to integrate and maintain structure in verbal tasks as well as in visual ones. Because it can occur in non-neglected space, be almeliorated by cueing, and be influenced by attentional demands, neglect itself can be considered as a symptom of a pervasive RHD deficit in attentional scanning, awareness, maintenance, and selectivity.

It is difficult to know if or how prosodic deficits fit into this picture. Prosodic comprehension deficits might be symptomatic of a wide range of impairments in attending to extralinguistic information. However, there is evidence that impaired pitch perception and reduced control over pitch in prosodic production may be significant factors in the prosodic deficits associated with RHD. When present, these deficits add to the picture of communicative disconnection, but they may not otherwise be related to the central or core cognitive and communicative impairments associated with RHD.

It is premature to use the term "RHD syndrome." Yet, it is not unreasonable to expect that there is an as yet unidentified set of core deficits that contribute to a central RHD communication disorder. It goes without saying that rehabilitation efforts are enhanced by taking the whole patient into account. So, too, efforts at understanding the mechanisms underlying cognitive and communicative impairments associated with RHD are enhanced by attention to their shared characteristics and features.

FUTURE DIRECTIONS

The management of RHD communicative impairments is relatively new. Treatment studies are clearly needed to guide our clinical efforts. Learning what does not work is as important as learning what does. Such studies also can help inform us about the underlying nature of the deficits treated. Studies that address generalization of treatment of a single deficit to untreated behaviors may be particularly helpful in identifying which RHD deficits are linked to one another and which ones are dissociated. In addition, treatment efficacy studies and treatment studies that demonstrate improved functional performance in everyday activities are very much needed.

Clinical and experimental research will continue to provide us with information about deficits associated with RHD. Future research on the nature of a given RHD disorder obviously would be enhanced if subjects under study had the disorder of interest. Just as nonaphasic patients with LHD are not included in studies of the nature of aphasia, so, too, RHD patients without the disorder in question should not be included in the subject pool simply because they have lesion or disease process in the right hemisphere. We also need studies that compare RHD subjects with a given disorder to RHD subjects without the disorder. What characteristics do they have in common and what, aside from the deficit in question, distinguishes them from one another?

Research on RHD communication disorders needs to describe subject characteristics more adequately, including performance on tests of neglect and communication. A major stumbling block to the interpretation of findings among studies of RHD patients has been the lack of measures of severity. Available tests do not provide overall severity scores, and little is known about which subtests are the best predictors of recovery. We need to identify the tasks and tests that define severity across a range of deficits, and tasks and tests that best predict level of overall functional communication. This effort has obvious benefits for patient care as well as for research. At this point we know, for example, that the presence of neglect is detrimental to recovering

independence in daily life, but, beyond the obvious visuospatial symptoms, we lack information on why this is so. What is the predictive value of attentional deficits, of specific semantic and cognitive deficits, and of various discourse impairments for recovery of communicative performance?

We need more information on the natural history of the various disorders associated with RHD. Until now research has focused on deficit description, and there are almost no longitudinal studies of recovery of cognitive and communicative disorders. Information about recovery would be a valuable contribution to prognostic efforts and would further our understanding of the deficits themselves.

It is hoped that the commerce between laboratory science and clinical reality will continue to expand. Clinical work that is informed by new research findings is the stronger for it. Research should not lose sight of the larger picture of RHD deficits and disorders that are apparent in clinical work. Hopefully, future research not only will address narrowly defined deficits, but will focus as well on discovering commonalities among deficits. By so doing, the day may come when we can exchange the location-as-disorder designation for a label that meaningfully identifies the core cognitive and communicative disorders associated with RHD as we continue to work toward improving the lives of patients with those disorders.

References

Adamovich, B., & Brooks, R. (1981). A diagnostic protocol to assess the communication deficits of patients with right hemisphere damage. In R. Brookshire (Ed.), *Clinical Aphasiology: Conference Proceedings* (pp. 244–253). Minneapolis: BRK.

Albert, M. C. (1973). A simple test of visual neglect. *Neurology, 23,* 658–664.

Alexander, M. P., Stuss, D. T., & Benson, D. F. (1979). Capgras syndrome: A reduplicative phenomenon. *Neurology, 29,* 334–339.

Allport, A. (1993). Attention and control: Have we been asking the wrong questions? A critical review of twenty-five years. In D. E. Meyer & S. Kornblum (Eds.), *Attention and performance, XIV: Synergies in experimental psychology, artificial intelligence, and cognitive neuroscience* (pp. 183–218). Cambridge: MIT.

Alpert, M., & Rosen, A. (1990). A semantic analysis of the various ways that the terms "affect," "emotion," and "mood" are used. *Journal of Communication Disorders, 23,* 273–246.

Andersen, G., Vestergaard, K., Ingemann-Nielsen, M., & Lauritzen, L. (1995). Risk factors for post-stroke depression. *Acta Psychiatrica Scandanavica, 92,* 193–198.

Andersen, G., Vestergaard, K., Riis, J. O., & Lauritzen, L. (1994). Incidence of post-stroke depression during the first year in a large unselected stroke population determined using a valid standardized rating scale. *Acta Psychiatrica Scandinavica, 90,* 190–195.

Anzola, G. P., & Vignolo, L. A. (1992). Simple reaction time to lateralized visual stimuli is not related to the hemispheric side of lesion. *Cortex, 28,* 401–409.

Apel, K., & Pospisil, A. (1997). *Narrative skills of individuals with right and left hemisphere damage.* Presented at the American Speech-Language-Hearing Association Annual Convention, Boston, MA.

Ardilla, A., & Rosselli, M. (1993). Spatial agraphia. *Brain and Cognition, 22,* 137–147.

Arguin, M., & Bub, D. (1993). Evidence for an independent stimulus-centered spatial reference frame from a case of visual hemineglect. *Cortex, 29,* 349–357.

Aronson, A. E. (1990). *Clinical voice disorders.* New York: Thieme.

Aston-Jones, G., & Bloom, F. E. (1981). Norepinephrine-containing locus coeruleus neurons in behaving rats exhibit pronounced responses to non-noxious environmental stimuli. *Journal of Neuroscience, 1,* 887–900.

Babinski, M. J. (1914). Contribution a l'etude des troubles mentaux dans l'hemiplegie organique cerebrale (Anosognosia). [contribution to the study of mental disturbance in organic cerebral hemiplegia (Anosognosia).] *Revue Neurologique, 12,* 845–848.

Baddeley, A. (1986). *Working memory.* Oxford: Oxford University Press.

Barbieri, C., & De Renzi, E. (1989). Patterns of neglect dissociations. *Behavioral Neurology, 2,* 13–24.

Baron-Cohen, S. (1988). Social and pragmatic deficits in autism: Cognitive or affective? *Journal of Autism and Developmental Disorders, 18,* 379–402.

Baron-Cohen, S. (1989). The autistic child's theory of mind: A case of specific developmental delay. *Journal of Child Psychology and Psychiatry, 30,* 285–297.

Baron-Cohen, S., Leslie, A. M., & Frith, U. (1985). Does the autistic child have a "theory of mind?" *Cognition, 21,* 37–46.

Bartolomeo, P., D'Erme, P., & Gainotti, G. (1994). The relationship between visuospatial and representational neglect. *Neurology, 44,* 1710–1714.

Battersby, W. S., Bender, M. B., Pollack, M., & Kahn, R. L. (1956). Unilateral "spatial agnosia" ("inattention") in patients with cerebral lesions. *Brain, 79,* 68–93.

Bauer, R. M. (1984). Autonomic recognition of names and faces: A neuropsychological application of the Guilty Knowledge Test. *Neuropsychologia, 22,* 457–469.

Bear, D. M. (1983). Hemispheric specialization and the neurology of emotion. *Archives of Neurology, 40,* 195–202.

Bear, D. M., & Fedio, P. (1977). Quantitative analysis of interictal behavior in temporal lobe epilepsy. *Archives of Neurology, 34,* 454–467.

Beeman, M. (1993). Semantic processing in the right hemisphere may contribute to drawing inferences from discourse. *Brain and Language, 44,* 80–120.

Behrens, S. J. (1985). The perception of stress and the lateralization of prosody. *Brain and Language, 26,* 332–348.

Behrens, S. J. (1988). The role of the right hemisphere in the production of linguistic stress. *Brain and Language, 33,* 104–127.

Behrens, S. J. (1989). Characterizing sentence intonation in a right hemisphere-damaged population. *Brain and Language, 37,* 181–200.

Behrmann, M., Moscovitch, M., Black, S. E., & Mozer, M. C. (1990). Perceptual and conceptual mechanisms in neglect dyslexia. *Brain, 113,* 1163–1183.

Bellas, D. N., Novelly, R. A., Eskenazi, B., & Wasserstein, J. (1988a). The nature of unilateral neglect in the olfactory sensory system. *Neuropsychologia, 26,* 45–52.

Bellas, D. N., Novelly, R. A., Eskenazi, B., & Wasserstein, J. (1988b). Unilateral displacement in the olfactory sense: A manifestation of the unilateral neglect syndrome. *Cortex, 24,* 267–275.

Bench, C. J., Frith, C. D., Grasby, P. M., Friston, K. J., Paulesu, E., Frackowiak, R. S. J., & Dolan, R. J. (1993). Investigations of the functional anatomy of attention using the Stroop Test. *Neuropsychologia, 31,* 907–922.

Benowitz, L. I., Bear, D. M., Rosenthal, R., Mesulam, M. -M., Zaidel, E., & Sperry, R. W. (1983). Hemispheric specialization in nonverbal communication. *Cortex, 19,* 5–11.

Benowitz, L. I., Moya, K. L., & Levine, D. N. (1990). Impaired verbal reasoning and constructional apraxia in subjects with right hemisphere damage. *Neuropsychologia, 28,* 231–241.

Benson, D. F. (1979). *Aphasia, alexia, and agraphia.* New York: Churchill Livingstone.

Benson, D. F. (1989). Disorders of visual gnosis. In J. W. Brown (Ed.), *Neuropsychology of visual perception.* Hillsdale, NJ: Lawrence Erlbaum.

Benson, D. F., Gardner, H., & Meadows, J. C. (1976). Reduplicative paramnesia. *Neurology, 26,* 147–151.

Benton, A. (1986). Reaction time in brain disease: Some reflections. *Cortex, 22,* 129–140.

Benton, A., & Joynt, R. J. (1959). Reaction time in unilateral cerebral disease. *Confinia Neurologica, 19,* 247–256.

Bidault, E., Luaute, J. P., & Tzavaras, A. (1986). Prosopagnosia and the delusional misidentification syndromes. *Bibliotheca Psychiatrica, 164,* 80–91.

Bihrle, A. M., Brownell, H. H., Powelson, J. A., & Gardner, H. (1986). Comprehension of humorous and nonhumorous materials by left and right brain damaged patients. *Brain and Cognition, 5,* 399–411.

Bisiach, E. (1988). Language without thought. In L. Weiskrantz (Ed.), *Thought without Language* (pp. 464–484). Oxford, UK: Clarendon Press.

Bisiach, E., Capitani, E., Luzzatti, C., & Perani, D. (1981). Brain and conscious representation of outside reality. *Neuropsychologia, 19,* 543–551.

Bisiach, E., Cornacchia, L., Sterzi, R., & Vallar, G. (1984). Disorders of perceived auditory lateralization after lesions of the right hemisphere. *Brain, 107,* 37–52.

Bisiach, E., Geminiani, G., Berti, A., & Rusconi, M. L.(1990). Perceptual and premotor factors of unilateral neglect. *Neurology, 40,* 1278–1281.

Bisiach, E., & Luzzatti, C. (1978). Unilateral neglect of representational space. *Cortex, 14,* 129–133.

Bisiach, E., Luzzatti, C., & Perani, D. (1979). Unilateral neglect, representational schema and consciousness. *Brain, 102,* 609–618.

Bisiach, E., & Rusconi, M .L. (1990). Break-down of perceptual awareness in unilateral neglect. *Cortex, 26*, 643–649.

Bisiach, E., Rusconi, M. L., & Vallar, G. (1991). Remission of somatoparaphrenic delusion through vestibular stimulation. *Neuropsychologia, 29*, 1029–1031.

Bisiach, E., Vallar, G., Perani, D., Papagno, C., & Berti, A. (1986). Unawareness of disease following lesions of the right hemisphere: Anosognosia for hemiplegia and anosognosia for hemianopia. *Neuropsychologia, 24*, 471–482.

Bloise, C. G. R., & Tompkins, C. A. (1993). Right brain damage and inference revision revisited. *Clinical Aphasiology, 21*, 145–155.

Blonder, L. X., Bowers, D., & Heilman, K. M. (1991). The role of the right hemisphere in emotional communication. *Brain, 114*, 1115–1127.

Blonder, L. X., Burns, A. F., Bowers, D., Moore, R. W., & Heilman, K. M. (1993). Right hemisphere facial expressivity during natural conversation. *Brain and Cognition, 21*, 44–56.

Blonder, L. X., Burns, A. F., Bowers, D., Moore, R. W., & Heilman, K. M. (1995). Spontaneous gestures following right hemisphere infarct. *Neuropsychologia, 33*, 203–213.

Blonder, L. X., Gur, R. E., & Gur, R. C. (1989). The effects of left and right hemiparkinsonism on prosody. *Brain and Language, 36*, 193–207.

Bloom, F. A. (1979). Chemical integrative processes in the central nervous system. In F. O. Schmitt & F. G. Worden (Eds.), *The neurosciences: Fourth study program.* Cambridge, MA: MIT Press.

Bloom, R. L., Borod, J. C., Obler, L. K., & Gerstman, L. J. (1992). Impact of emotional content on discourse production in patients with unilateral brain damage. *Brain and Language, 42*, 153–164.

Bloom, R. L., Borod, J. C., Obler, L. K., & Gerstman, L. J. (1993). Suppression and facilitation of pragmatic performance: Effects of emotional content on discourse following right and left brain damage. *Journal of Speech and Hearing Research, 36*, 1227–1235.

Bloom, R. L., Carozza, L. S., Berg, H., & Curran-Curry, C. (1997). *"Theory of Mind" in patients with left and right brain damage.* Presented at the American Speech-Language-Hearing Association Convention, Boston, MA.

Bogousslavsky, J., & Regli, F., (1988). Response-to-next-patient-stimulation: A right hemisphere syndrome. *Neurology, 38*, 1125–1127.

Bornstein, B., Sroka, H., & Munitz, H. (1969). Prosopagnosia with animal face agnosia. *Cortex, 5*, 164–169.

Borod, J. C. (1992). Interhemispheric and intrahemispheric control of emotion: A focus on unilateral brain damage. *Journal of Consulting and Clinical Psychology, 60*, 339–348.

Borod, J. C., Andelman, F., Obler, L. K., Tweedy, J. R., & Welkowitz, J. (1992). Right hemisphere specialization for the identification of emotional words and sentences: Evidence from stroke patients. *Neuropsychologia, 30*, 827–844.

Borod, J. C., Caron, X., & Koff, E. (1981). Facial asymmetry for positive and negative expressions: Sex differences. *Neuropsychologia, 19*, 819–824.

Borod, J. C., Kashemi, D. R., Haywood, C. S., Andelman, F., Obler, L. K., Welkowitz, J., Bloom, R. L., & Tweedy, J. R. (1996). Hemispheric specialization for discourse reports of emotional experiences: Relationships to demographic, neurologicial, and perceptual variables. *Neuropsychologia, 34*, 351–359.

Borod, J. C., Koff, E., Lorch, M. P., & Nicholas, M. (1985). Channels of emotional expression in patients with unilateral brain damage. *Archives of Neurology, 42*, 345–348.

Borod, J. C., Koff, E., Lorch, M. P., & Nicholas, M. (1986). The expression and perception of facial emotion in brain-damaged patients. *Neuropsychologia, 24*, 169–180.

Borod, J. C., Koff, E., Lorch, M. P., Nicholas, M., & Welkowitz, J. (1988). Emotional and nonemotional facial behavior in patients with unilateral brain damage. *Journal of Neurology, Neurosurgery, and Psychiatry, 51*, 826–832.

Borod, J. C., Welkowitz, J., Alpert, M., Brozgold, A. Z., Martin, C., Peselow, E., & Diller, L. (1990). Parameters of emotional processing in neuropsychiatric disorders: Conceptual issues and a battery of tests. *Journal of Communication Disorders, 23*, 247–271.

Bowers, D., Bauer, R. M., Coslett, H. B., & Heilman, K. M. (1985). Processing of faces by patients with unilateral hemisphere lesions: I. Dissociation between judgements of facial affect and facial identity. *Brain and Cognition, 4*, 258–272.

Bowers, D., Coslett, H. B., Bauer, R. M., Speedie, L., & Heilman, K. M. (1987). Comprehension of emotional prosody following unilateral hemispheric lesions: Processing defect versus distraction defect. *Neuropsychologia, 25*, 317–328.

Bradvik, B., Dravins, C., Holtas, S., Rosen, I., Ryding, E., & Ingvar, D. H. (1991). Disturbances of speech prosody following right hemisphere infarcts. *Acta Scandinavica, 84,* 114–126.

Brain, W. R. (1941). Visual disorientation with special reference to lesions of the right cerebral hemisphere. *Brain, 64,* 244–272.

Brookshire, R. H., & Nicholas, L. E. (1984). Comprehension of directly and indirectly stated main ideas and details in discourse by brain-damaged and non-brain-damaged listeners. *Brain and Language, 21,* 21–36.

Brookshire, R. H., & Nicholas, L. E. (1993). *The discourse comprehension test.* Tucson, AZ: Communication Skill Builders.

Brownell, H. H., Blum, A., & Winner, E. (1994). Attributional bias in RHD patients with impaired discourse comprehension. *Brain and Language, 43,* 476–478.

Brownell, H. H., Carroll, J. J., Rehak, A., & Wingfield, A. (1992). The use of pronoun anaphora and speaker mood in the interpretation of conversational utterances by right hemisphere brain-damaged patients. *Brain and Language, 43,* 121–147.

Brownell, H. H., Gardner, G., Prather, P., & Martino, G. (1995). Language, communication and the right hemisphere. In H. S. Kirshner (Ed.), *Handbook of neurological speech and language disorders,* 325–349. New York: Marcel Dekker.

Brownell, H. H., & Martino, G. (1998). Deficits in inference and social cognition: The effects of right hemisphere brain damage on discourse. In M. Beeman & C. Chiarello (Eds.), *Right hemisphere language comprehension: Perspectives from cognitive neuroscience.* Mahwah, NJ: Lawrence Erlbaum.

Brownell, H. H., Michel, D., Powelson, J., & Gardner, H. (1983). Surprise but not coherence: Sensitivity to verbal humor in right-hemisphere patients. *Brain and Language, 18,* 20–27.

Brownell, H. H., Pincus, D., Blum, A., Rehak, A., & Winner, E. (1997). The effects of right-hemisphere brain damage on patients' use of terms of personal reference. *Brain and Language, 57,* 60–79.

Brownell, H. H., Potter, H. H., Bihrle, A. M., & Gardner, H. (1986). Inference deficits in right brain-damaged patients. *Brain and Language, 27,* 310–321.

Brownell, H. H., Potter, H. H., Michelow, D., & Gardner. (1984). Sensitivity to lexical denotation and connotation in brain damaged patients: A double dissociation? *Brain and Language, 22,* 253–265.

Brownell, H. H., Simpson, T. L., Bihrle, A. M., Potter, H. H., & Gardner, H. (1990). Appreciation of metaphoric alternative word meanings by left and right brain-damaged patients. *Neuropsychologia, 28,* 375–383.

Brunn, J. L., & Farah, M. J. (1991). The relation between spatial attention and reading: Evidence from the neglect syndrome. *Cognitive Neuropsychology, 8,* 59–75.

Bryan, K. L. (1988). Assessment of language disorders after right hemisphere damage. *British Journal of Disorders of Communication, 23,* 111–125.

Bryan, K. L. (1989). Language prosody and the right hemisphere. *Aphasiology, 3,* 285–299.

Bryan, K.L. (1995). *Right Hemisphere Language Battery* (2nd ed.). London: Whurr Publishers.

Bryer, J. B., Starkstein, S. E., Votypka, V., Parikh, R. M., Price, T. R., & Robinson, R. G. (1992). Reduction of CSF monoamine metabolites in poststroke depression: A preliminary report. *Journal of Neuropsychiatry and Clinical Neuroscience, 4,* 440–442.

Bub, D., Audet, T., & Lecours, A. R. (1990). Re-evaluating the effect of unilateral brain damage on simple reaction time to auditory stimulation. *Cortex, 26,* 227–237.

Buck, R., & Duffy, R. J. (1980). Nonverbal communication of affect in brain-damaged patients. *Cortex, 16,* 351–362.

Burgess, C., & Simpson, G. B. (1988). Cerebral hemispheric mechanisms in the retrieval of ambiguous word meanings. *Brain and Language, 33,* 86–103.

Burns, M. (1997). *The Burns Brief Inventory of Communication and Cognition.* San Antonio: Psychological Corporation.

Butter, C. M. (1992). Effect of stimuli in right hemispace on left-sided neglect in a line cancellation task. *Neuropsychologia, 30,* 859–864.

Calvanio, R., Petrone, P. N., & Levine, D. N. (1987). Left visual spatial neglect is both environment-centered and body-centered. *Neurology, 37,* 1179–1183.

Campbell, D. C., & Oxbury, J. M. (1976). Recovery from unilateral visuo-spatial neglect? *Cortex, 12,* 303–312.

Cancelliere, A. E. B., & Kertesz, A. (1990). Lesion localization in acquired deficits of emotional expression and comprehension. *Brain and Cognition, 13,* 133–147.

Capgras, J., & Reboul-Lachaux, J. (1923). L'illusion des soises dans un delire systematise chronique. *Bulletin de la Societe Clinique de Medecine Mentale, 2,* 6–16.

Caplan, B. (1987). Assessment of unilateral neglect: A new reading test. *Journal of Clinical and Experimental Neuropsychology, 9,* 359–364.

Caplan, L. R., Kelly, M., Kase, C. S., Hier, D. B., White, J. L., Tatemichi, T., Mohr, J., Price, T., & Wolf, P. (1986). Infarcts of the inferior division of the right middle cerebral artery: Mirror image of Wernicke's aphasia. *Neurology, 36,* l015–1020.

Cappa, S., Papagno, C., & Vallar, G. (1990). Language and verbal memory after right hemispheric stroke: A clinical-CT scan study. *Neuropsychologia, 28,* 503–509.

Cappa, S., Sterzi, R., Vallar, G., & Bisiach, E. (1987). Remission of hemineglect and anosognosia during vestibular stimulation. *Neuropsychologia, 25,* 775–782.

Caramazza, A., & Hillis, A. E. (1990). Levels of representation, co-ordinate frames, and unilateral neglect. *Cognitive Neuropsychology, 7,* 391–446.

Carmon, A., & Nachshon, I. (1971). Effect of unilateral brain damage on perception of temporal order. *Cortex, 7,* 410–418.

Chatterjee, A., Mennemeier, M., & Heilman, K. M. (1992). Search patterns and neglect: A case study. *Neuropsychologia, 30,* 657–672.

Chedru, F., Leblanc, M., & L'hermitte, F. (1973). Visual searching in normal and brain-damaged subjects (Contribution to the study of unilateral inattention). *Cortex, 9,* 95–111.

Cherney, L. R., & Canter, G. J. (1993). Informational content in the discourse of patients with probable Alzheimer's disease and patients with right brain damage. *Clinical Aphasiology, 21,* 123–133.

Chiarello, C., Burgess, C., Richards, L., & Pollock, A. (1990). Semantic and associative priming in the cerebral hemispheres: Some words do, some words don't . . . Sometimes, some places. *Brain and Language, 38,* 75–104.

Chiarello, C., & Church, K. L. (1986). Lexical judgements after right or left-hemisphere injury. *Neuropsychologia, 24,* 623–640.

Chobor, K. L., & Brown, J. W. (1987). Phoneme and timbre monitoring in left and right cerebrovascular accident patients. *Brain and Language, 30,* 278–284.

Cicone, M., Wapner, W., & Gardner, H. (1980). Sensitivity to emotional expressions and situations in organic patients. *Cortex, 16,* 145–158.

Cimino, C. R., Verfaellie, M., Bowers, D., & Heilman, K. (1991). Autobiographical memory: Influence of right hemisphere damage on emotionality and specificity. *Brain and Cognition, 15,* 106–118.

Clark, C. R., Geffen, G. M., & Geffen, L. B. (1987). Catecholamines and attention. I: Animal and clinical studies. *Neuroscience and Biobehavioral Reviews, 11,* 341–352.

Clark, C. R., Geffen, G. M., & Geffen, L. B. (1989). Catecholamines and the covert orientation of attention in humans. *Neuropsychologia, 27,* 131–139.

Clark, H. H., & Haviland, S. E. (1977). Comprehension and the given-new contract. In R. O. Freddle (Ed.), *Discourse production and comprehension* (pp. 1–40). Norwood, NJ: Ablex.

Cohen, R. M., Semple, W. E., Gross, M., Holcomb, H. J., Dowling, S. M., & Nordahl. (1988). Functional localization of sustained attention. *Neuropsychiatry, Neuropsychologogy, and Behavioral Neurology, 1,* 3–20.

Cohn, R. (1972). Eyeball movements in homonymous hemianopia following simultaneous bi-temporal object presentation. *Neurology, 22,* 12–14.

Collins, M. (1975). The minor hemisphere. In R. H. Brookshire (Ed.), *Clinical aphasiology conference proceedings.* Minneapolis, MN: BRK Publishers.

Collins, M. (1986). *Diagnosis and treatment of global aphasia.* San Diego: College-Hill Press.

Colombo, A., De Renzi, E., & Faglioni, P. (1976). The occurrence of visual neglect in patients with unilateral cerebral disease. *Cortex, 12,* 221–231.

Colsher, P. L., Cooper, W. E., & Graff-Radford, N. (1987). Intonation variability in the speech of right-hemisphere damaged patients. *Brain & Language, 32,* 379–383.

Corwin, J. V., Kanter, S. L., Watson, R. T., Heilman, K. M., Valenstein, E., & Hashimoto, A. (1986). Apomorphine has a therapeutic effect on neglect produced by unilateral dorsomedial prefrontal cortex lesions in rats. *Experimental Neurology, 94,* 683–689.

Coslett, H. B. (1997). Neglect in vision and visual imagery: a double dissociation. *Brain, 120,* 1163–1171.

Coslett, H. B., Bowers, D., Fitzpatrick, E., Haws, B., & Heilman, K. M. (1990). Directional hypokinesia and hemispatial inattention in neglect. *Brain, 113,* 475–486.

Coslett, H. B., Bowers, D., & Heilman, K. M. (1987). Reduction in cerebral activation after right hemisphere stroke. *Neurology, 37,* 957–962.

Coslett, H. B., & Heilman, K. M. (1989). Hemihypokinesia after right hemisphere stroke. *Brain and Cognition, 9,* 267–278.

Courbon, P., & Fail, G. (1927). Syndrome d'illusion de Fregoli et schizophrenie. *Bulletin de la Societe Clinique de Medecine Mentale, 15,* 121–124.

Crow, J. T. (1991). The origins of psychosis and the "Descent of Man." *British Journal of Psychiatry, 159,* 76–82.

Cummings, J. L. (1994). Depression in neurologic diseases. *Psychiatric Annals, 24,* 525–531.

Cummings, J. L. (1995). The neuroanatomy of depression. *Journal of clinical Psychiatry, 54,* 14–20.

Cutting, J. (1978). Study of anosognosia. *Journal of Neurology, Neurosurgery, and Psychiatry, 41,* 548–555.

Cutting, J. (1991). Delusional misidentification and the role of the right hemisphere in the appreciation of identity. *British Journal of Psychiatry, 159,* 70–75.

Damasio, A. R., Damasio, H., & Chui, H. C. (1980). Neglect following damage to frontal lobe or basal ganglia. *Neuropsychologia, 18,* 128–132.

Damasio, A. R., Damasio, H., & Van Hoesen, G. W. (1982). Prosopagnosia: Anatomic basis and behavioral mechanisms. *Neurology, 32,* 331–341.

Daneman, M., & Carpenter, P. A. (1983). Individual differences in integrating information between and within sentences. *Journal of Experimental Psychology: Learning, Memory, and Cognition, 9,* 561–584.

Davidson, R., Ekman, P., Saron, C. D., Senulis, J. A., & Friesen, W. V. (1990). Approach-withdrawal and cerebral asymmetry: Emotional expression and brain physiology I. *Journal of Personality and Social Psychology, 58,* 330–341.

Davidson, R. J., Fedio, P., Smith, B. D., Aurielle, E., & Martin, A. (1992). Lateralized mediation of arousal and habituation: Differential bilateral electrodermal activity in unilateral temporal lobectomy patients. *Neuropsychologia, 30,* 1053–1063.

Davidson, R. J., & Schwartz, G. E. (1976). Patterns of cerebral lateralization during cardiac biofeedback versus the self-regluation of emotion: Sex differences. *Psychophysiology, 13,* 62–68.

Davidson, R. J., Schwartz, G. E., Saron, C., Bennet, J., & Goleman, D. J. (1979). Frontal versus parietal EEG asymmetry during positive and negative affect. *Psychophysiology, 16,* 202–203.

Dee, H. L., & Van Allen, M. W. (1973). Speed of decision-making processing in patients with unilateral cerebral disease. *Archives of Neurology, 28,* 163–166.

DeKosky, S., Heilman, K. M., Bowers, D., & Valenstein, E. (1980). Recognition and discrimination of emotional faces and pictures. *Brain and Language, 9,* 206–214.

Delis, D. C., Wapner, W., Gardner, H., & Moses, J. A. (1983). The contribution of the right hemisphere to the organization of paragraphs. *Cortex, 19,* 43–50.

Denes, G., Caldognetto, E. M., Semenza, C., Vagges, K., & Zettin, M. (1984). Discrimination and identification of emotions in human voice by brain-damaged subjects. *Acta Neurologica Scandinavica, 69,* 154–162.

Denes, G., Semenza, C., Stoppa, E., & Lis, A. (1982). Unilateral spatial neglect and recovery from hemiplegia. *Brain, 105,* 543–552.

Denny-Brown, D., Meyer, J. S., & Horenstein, S. (1952). The significance of perceptual rivalry resulting from parietal lesion. *Brain, 75,* 433–471.

De Renzi, E., & Faglioni, P. (1965). The comparative efficiency of intelligence and vigilance tests detecting hemispheric change. *Cortex, 1,* 410–433.

De Renzi, E., Faglioni, P., & Scotti, G. (1970). Hemispheric contribution to exploration of space through the visual and tactile modality. *Cortex, 6,* 191–203.

De Renzi, E., Gentilini, M., & Barbieri, C. (1989). Auditory neglect. *Journal of Neurology, Neurosurgery, and Psychiatry, 52,* 613–617.

De Renzi, E., Gentilini, M., Faglioni, P., & Barbieri, C. (1989). Attentional shift towards the rightmost stimuli in patients with left visual neglect. *Cortex, 25,* 231–237.

DeRenzi, E., & Vignolo, L. A. (1962). The token test: A sensitive test to detect receptive disturbances in aphasics. *Brain, 85,* 665–678.

D'Erme, P., Robertson, I., Bartolomeo, P., Daniele, A., & Gainotti, G. (1992). Early rightwards orienting of attention on simple reaction time performance in patients with left-sided neglect. *Neuropsychologia, 30,* 989–1000.

Descarries, L., & Lapierre, Y. (1973). Norepinephrine and axon terminals in the cerebral cortex of the rat. *Brain Research, 51,* 141–160.

Deutsch, G., Papanicolaou, A. C., Bourbon, T., Eisenberg, H. M. (1987). Cerebral blood flow evidence of right cerebral activation in attention demanding tasks. *International Journal of Neuroscience, 36,* 23–28.

Diamond, S. J. (1976). Depletion of attentional capacity after total commissurotomy in man. *Brain, 99,* 347–356.

Diamond, S. J., & Beaumont, J. G. (1973). Difference in the vigilance performance of the right and left hemispheres. *Cortex, 9,* 259–265.

Diggs, C. C., & Basili, A. G. (1987). Verbal expression of right cerebrovascular accident patients: Convergent and divergent language. *Brain and Language, 30,* 130–146.

Diller, L., & Weinberg, J. (1977). Hemi-inattention in rehabilitation: The evolution of a rational remediation program. In E. A. Weinstein & R. P. Friedland (Eds.), *Advances in Neurology,* (Vol. 18, pp. 63–82). Philadelphia: Raven.

Divenyi, P. L., & Robinson, A. J. (1989). Nonlinguistic auditory compatabilities in aphasia. *Brain and Language, 37,* 290–396.

Doricchi, F., Guariglia, C., Paolucci, S., & Pizzamiglio, L. (1990). Severe reduction of leftwards REMs in patients with left unilateral heminattention. In J. Horne (Ed.), *Sleep 90.* Bochum: Pontenagel Press.

Duffy, J. R. (1994). Schuell's stimulation approach to rehabilitation. In X. Chapey (Ed.), *Language intervention strategies in adult aphasia* (3rd ed., pp. 146–177). Baltimore: Williams & Wilkins.

Duffy, J. R. (1995). *Motor speech disorders: Substrates, differential diagnosis, and management.* St Louis: Mosby.

Dupont, R. M., Cullum, C. M., & Jeste, D. V. (1988). Poststroke depression and psychosis. *Psychiatric Clinics of North America, 11,* 133–149.

Egelko, S., Gordon, W. A., Hibbard, M. R., Diller, L., Lieberman, A., Holliday, R., Ragnarsson, K., Shaver, M. S., & Orazem, J. (1988). Relationship among CT scans, neurological exam, and neuropsychological test performance in right brain-damaged stroke patients. *Journal of Clinical and Experimental Neuropsychology, 10,* 539–564.

Eisenson, J. (1962). Language and intellectual modifications associated with right cerebral damage. *Language and Speech, 5,* 49–53.

Ekman, P. (1973). Cross-cultural studies of facial expression. In P. Ekman (Ed.), *Darwin and fa-cial expression: A century of research in review.* New York: Academic Press.

Ellis, A. W., Flude, B. M., & Young, A. W. (1987). "Neglect dyslexia" and the early visual processing of letters in words and nonwords. *Cognitive Neuropsychology, 4,* 439–464.

Ellis, A. W., & Young, A. W. (1990). Accounting for delusional misidentifcations. *British Journal of Psychiatry, 157,* 239–248.

Ellis, H. D., Young, A. W., & Flude, B. M. (1993). Neglect and visual language. In I. Robertson & J. C. Marshall (Eds.), *Unilateral neglect: Clinical and experimental studies* (pp. 233–256). Hillsdale, NJ: Lawrence Erlbaum.

Emmory, K. D. (1987). The neurological substrates for prosodic aspects of speech. *Brain and Language, 30,* 305–320.

Faglioni, P., Scotti, G., & Spinnler, H. (1971). The performance of brain damaged patients in spatial localization of visual and tactile stimuli. *Brain, 94,* 443–454.

Farah, M. J., Brunn, J. L., Wong, A. B., Wallace, M. A., & Carpenter, P. A. (1990). Frames of reference for allocating attention to space: Evidence from the neglect syndrome. *Neuropsychologia, 28,* 335–347.

Farah, M. J., Monheit, M. A., & Wallace, M. A. (1991). Unconscious perception of "extinguished" visual stimuli: Reassessing the evidence. *Neuropsychologia, 29,* 949–985.

Farah, M. J., Wallace, M. A., & Vecera, S. P. (1993). "What" and "where" of visual attention: Evidence from the neglect syndrome. In I. Robertson & J. C. Marshall (Eds.), *Unilateral neglect: Clinical and experimental evidence* (pp. 123–138). Hillsdale, NJ: Lawrence Erlbaum.

Farah, M. J., Wong, A. B., Monheit, M. A., & Morrow, L. A. (1989). Parietal lobe mechanisms of spatial attention: Modality-specific or supramodal? *Neuropsychologia, 27,* 461–470.

Feinberg, T. E., Haber, L. D., & Stacy, C. B. (1990). Ipsilateral extinction in the hemineglect syndrome. *Archives of Neurology, 47,* 802–804.

Feinberg, T. E., & Shapiro, R. M. (1989). Misidentification-reduplication and the right hemisphere. *Neuropsychiatry, Neuropsychology and Behavioral Neurology, 2,* 38–39.

Ferro, J. M., Kertesz, A., & Black, S. E. (1987). Subcortical neglect: Quantication, anatomy, and recovery. *Neurology, 37,* 1487–1492.

Fisher, C. M. (1982). Disorientation for place. *Archives of Neurology, 39,* 33–36.

Fleet, W. S., Valenstien, E., Watson, R. T., & Heilman, K. M. (1987). Dopamine agonist therapy for neglect in humans. *Neurology, 37,* 1765–1770.

Foldi, N. S. (1987). Appreciation of pragmatic interpretations of indirect commands: Comparison of right and left hemisphere brain-damaged patients. *Brain and Language, 31,* 88–108.

Folstein, M. F., Maiberger, R., & McHugh, P. R. (1977). Mood disorder as a specific complication of stroke. *Journal of Neurology, Neurosurgery, and Psychiatry, 40,* 1018–1020.

Foote, S. L., & Bloom, F. E. (1979). Activity of norepinephrine-containing locus coeruleus neurons in the unanesthetized squirrel monkey. In E. Usdin, I. J. Kopin, & J. Barchas (Eds.), *Catecholamines: Basic and clinical frontiers, Vol. 1* (pp. 625–627). New York: Pergamon Press.

Foote, S. L., Feedman, R., & Oliver, A. P. (1975). Effects of putative neurotransmitters on neuronal activity in monkey auditory cortex. *Brain Research, 86,* 229–242.

Forstl, H., Almeida, O. P., Owen, A. M., Burns, A., & Howard, R. (1991). Psychiatric, neurological and medical aspects of misidentification syndromes: A review of 260 cases. *Psychological Medicine, 21,* 905–910.

Frederiks, J. A. M. (1969). Disorders of the body schema. In P. J. Vinken & G. W. Bruyn (Eds.), *Handbook of clinical neurology, Vol.4* (pp. 373–393). Amsterdam: Elsvier.

Freedman, M., Leach, L., Kaplan, E., Winocur, G., Shulman, K. L., & Delis, D. C. (1994). *Clock drawing: A neuropsychological analysis.* New York: Oxford University.

Friberg, L., Olsen, T. S., Roland, P. E., Paulson, O. B., & Lassen, N. A. (1985). Focal increase of blood flow in the cerebral cortex of man during vestibular stimulation. *Brain, 108,* 609–623.

Friedland, R. P., & Weinstein, E. A. (1977). Hemi-inattention and hemisphere specialization: Introduction and historical review. *Advances in Neurology, 18,* 1–26.

Frith, U. (1989). A new look at language and communication in autism. *British Journal of Disorders of Communication, 24,* 123–150.

Fromm, D., Holland, A. J., Swindell, C. S., & Reinmuth O. M. (1985). Various consequences of subcortical stroke: Prospective study of 16 consecutive cases. *Archives of Neurology, 42,* 943–950.

Gainotti, G. (1972). Emotional behavior and hemispheric side of lesion. *Cortex, 8,* 41–55.

Gainotti, G., Caltagrione, C., & Miceli, G. (1983).

Selective semantic-lexical discrimination in right-brain-damaged patients. In E. Perecman (Ed.), *Cognitive processing in the right hemisphere* (pp. 149–167). New York: Academic Press.

Gainotti, G., Caltagrione, C., Miceli, G., & Masullo, C. (1981). Selective semantic-lexical impairment of language comprehension in right-brain-damaged patients. *Brain and Language, 13,* 201–211.

Gainotti, G., D'Erme, P., & Bartolomeo, P. (1991). Early orientation of attention toward the half of space ipsilateral to the lesion in patients with unilateral brain damage. *Journal of Neurology, Neurosurgery, and Psychiatry, 54,* 1082–1089.

Gainotti, G., D'Erme, P., Monteleone, D., & Silveri, M. C. (1986). Mechanisms of unilateral spatial neglect in relation to laterality of cerebral lesions. *Brain, 109,* 599–612.

Gardner, H., Brownell, H. H., Wapner, W., & Michelow, D. (1983). Missing the point: The role of the right hemisphere in the processing of complex linguistic materials. In E. Perecman (Ed.), *Cognitive processing in the right hemisphere* (pp. 169–191). New York: Academic Press.

Gardner, H., & Denes, G. (1973). Connotative judgements by aphasic patients on a pictorial adaptation of semantic differential. *Cortex, 9,* l83–196.

Gardner, H., Ling, P. K., Flamm, L., & Silverman, J. (1975). Comprehension and appreciation of humorous material following brain damage. *Brain, 98,* 399–412.

Gazzaniga, M. S. (1970). *The bisected brain.* New York: Appleton-Centruy-Crofts.

Gazzaniga, M. S. (1983a). Reply to Levy and to Zaidel. *American Psychologist,* 547–549.

Gazzaniga, M. S. (1983b). Right hemisphere language following commissurotomy: A twenty year perspective. *Annals of Psychology, 38,* 525–537.

Gazzaniga, M. S., Bogen, J. E., & Sperry, R. W. (1962). Some functional effects of sectioning the cerebral commissures in man. *Proceedings of the National Academy of Sciences, 48,* 1765–1769.

Gentilini, M., Barbieri, C., De Renzi, E., & Faglioni, P. (1989). Space exploration with and without the aid of vision in hemisphere-damaged patients. *Cortex, 25,* 643–651.

Gernsbacher, M. A. (1990). *Comprehension as structure building.* Hillsdale, NJ: Lawrence Erlbaum.

Gernsbacher, M. A., & Faust, M. E. (1991). The mechanism of suppression: A component of general comprehension skill. *Journal of Experimental Psychology: Learning, Memory, and Cognition, 17,* 245–262.

Gernsbacher, M. A., Varner, K. R., & Faust, M. E. (1990). Investigating differences in general comprehension skill. *Journal of Experimental Psychology: Learning, Memory, and Cognition, 16,* 430–445.

Gerstmann, J. (1942). Problem of imperception of disease and of impaired body territories with organic lesions: Relation to body scheme and its disorders. *Archives of Neurology and Psychiatry, 48,* 890–914.

Girotti, F., Casazza, M., Musicco, M., & Avanzini, G. (1983). Oculomotor disorders in cortical lesions in man: The role of unilateral neglect. *Neuropsychologia, 21,* 543–553.

Gloning, I., Gloning, K., Hoff, H., & Tschabitscher, H. (1966). Zur prosopagnosie. *Neuropsychologia, 4,* 113–132.

Goldberg, E., & Costa, L. D. (1981). Hemispheric differences in the acquisition and use of descriptive systems. *Brain and Language, 14,* 144–173.

Goodglass, H., & Kaplan, E. (1983). *The Boston Diagnostic Aphasia Examination.* Philadelphia: Lea & Febiger.

Gordon, H. W. (1970). Hemispheric asymmetries in the perception of musical chords. *Cortex, 6,* 387–398.

Gorelick, P. B., & Ross, E. D. (1987). The aprosodias: further functional-anatomical evidence for the organization of affective language in the right hemisphere. *Journal of Neurology, Neurosurgery, and Psychiatry, 50,* 553–560.

Green, J. B., & Hamilton, W. J. (1976). Anosognosia for hemiplegia: Somatosensory evoked potential studies. *Neurology, 26,* 1141–1144.

Grice, H. P. (1975). Logic and conversation. In P. Cole & J. L. Morgan (Eds.), *Syntax and semantics* (Vol. III, pp. 41–58). New York: Academic Press.

Gronwall, D. M. A. (1977). Paced auditory serial-addition task: A measure of recovery from concussion. *Perceptual and Motor Skills, 44,* 367–373.

Grossman, M. (1981). A bird is a bird is a bird: Making reference within and without superordinate categories. *Brain and Language, 12,* 313–331.

Guariglia, C., & Antonucci, G., (1992). Personal and extrapersonal space: A case of neglect dissociation. *Neuropsychologia, 30,* 1001–1009.

Guariglia, C., Padovani, A., Pantano, P., & Pizzamiglio, L. (1993). Unilateral neglect restricted to visual imagery. *Nature, 364,* 235–237.

Gur, R. C., Packer, I. K., Hungerbuhler, J. P., Reivich, M., Obrist, W. D., Amarnek, W. S., & Sackeim, H. A., (1980). Differences in the distribution of gray and white matter in human cerebral hemispheres. *Science, 207,* 1226–1228.

Hakim, H., Verma, N., & Greiffenstein, M. (1988). Pathogenesis of reduplicative paramnesia. *Journal of Neurology, Neurosurgery, and Psychiatry, 51,* 839–841.

Halligan, P. W., Manning, L., & Marshall, J. C. (1990). Individual variations in line bisection: A study of four patients with right hemisphere damage and normal controls. *Neuropsychologia, 28,* 1043–1051.

Halligan, P. W., Manning, L., & Marshall, J. C. (1991). Hemispheric activation vs. spatiomotor cueing in visual neglect: A case study. *Neuropsychologia, 29,* 165–176.

Halligan, P. W., & Marshall, J. C. (1989). Is neglect (only) lateral? A quadrant analysis of line cancellation. *Journal of Clinical and Experimental Neuropsychology, 11,* 793–798.

Halligan, P. W., & Marshall, J. C. (1993). The history and clinical presentation of neglect. In I. Robertson & J. C. Marshall (Eds.), *Unilateral neglect: Clinical and experimental studies* (pp. 3–26). Hillsdale, NJ: Lawrence Erlbaum.

Halligan, P. W., & Marshall, J. C. (1994). Focal and global attention modulate the expression of visuospatial neglect: A case study. *Neuropsychologia, 32,* 13–21.

Halligan, P. W., Marshall, J. C., & Wade, D. T. (1989). Visuospatial neglect: Underlying factors and test sensitivity. *The Lancet, October 14,* 908–910.

Halligan, P. W., Marshall, J. C., & Wade, D. T. (1990). Do visual field deficits exacerbate visuo-spatial neglect? *Journal of Neurology, Neurosurgery, and Psychiatry, 53,* 487–491.

Halligan, P. W., Marshall, J. C., & Wade, D. T. (1995). Unilateral somatoparaphrenia after right hemisphere stroke: A case description. *Cortex, 31,* 173–182.

Halper, A., Cherney, L. R., & Burns, M. S. (1996). *Clinical management of right hemisphere dysfunction* (2nd ed.). Gaithersburg, MD: Aspen.

Happe, F. G. E. (1994). An advanced test of theory of mind: Understanding of story characters' thoughts and feelings by able autistic, mentally handicapped, and normal children and adults. *Journal of Autism and Developmental Disorders, 24,* 129–154.

Harley, C. W. (1987). A role for norepinephrine in arousal, emotion, and learning?: Limbic modulation by norepinephrine and the Kety hypothesis. *Progress in Neuro-Psychopharmacology and Biological Psychiatry, 11,* 419–458.

Hecaen, H. (1962). Clinical symptomotology in right and left hemisphere lesions. In V. B. Mountcastle (Ed.), *Interhemispheric relations and cerebral dominance.* Baltimore: Johns Hopkins Press.

Heilman, K. M. (1979). Neglect and related disorders. In K. M. Heilman & E. Valenstein (Eds.), *Clinical neuropsychology* (pp. 268–307). New York: Oxford.

Heilman. K. M., Bowers, D., Coslett, H. B., Whelan, H., & Watson, R. T. (1985). Directional hypokinesia: Prolonged reaction times for leftward movements in patients with right hemisphere lesions and neglect. *Neurology, 35,* 855–859.

Heilman, K. M., Bowers, D., Speedie, L., & Coslett, H. B. (1984). Comprehension of affective and nonaffective prosody. *Neurology, 34,* 917–921.

Heilman, K. M., Bowers, D., Valenstein, E., & Watson, R. T. (1987). Hemispace and hemispatial neglect. In M. Jeannerod (Ed.), *Neurophysiological and neuropsychological aspects of spatial neglect* (pp. 115–182). Amsterdam: Elsevier.

Heilman, K. M., Scholes, R., & Watson, R. T. (1975). Auditory affective agnosia: Disturbed comprehension of affective speech. *Journal of Neurology, Neurosurgery, and Psychiatry, 38,* 69–72.

Heilman, K. M., Schwartz, H. D., & Watson, R. T. (1978).Hypoarousal in patients with the neglect syndrome and emotional indifference. *Neurology, 28,* 229–232.

Heilman, K. M., & Valenstein, E. (1972a). Auditory neglect in man. *Archives of Neurology, 26,* 32–35.

Heilman, K. M., & Valenstein, E. (1972b). Frontal lobe neglect in man. *Neurology, 22,* 660–664.

Heilman, K. M., Valenstein, E., & Watson, R. T. (1984). Neglect and related disorders. *Seminars in Neurology, 4,* 209–219.

Heilman, K. M., & Van Den Abell, T. (1980). Right hemisphere dominance for attention: The mechanism underlying hemispheric asymmetries of inattention (neglect). *Neurology, 30:* 327–330.

Heilman, K. M., & Watson, R. T. (1977). Mechanisms underlying the unilateral neglect syndrome. In E. A. Weinstein & R. P. Friedland (Eds.), *Advances in Neurology, 18,* 91–106.

Helm-Estabrooks, N. (1995). *Cognitive linguistic task book.* Cape Cod, MA: Cape Cod Institute for Communication Disorders.

Hier, D. B., & Kaplan, J. (1980). Verbal comprehension deficits after right hemisphere damage. *Applied Psycholginguistics, 1,* 279–294.

Hier, D. B., Mondlock, J., & Caplan, L. R. (1983). Behavioral abnormalities after right hemisphere stroke. *Neurology, 33,* 337–344.

Hird, K., & Kirsner, K. (1993). Dysprosody following acquired neurogenic impairment. *Brain and Language, 48,* 46–60.

Hirst, W., LeDoux, J., & Stein, S. (1984). Constraints on the processing of indirect speech acts: Evidence from aphasiology. *Brain and Language, 23,* 26–33.

Hooper Visual Organization Test. (1983). Los Angeles: Western Psychological Services.

Hornak, J. (1992). Ocular exploration in the dark by patients with visual neglect. *Neuropsychologia, 30,* 547–552.

Horner, J., Massey, E. W., Woodruff, W. W., Chase, K. N., & Dawson, D. V. (1989). Task-dependent neglect: Computed tomography size and locus correlations. *Journal of Neurologic Rehabilitation, 3,* 7–13.

Hough, M. S. (1990). Narrative comprehension in adults with right and left hemisphere brain-damage: Theme organization. *Brain and Language, 38,* 253–277.

Hough, M. S., Pabst, M. J., & DeMarco, S. (1994). Categorization skills in right hemisphere brain damage for common and goal-derived categories. *Clinical Aphasiology, 22,* 35–51.

Hough, M. S., & Pierce, R. S. (1988, November). *Word fluency revisited: Common and functional category structure in aphasic adults.* Paper presented at the annual American Speech-Language-Hearing Association Convention, St. Louis, MO.

Hough, M. S., & Pierce, R. S. (1993). Contextual and thematic influences on narrative comprehension of left and right hemisphere brain-damaged patients. In H. H. Brownell & Y. Joanette (Eds.), *Narrative discourse in neurologically impaired and normal aging adults* (pp. 213–238). San Diego: Singular Publishing Group.

Hough, M. S., & Snow, M. S. (1989, November). *Category structure for goal-derived and common categories in aging.* Paper presented at the annual American Speech-Language-Hearing Association Convention, St. Louis.

House, A., Dennis, M., Warlow, C., Hawton, K., & Molyneux, A. (1990). Mood disorders after stroke and their relation to lesion location. *Brain, 113,* 1113–1129.

House, A., Rowe, D., & Standen, P. J. (1987). Affective prosody in the reading voice of stroke patients. *Journal of Neurology, Neurosurgery, and Psychiatry, 50,* 910–912.

Howes, D., & Boller, F. (1975). Simple reaction time: Evidence for focal impairment from lesions of the right hemisphere. *Brain, 98,* 317–322.

Huber, W. (1990). Text comprehension and production in aphasia: Analysis in terms of micro- and macroprocessing. In Y. Joanette & H. H. Brownell (Eds.), *Discourse ability and brain damage: Theoretical and empirical perspectives* (pp. 154–179). New York: Springer-Verlag.

Huber, W., & Gleber, J. (1982). Linguistic and nonlinguistic processing of narratives in aphasia. *Brain and Language, 16,* 1–18.

Humphreys, G. W., & Riddoch, M. J. (1993). Interactive attentional systems and unilateral visual neglect. In I. Robertson & J. C. Marshall (Eds.), *Unilateral neglect: Clinical and experimental studies* (pp. 139–168). Hillsdale, NJ: Lawrence Erlbaum.

Iacoboni, M., Padovani, A., DiPiero, V., & Lenzi, G. L. (1995). Post-stroke depression: Relationships with morphological damage and cognition over time. *International Journal of Neurological Science, 16,* 209–216.

Ishiai, S., Furukawa, T., & Tsukagoshi, H. (1989). Visuo-spatial processes of line bisection and the mechanisms underlying unilateral spatial neglect. *Brain, 112,* 1485–1502.

Ishiai, S., Sugishita, M., Mitani, K., & Ishizawa, M. (1992). Leftward search in left unilateral spatial neglect. *Journal of Neurology, Neurosurgery, and Psychiatry, 55,* 40–44.

Ito, K., Tanabe, H., Ikejiri, Y., Okuda, J., Sawada, T., & Shiraishi, J. (1989). Tactile extinction to simple (elementary) and complex stimuli. *Acta Neurologica Scandanavia, 80,* 68–77.

Iversen, S. D. (1977). Brain dopamine systems and behavior. In L. L. Iversen, S. D. Iversen, & S. H. Snyder (Eds.), *Handbook of psychopharmacology, Vol. 8. Drugs, neurotransmitters and behavior* (pp. 333–384). New York: Plenum Press.

Janer, K. W., & Pardo, J. V. (1991). Deficits in selective attention following bilateral Ante-rior cingulotomy. *Journal of Cognitive Neuroscience, 3,* 231–241.

Jennings, J. R. (1986). Bodily changes during attention. In M. G. H. Coles, E. Donchin, & S. W. Porges, *Psychophysiology: Systems, processes, and application* (pp. 268–289). New York: Guilford Press.

Joanette, Y., Brouchon, M., Gauthier, L., & Samson, M. (1986). Pointing with the left versus right hand in left visual field neglect. *Neuropsychologia, 24,* 391–396.

Joanette, Y., & Goulet, P. (1986). Criterion-specific reduction of verbal fluency in right brain-damaged right-handers. *Neuropsychologia, 24,* 875–879.

Joanette, Y., Goulet, P., & Hannequin, D. (1990). *Right hemisphere and verbal communication.* New York: Springer-Verlag.

Joanette, Y., Goulet, P., & Le Dorze, G. (1988). Impaired word naming in right-brain-damaged right-handers: Error types and time-course analyses. *Brain and Language, 34,* 54–64.

Joanette, Y., Goulet, P., Ska, B., & Nespoulous, J. L. (1986). Informative content of narrative discourse in right brain-damaged right-handers. *Brain and Language, 29,* 81–105.

Joanette, Y., LeCours, A. R., Lepage, Y., & Lamoureaux, M. (1983). Language in right-handers with right-hemisphere lesions: A preliminary study including anatomical, genetic, and social factors. *Brain and Language, 20,* 217–248.

Jocic, A., & Staton, D. R. (1993). Reduplication after right middle cerebral artery infarction. *Brain and Cognition, 23,* 222–230.

Jongbloed, L. (1986). Prediction of function after stroke: A critical review. *Stroke, 17,* 765–776.

Just, M. A., & Carpenter, P. A. (1992). A capacity theory of comprehension: Individual differences in working memory. *Psychological Review, 99,* 122–149.

Kaplan, J. A., Brownell, H. H., Jacobs, J. R., & Gardner, H. (1990). The effects of right hemisphere damage on the pragmatic interpretation of conversational remarks. *Brain and Language, 38,* 315–333.

Kaplan, J. A., Goodglass, H., & Weintraub, S. (1983). *The Boston Naming Test.* Philadelphia: Lea & Febiger.

Kaplan, R. F., Verfaillie, M., Meadows, M. E., Caplan, L. R., Peasin, M. S., & De Witt, D. (1991). Changing attentional demands in left hemispatial neglect. *Archives of Neurology, 48,* 1263–1266.

Karnath, H. -O., & Huber, W. (1992). Abnormal eye movement behaviour during text reading in neglect syndrome: A case study. *Neuropsychologia, 30,* 593–598.

Kartsounis, L. D., & Warrington, E. K. (1989). Unilateral visual neglect overcome by cues implicit in stimulus arrays. *Journal of Neurology, Neurosurgery, and Psychiatry, 52,* 1253–1259.

Kennedy, M. R. T., Strand, E. A., Burton, W., Peterson, C. (1994). Analysis of first-encounter conversations of right-hemisphere-damaged adults. *Clinical Aphasiology, 22,* 67–80.

Kent, R. D., & Rosenbek, J. C. (1982). Prosodic disturbance and neurologic lesion. *Brain and Language, 15,* 259–291.

Kertesz, A. (1979). *Aphasia and associated disorders.* New York: Grune & Stratton.

Kertesz, A. (1982). *Western Aphasia Battery.* New York: Grune & Stratton.

Kertesz, A., & Dobrowolski, S. (1981). Right-hemisphere deficits, lesion size and location. *Journal of Clinical Neuropsychology, 3,* 283–299.

Kimura, D. (1964). Left-right differences in the perception of melodies. *Quarterly Journal of Experimental Psychology, 16,* 355–358.

King, F. L., & Kimura, D. (1972). Left ear superiority in dichotic perception of vocal and nonverbal sounds. *Canadian Journal of Psychology, 26,* 111–116.

Kinsbourne, M. (1987). Mechanisms of unilateral neglect. In M. Jeanerrod (Ed.), *Neurophysiological and neuropsychological aspects of spatial neglect* (pp. 68–86). Amsterdam: Elsevier.

Kinsbourne, M. (1993). Orientational bias model of unilateral neglect: Evidence from attentional gradients within hemisphere. In I. Robertson & J. C. Marshall (Eds.), *Unilateral neglect: Clinical and experimental studies* (pp. 63–86). Hillsdale, NJ: Lawrence Erlbaum.

Kinsbourne, M., & Warrington, E. (1962). A variety of reading disability associated with right-hemisphere lesions. *Journal of Neurology, Neurosurgery and Psychiatry, 25,* 339–344.

Kinsella, G., & Ford, B., (1980). Acute recovery patterns instroke. *Medical Journal of Australia, 2,* 663–666.

Kinsella, G., Olver, J., Ng, K., Packer, S. & Stark, R. (1993). Analysis of the syndrome of Unilateral neglect. *Cortex, 29,* 135–140.

Koella, W. P. (1982). A modern neurobiological concept of vigilance. *Experientia, 38,* 1426–1437.

Kooistra, C. A., & Heilman, K. M. (1989). Hemispatial visual inattention masquerading as hemianopia. *Neurology, 39,* 1125–1127.

Lacey, B. C., & Lacey, J. I. (1974). Studies of heart rate and other bodily processes in sensorimotor behavior. In P. A. Obrist, A. Black, J. Bruner, & L. DiCara (Eds.), *Cardiovascular psychophysiology: Current issues in response mechanisms, biofeedback, and methodology.* Chicago: Aldine-Ahterton.

Ladavas, E. (1987). Is the hemispatial deficit produced by right parietal lobe damage associated with retinalor gravitational coordinates? *Brain, 110,* 167–180.

Ladavas, E. (1990). Selective spatial attention in patients with visual extinction. *Brain, 113,* 1527–1538.

Ladavas, E. (1993). Spatial dimensions of automatic and voluntary orienting components of attention. In I. Robertson & J. C. Marshall (Eds.), *Unilateral neglect: Clinical and experimental studies* (pp. 193–210). Hillsdale, NJ: Lawerence Erlbaum.

Ladavas, E., Del Pesce, M., & Provinciali, L. (1989). Unilateral attention deficits and hemispheric asymmetries in the control of visual attention. *Neuropsychologia, 27,* 353–366.

Ladavas, E., Petronion, A., & Umilta, C. (1990). The deployment of visual attention in the intact field of hemineglect patients. *Cortex, 26,* 307–317.

Lalande, S., Braun, C. M. J., Charlebois, N., & Whitaker, H. A. (1992). Effects of right and left hemisphere cerebrovascular lesions on discrimination of prosodic and semantic aspects of affect in sentences. *Brain and Language, 42,* 165–186.

Landis, T., Assal, G., & Perret, C. (1979). Opposite cerebral hemispheric superiorities for visual associative processing of emotional facial expressions and objects. *Nature, 278,* 739–740.

Landis, T., Cummings, J. G., Christen, L., Bogen, J. E., & Imhof, H. G. (1986). Are unilateral right posterior cerebral lesions sufficient to cause prosopagnosia? Clinical and radiological findings in six additional patients. *Cortex, 22,* 243–252.

Langer, K. G. (1995). Depression and physical disability: Relationship of self-rated and observer-rated disability to depression. *Neuropsychiatry, Neuropsychology and Behavioral Neurology, 8,* 271–276.

Laplane, D., & Degos, J. D. (1983). Motor neglect. *Journal of Neurology, Neurosurgery, and Psychiatry, 46,* 152–158.

Leslie, A. M. (1987). Pretense and representation: The origins of "Theory of Mind." *Psychological Review, 94,* 412–426.

Lesser, R. (1974). Verbal comprehension in aphasia: An English version of three Italian tests. *Cortex, 10,* 247–263.

Levine, D. N., & Finklestein, S. (1982). Delayed psychosis after right temporoparietal stroke or trauma: Relation to epilepsy. *Neurology, 32,* 267–273.

Levine, D. N., & Grek, A. (1984). The anatomic basis of delusions after right cerebral infarction. *Neurology, 34,* 577–582.

Levine, D. N., & Kinsbourne, M. (1986). Neurobehavior. In S. H. Appel (Ed.), *Current neurology* (Vol. 6, pp. 325–346). Chicago: Year Book Medical Publishers, Inc.

Ley, R. G., & Bryden, M. P. (1979). Hemispheric differences in processing emotions and faces. *Brain and Language, 7,* 127–138.

Lipsey, J. R., Robinson, R. G., Pearlson, G. D., Rao, K., & Price, T. R. (1984, February). Nortriptyline treatment for post-stroke depression: A double blind study. *Lancet,* 297–300.

Logan, G. D. (1988). Toward an instance theory of automatization. *Psychological Review, 95,* 492–527.

Lojek-Osiejuk, E. (1996). Knowledge of scripts reflected in discourse of aphasics and right-brain-damaged patients. *Brain and Language, 53,* 58–80.

Luria, A. (1973). *The working brain: An introduction to neuropsychology.* Harmondsworth: Penguin Books.

Mackisack, E. L., Myers, P. S., & Duffy, J. R. (1987). Verbosity and labeling behavior: The performance of right hemisphere and non-brain-damaged adults on an inferential picture description task. In R. H. Brookshire (Ed.), *Clinical Aphasiology* (Vol. 17, pp. 143–151). Minneapolis: BRK Publishers.

Magnun, G. R., Luck, S. J., Plager, R., Loftus, W., Hillyard, S. A., Handy, T., Clark, V. P., & Gazzaniga, M. S. (1994). Monitoring the visual world: Hemispheric asymmetries and subcortical processes in attention. *Journal of Cognitive Neuroscience, 6,* 267–275.

Mammucari, A., Caltagirone, C., Ekman, P., Friesen, W., Gainotti, G., Pizzamiglio, L., & Zoccolotti, P. (1988). Spontaneous facial expression of emotions in brain-damaged patients. *Cortex, 24,* 521–533.

Manning, L., Halligan, P. W., & Marshall, J. C. (1990). Individual variation in line bisection.

A study of normal subjects with application to the interpretation of visual neglect. *Neuropsychologia, 28,* 647–655.

Mark, V. W., & Heilman, K. M. (1988). Does fatigue account for left peripersonal neglect? [Abstract]. *Journal of Clinical and Experimental Neuropsychology, 10,* 335.

Mark, V. W., Kooistra, C. A., & Heilman, K. M. (1988). Hemispatial neglect affected by non-neglected stimuli. *Neurology, 38,* 1207–1211.

Marquardsen, J. (1969). The natural history of acutecerebrovascular disease: A retrospective study of 769 patients. *Acta Neurologica Scandinavica, 38*(Suppl.), 1–192.

Marr, D. (1982). *Vision.* San Francisco: Freeman.

Marshall, J. C., & Halligan, P. W. (1988). Blindsight and insight in visuo-spatial neglect. *Nature, 336,* 766–767.

Marshall, J. F., & Gotthelf, T. (1979). Sensory inattention in rats with 6–hydroxydopamine-induced degeneration of ascending dopaminergic neurons: Apomorphine-induced reversal of deficits. *Experimental Neurology, 65,* 398–411.

Martin, C. C., Borod, J. C., Alpert, M., Brozgold, A., & Welkowitz, J. (1990). Spontaneous expression of facial emotion in schizophrenic and right-brain-damaged patients. *Journal of Communicaiton Disorders. 23,* 287–301.

McDonald, S. (1993). Viewing the brain sideways? Frontal versus right hemisphere: Explanations of non-aphasic language disorders. *Aphasiology, 7,* 535–549.

McDonald, S., & Pearce, S. (1996). Clinical insights into pragmatic theory: Frontal lobe deficits and sarcasm. *Brain and Language, 53,* 81–104.

McDonald, S., & Wales, R.(1986). An investigation of the ability to process inferences in language following right hemisphere brain damage. *Brain and Language, 29,* 68–80.

McGlynn, S. M., & Schacter, D. L. (1989). Unawareness of deficits in neuropsychological syndromes. *Journal of Clinical and Experimental Neuropsychology, 11,* 143–205.

McGuinness, D., & Pribram, K. (1980). The neuropsychology of attention: Emotional and motivational controls. In M. C. Wittrock (Ed.), *The brain and psychology.* New York: Academic Press.

McNeil, M. R., & Prescott, T. E. (1978), *The Revised Token Test.* Austin, TX: Pro-Ed.

Meador, K. J., Loring, D. W., Bowers, D., & Heilman, K. M. (1987). Remote memory and neglect syndrome. *Neurology, 37,* 522–526.

Meinberg, O., Zangemeister, W. H., Rosenberg, M., Hoyt, W. F., & Stark, L. (1981). Saccadic eye movement strategies in patients with homonymous hemianopia. *Annals of Neurology, 9,* 537–544.

Merewether, F. C., & Alpert, M. (1990). The components and neuroanatomic basis of prosody. *Journal of Communication Disorders, 31,* 325–336.

Mesulam, M. -M. (1981). A cortical network for directed attention and unilateral neglect. *Annals of Neurology, 10,* 309–325.

Mesulam, M. -M (1985). Attention, confusional states, and neglect. In M. -M Mesulam (Ed.), *Principles of behavioral neurology* (pp. 125–168). Philadelphia: F. A. Davis.

Mesulam, M. -M., Waxman, S. G., Geschwind, N., & Sabin, T. D. (1976). Acute confusional states with right middle cerebral artery infarctions. *Journal of Neurology, Neurosurgery and Psychiatry, 39,* 84–89.

Mijovic, D. (1991). Mechanisms of visual spatial neglect: Absence of directional hypokinesia in spatial exploration. *Brain, 114,* 1575–1593.

Miller, L. (1994). Unusual head injury syndromes: Clinical, neuropsychological, and forensic considerations. *The Journal of Cognitive Rehabilitation, 12,* 12–22.

Monrad-Krohn, G. H. (1947). Dysprosody or altered "melody of language." *Brain, 70,* 405–415.

Morrow, L., Vrtunski, P. B., Kim, Y., & Boller, F. (1981). Arousal responses to emotional stimuli and laterality of lesion. *Neuropsychologia, 19,* 65–71.

Moya, K. L., Benowitz, L. I., Levine, D. N., & Finklestein, S. P. (1986). Covariant deficits in visuospatial abilities and recall of verbal narrative after right hemisphere stroke. *Cortex, 22,* 381–397.

Myers, P. S. (1978). Analysis of right hemisphere communication deficits: Implications for speech pathology. In R. H. Brookshire (Ed.), *Clinical aphasiology: Conference Proceedings* (pp. 49–57). Minneapolis, MN: BRK Publishers.

Myers, P. S. (1979). Profiles of communication deficits in patients with right cerebral hemisphere damage. In R. H. Brookshire (Ed.), *Clinical aphasiology: Conference proceedings* (pp. 38–46). Minneapolis: BRK Publishers.

Myers, P. S. (1994). Communication disorders associated with right hemisphere brain damage. In R. Chapey (Ed.), *Language intervention strategies in adult aphasia* (3rd ed., pp. 514–534). Baltimore: Wiliams & Wilkins.

Myers, P. S. (1997). Right hemisphere syndrome. In L. LaPointe (Ed.), *Aphasia and related neurogenic disorders* (pp. 201–225). New York: Thieme Medical Publishers.

Myers, P. S., & Brookshire, R. H. (1994). The effects of visual and inferential complexity on the picture descriptions of non-brain-damaged and right-hemisphere-damaged adults. *Clinical Aphasiology, 22,* 25–34.

Myers, P. S., & Brookshire, R. H. (1995). Effects of noun type on naming performance of right-hemisphere-damaged and non-brain-damaged adults. *Clinical Aphasiology, 23,* 195–206.

Myers, P. S., & Brookshire, R. H. (1996). Effect of visual and inferential variables on scene descriptions by right-hemisphere-damaged and non-brain-damaged adults. *Journal of Speech and Hearing Research, 39,* 870–880.

Myers, P. S., & Linebaugh, C. W. (1981). Comprehension of idiomatic expressions by right-hemisphere-damaged adults. In R. H. Brookshire (Ed.), *Clinical aphasiology: Conference Proceedings* (pp. 254–261). Minneapolis: BRK Publishers.

Myers, P. S., Linebaugh, C. W., & Mackisack-Morin, E. L. (1985). Extracting implicit meaning: Right versus left hemisphere damage. *Clinical Aphasiology, 15,* 72–80.

Myers, P. S., & Mackisack, E. L. (1986). Defining single and dual definition idioms: The performance of right hemisphere and non-brain-damaged adults. *Clinical Aphasiology, 17,* 267–274.

Myers, P. S., & Mackisack, E. L. (1990). Right hemisphere syndrome. In L. LaPointe (Ed.), *Aphasia and related neurogenic disorders* (1st ed., pp. 196–209). New York: Thieme Medical Publishers.

Nagel-Leiby, S., Buchtel, H. A., & Welch, K. M. A. (1990). Cerebral control of directed visual attention and orienting saccades. *Brain, 113,* 237–276.

Natale, M., Gur, R. E., & Gur, R. C. (1983). Hemispheric asymmetries in processing emotional expressions. *Neuropsychologia, 21,* 555–565.

Nebes, R. D. (1972). Dominance of the minor hemisphere in commissurotomized man. *Brain, 95,* 633–638.

Nelson, L. D., Cicchetti, D., Satz, P., Sowa, M., & Mitrushina, M. (1994). Emotional sequelae of stroke: A longitudinal perspective. *Journal of*

Clinical and Experimental Neuropsychology, 16, 796–806.

Ng, K. C., Chan, K. L., & Straughan, P. T. (1995). A study of post-stroke depression in a rehabilitative center. *Acta Psychiatrica Scandinavia, 92,* 75–79.

Nichelli, P., Rinaldi, M., & Cubelli, R. (1989). Selective spatial attention and length representation in normal subjects and in patients with unilateral spatial neglect. *Brain and Cognition, 9,* 57–70.

Nichelli, P., Venneri, A., Pentore, R., & Cubelli, R. (1993). Horizontal and vertical neglect dyslexia. *Brain and Language, 44,* 264–283.

Nicholas, L. E., & Brookshire, R. H. (1993). A system for quantifying the informativeness and efficiency of the connected speech of adults with aphasia. *Journal of Speech and Hearing Research, 36,* 338–350.

Nicholas, L. E., & Brookshire, R. H. (1995). Presence, completeness, and accuracy of main concepts in the connected speech of non-brain-damaged adults and adults with aphasia. *Journal of Speech and Hearing Research, 38,* 145–157.

Norman, D. A., & Shallice, T. (1986). Attention to action: Willed and automatic control of behavior. In R. J. Davidson, G. E. Schwartz, & D. Shapiro (Eds.), *Consciousness and self-regulation. Vol. 4.* New York: Plenum Press.

Ogden, J. A. (1985a). Anterior-posterior interhemispheric differences in the loci of lesions producing visual hemineglect. *Brain and Cognition, 4,* 59–75.

Ogden, J. A. (1985b). Contralesional neglect of constructed visual images in right and left brain-damaged patients. *Neuropsychologia, 23,* 273–277.

Ogden, J. A. (1987). The "neglected" left hemisphere and its contribution to visuospatial neglect. In M.Jeannerod (Ed.), *Neurophysiological and neuropsychological aspects of spatial neglect* (pp. 215–234). Amsterdam: Elsevier.

Oke, A., Keller, R., Mefford, I., & Adams, R. (1978). Lateralization of norepinephrine in human thalamus. *Science, 200,* 1411–1413.

Oke, A., Lewis, R., & Adams, R. N. (1980). Hemispheric asymmetry of norepinephrine distribution in rat thalamus. *Brain Research, 188,* 269–272.

Ostrove, J. M., Simpson, T., & Gardner, H. (1990). Beyond scripts: A note on the capacity of right hemisphere-damaged patients to process social and emotional content. *Brain and Cognition, 12,* 144–154.

Pardo, J. V., Fox, P. T., & Raichle, M. E. (1991). Localization of a human system for sustained attention by positron emission tomography. *Nature, 349,* 61–64.

Pardo, J. V., Pardo P. J., Janer K. W., & Raichle, M. E. (1990). The anterior cingulate cortex mediates processing selection in the Stroop attentional conflict paradigm. *Proceedings of the National Academy of Science, 87,* 256–259.

Parisi, D., & Pizzamiglio, L. (1970). Syntactic comprehension in aphasia. *Cortex, 6,* 204–215.

Pearlson, G. D., & Robinson, R. G. (1981). Suction lesions of the frontal cerebral cortex in the rat induce asymmetrical behavioral and catecholaminergic responses. *Brain Research, 218,* 233–242.

Penn, C. (1988). The profiling of syntax and pragmatics in aphasia. *Clinical Linguisitics and Phonetics, 2,* 179–208.

Perani, D., Vallar, G., Paulesu, E., Alberoni, M., & Fazio, F. (1993). Left and right hemisphere contribution to recovery from neglect after right hemisphere damage an [18 F] FDG PET study of two cases. *Neuropsychologia, 31,* 115–125.

Pick, A. (1903). Clinical studies III: On reduplicative paramnesia. *Brain, 26,* 260–267.

Pimental, P. A., & Kingsbury, N. A. (1989). *Mini inventory of right brain injury.* Austin: Pro-Ed.

Pinek, B., Duhamel, J. R., Cave, C., & Brouchon, M. (1989). Audio-spatial deficit in humans: Differential effects associated with left versus right hemisphere parietal damage. *Cortex, 25,* 175–186.

Pizzamiglio, L., Antonucci, G., Judica, A., Montenero, P., Razzano, C., & Zoccolotti, P. (1992). Cognitive rehabilitation of the hemineglect disorder in chronic patients with unilateral right brain damage. *Journal of Clinical and Experimental Neuropsychology, 14,* 901–923.

Pizzamiglio, L., Cappa, S., Vallar, G., Zoccolotti, P., Bottini, G., Ciurli, P., Guariglia, C., & Antonucci, G., (1989). Visual neglect for far and near extra-personal space in humans. *Cortex, 25,* 471–477.

Plourde, G., Joanette, Y., Fontaine, F. S., LaPlante, L., & Renaseau-Leclerc, C. (1993). The severity of visual hemineglect follows a bimodal frequency distribution. *Brain and Cognition, 21,* 131–139.

Ponsford, J. L., & Kinsella, G. (1988). Evaluation of a remedial programme for attentional deficits following closed-head injury. *Journal of*

Clinical and Experimental Neuropsychology, 10, 693–708.

Posner, M. I., Inhoff, A., Friedrich, F. J., & Cohen, A. (1987). Isolating attentional systems: A cognitive anatomical analysis. *Psychobiology, 15,* 107–121.

Posner, M. I., & Petersen, S. E. (1990). The attention system of the human brain. *Annual Review of Neuroscience, 13,* 25–42.

Posner, M. I., Walker, J. A., Friedrich, F. A., & Rafal, R. D. (1984). Effects of parietal lobe injury on covert orienting of visual attention. *Journal of Neuroscience, 4,* 1863–1874.

Posner, M. I., Walker, J. A., Friedrich, F. A., & Rafal, R. D. (1987). How do the parietal lobes direct covert attention? *Neuropsychologia, 25,* 135–145.

Premack, D., & Woodruff, G. (1975). Problem-solving in chimpanzee: Test for comprehension. *Science, 202,* 532–535.

Premack, D., & Woodruff, G. (1978). Does the chimpanzee have a theory of mind? *The Behavioral and Brain Sciences, 1,* 515–526.

Pribram, K. H., & McGuinness, D. (1975). Arousal, activation, and effort in the control of attention. *Psychological Review, 82,* 116–149.

Price, B. H., & Mesulam, M. (1985). Psychiatric manifestations of right hemisphere infarctions. *Journal of Nervous and Mental Disease, 173,* 610–614.

Prutting, C. A., & Kirchner, D. M. (1987). A clinical appraisal of the pragmatic aspects of language. *Journal of Speech and Hearing Disorders, 52,* 105–119.

Purdy, M. (1997, November). *Script knowledge in right brain-damaged adults.* Paper presented to the American Speech-Language-Hearing Association Convention, Boston, MA.

Rafal, R. D., & Posner, M. I. (1987). Deficits in human visual spatial attention following thalamic lesions. *Proceedings of the National Academy of Science, 84,* 7349–7353.

Ramasubbu, R., & Kennedy, S. H. (1994). Factors complicating the diagnosis of depression in cerebrovascular disease Part I: Phenomenological and nosological issues. *Canadian Journal of Psychiatry, 39,* 596–607.

Rapcsak, S. Z., Cimino, C. R., & Heilman, K. M. (1988). Altitudinal neglect. *Neurology, 38,* 277–281.

Rapcsak, S. Z., Verfaellie, M., Fleet, W. S., & Heilman, K. M. (1989). Selective attention in hemispatial neglect. *Archives of Neurology, 46,* 178–182.

Reding, M. J., Orto, L. A., Winter, S. W., Fortuna,

I. M., Di Ponte, P. M., & McDowell, F. H. (1986). Antidepressant therapy after stroke: A double-blind trial. *Archives of Neurology, 43,* 763–765.

Rehak, A., Kaplan, J. A., & Gardner, H. (1992). Sensitivity to conversational deviance in right-hemisphere-damaged patients. *Brain and Language, 42,* 203–217.

Rehak, A., Kaplan, J. A., Weylman, S. T., Kelly, B., Brownell, H. H., & Gardner, H. (1992). Story processing in right-hemisphere brain-damaged patients. *Brain and Language, 42,* 320–336.

Reitan, R. M. (1958). Validity of the Trail Making Test as an indicator of organic brain damage. *Perceptual and Motor Skills, 8,* 271–276.

Reitan, R. M., & Wolfson, D. (1985). *The Halstead-Reitan Neuropsychological Test Battery.* Tucson, AZ: Neuropsychology Press.

Reuter-Lorenz, P. A., & Posner, M. I. (1990). Components of neglect from right-hemisphere damage: An analysis of line bisection. *Neuropsychologia, 28,* 321–333.

Riddoch, M. J., & Humphreys, G. W. (1987). Perceptual action systems in unilateral neglect. In M. Jeannerod (Ed.), *Neurophysiological and neuropsychological aspects of spatial neglect* (pp. 151–181). Amsterdam: Elsevier.

Riddoch, M. J., Humphreys, G. W., Cleton, P., & Fery, P. (1990). Interaction of attentional and lexical processes in neglect dyslexia. *Cognitive Neuropsychology, 7,* 479–518.

Rivers, D. L., & Love, R. J. (1980). Language performance on visual processing tasks in right hemisphere lesion cases. *Brain and Language, 10,* 348–366.

Rizzo, M., & Robin, D. A. (1990). Simultagnosia: A defect of sustained attention yields insights on visual information processing. *Neurology, 40,* 447–455.

Rizzo, M., & Robin, D. A. (1996). Bilateral effects of unilateral visual cortex lesions. *Brain, 119,* 951–963.

Rizzolatti, G., & Berti, A. (1993). Neural mechanisms of spatial neglect. In I. H. Robertson & J. C. Marshall (Eds.), *Unilateral neglect: Clinical and experimental studies* (pp. 87–106). Hillsdale, NJ: Lawrence Erlbaum.

Rizzolatti, G., & Camarda, R. (1987). Neural circuits for spatial attention and unilateral neglect. In M. Jeannerod (Ed.) *Neurophysiological and neuropsychological aspects of neglect* (pp. 289–313). Amsterdam: Elsevier.

Rizzolatti, G., Riggio, L., Dascola, I., & Umilta, C. (1987). Reorienting attention across the horizontal and vertical meridians: Evidence in favor of a premotor theory of attention. *Neuropyschologia, 25,* 55–71.

Robbins, T. W., & Everett, B. J. (1982). Functional studies of the central catecholamines. *International Review of Neurobiology, 23,* 303–365.

Robertson, I. (1989). Anomalies in the laterality of omissions in unilateral left visual neglect: Implications for an attentional theory of neglect. *Neuropsychologia, 27,* 157–165.

Robertson, I. (1990). Digit span and visual neglect: A puzzling relationship. *Neuropsychologia, 28,* 217–222.

Robertson, I. H., Gray, J. M., Pentland, B., & Waite, M. A. (1989). Microcomputer-based rehabilitation for unilateral left visual neglect: A randomized controlled trial. *Archives of Physical Medicine and Rehabilitation, 71,* 663–668.

Robertson, I. H., Halligan, P. W., & Marshall, J. C. (1993). Prospects for the rehabilitation of unilateral neglect. In I. H. Robertson & J. C. Marshall (Eds.), *Unilateral neglect: Clinical and experimental studies* (pp. 279–292). Hillsdale, NJ: Lawrence Erlbaum.

Robertson, I., & North, N. (1992). Spatio-motor cueing in unilateral left neglect: The role of hemispace, hand and motor activation. *Neuropsychologia, 30,* 553–563.

Robertson, I., & North, N. (1993). Active and passive activation of left limbs: Influence on visual and sensory neglect. *Neuropsychologia, 31,* 293–300.

Robertson, I., Ward, T., Ridgeway, V., & Nimmo-Smith, I. (1994). *Test of Everyday Attention.* London: Thames Valley Test Company.

Robertson, L. C., & Delis, D. C. (1986). "Part-whole" processing in unilateral brain-damaged patients: Dysfunction of hierarchical organization. *Neuropsychologia, 24,* 363–370.

Robin, D. A., Tranel, D., & Damasio, H. (1990). Auditory perception of temporal and spectral events in patients with focal left and right cerebral lesions. *Brain and Language, 39,* 539–555.

Robinson, R. G. (1985). Lateralized behavioral and neurochemical consequences of Unilateral brain injury in rats. In S. G. Glick (Ed.), *Cerebral lateralization in nonhuman species* (pp. 135–156). Orlando, FL: Academic Press.

Robinson, R. G., Kubos, K. L., Starr, L. B., Rao, K., & Price, T. R. (1984). Mood disorders in stroke patients: Importance of location of lesion. *Brain, 107,* 81–93.

Robinson, R. G., & Price, T. R. (1982). Post-stroke depressive disorders: A follow-up study of 103 patients. *Stroke, 13,* 635–641.

Robinson, R. G., Starr, L. B., Kubos, K. L., & Price, T. R. (1983). A two year longitudinal study of post-stroke mood disorders: Findings during the initial evaluation. *Stroke, 14,* 736–741.

Robinson, R. G., Starr, L. B., Lipsey, J. R., Rao, K., & Price, T. R. (1984). A two year longitudinal study of post-stroke mood disorders: Dynamic changes in associated variables over the first six months of follow-up. *Stroke, 15,* 510–517.

Rode, G., Charles, N., Perenin, M. T., Vighetto, A., Trillet, M., Aimard, G. (1992). Partial remission of hemiplegia and somatoparaphrenia through vestibular stimulation in a case of unilateral neglect. *Cortex, 28,* 203–208.

Roman, M., Brownell, H. H., Potter, H. H., Seibold, M. S., & Gardner, H. (1987). Script knowledge in right hemisphere-damaged and normal elderly adults. *Brain and Language, 31,* 151–170.

Rosenthal, R., Hall, J. A., DiMatteo, M. R., Rogers, P. L., & Archer, D. (1979). *Profile of nonverbal sensitivity (PONS).* Baltimore: Johns Hopkins University

Ross, E. D. (1981). The aprosodias. *Archives of Neurology, 38,* 561–569.

Ross, E. D. (1985). Modulation of affect and nonverbal communication by the right hemisphere. In M. -M. Mesulam, (Ed.), *Principles of behavioral neurology* (pp. 239–257). Philadelphia: F. A. Davis.

Ross, E. D. (1988). Prosody and brain lateralization: Fact vs. fancy or is it all just semantics? *Archives of Neurology, 45,* 338–339.

Ross, E. D. (1993). Nonverbal aspects of language. *Behavioral Neurology, 11,* 9–23.

Ross, E. D., Edmondson, J. A., Seibert, G. B., & Homan, R. W. (1988). Acoustic analysis of affective measures of prosody during right-sided Wada test: A within-subjects verification of the right hemisphere's role in language. *Brain and Language, 33,* 128–145.

Ross, E. D., Harney, J. H., deLacoste-Utamsing, C., & Purdy, P. D. (1981). How the brain integrates affective and propositional language into a unified behavioral function. *Archives of Neurology, 38,* 745–748.

Ross, E. D., & Mesulam, M. -M. (1979). Dominant language functions of the right hemisphere? Prosody and emotional gesturing. *Archives of Neurology, 36,* 144–148.

Ross, E. D., & Rush, A. J. (1981). Diagnosis and neuroanatomical correlates of depression in brain-damaged patients: Implications for a neurology of depression. *Archives of General Psychiatry, 36,* 144–148.

Rubens, A. B. (1985). Caloric stimulation and unilateral visual neglect. *Neurology, 35,* 1019–1024.

Ruff, R. M., Evans, R. W., & Light, R. H. (1986). Automatic detection vs. controlled search: A paper-and-pencil approach. *Perceptual and Motor Skills, 62,* 407–416.

Ruff, R. M., Hersh, N. A., & Pribram, K. H. (1981). Auditory spatial deficits in the personal and extrapersonal frames of reference due to cortical lesions. *Neuropsychologia, 19,* 435–443.

Ruff, R. M., Nieman, H., Allen, C. C., Farrow, C. E., & Wylie, T. (1992). The Ruff 2 and 7 selective attention test: A neuropsychological application. *Perceptual and Motor Skills, 75,* 1311–1319.

Ruff, R., & Volpe, B. T. (1981). Environmental reduplication associated with right frontal and parietal lobe injury. *Journal of Neurology, Neurosurgery, and Psychiatry, 44,* 382–386.

Ryalls, J. H. (1982). Intonation in Broca's aphasia. *Neuropsychologia, 20,* 366–360.

Ryalls, J. H. (1986). What constitutes a primary disturbance of speech prosody? A reply to Shapiro and Danly. *Brain and Language, 29,* 183–187.

Ryalls, J. H., & Behrens, S. J. (1988). An overview of changes in fundamental frequency associated with cortical insult. *Aphasiology, 2,* 107–115.

Ryalls, J., Joanette, Y., & Feldman, L. (1987). An acoustic comparison of normal and right-hemisphere-damaged speech prosody. *Cortex, 23,* 685–694.

Sakeim, H. A., Greenberg, M. S., Weiman, A. L., Gur, R. C., Hungerbuhler, J. P., & Geschwind, N. (1982). Hemispheric asymmetry in the expression of positive and negative emotions. *Archives of Neurology, 39,* 210–218.

Sargent, J. (1987). Information processing and laterality effects for object and face perception. In G. W. Humphreys & M. J. Riddoch (Eds.), *Visual object processing: A cognitive neuropsychological approach* (pp. 145–174). Hillsdale, NJ: Lawrence Erlbaum.

Schenkenberg, T., Bradford, D. C., & Ajax, E. T. (1980). Line bisection and unilateral visual neglect in patients with neurologic impairment. *Neurology, 30:* 509–517.

Schlanger, B. B., Schlanger, P., & Gerstman, L. J. (1976). The perception of emotionally toned sentences by right-hemisphere-damaged and aphasic subjects. *Brain and Language, 3,* 396–403.

Schmidley, J. W., & Messing, R. O. (1984). Agitated confusional states in patients with right hemisphere infarctions. *Stroke, 15,* 883–885.

Schneiderman, E. I., Murasugi, K. G., & Saddy, J. D. (1992). Story arrangement ability in right brain-damaged patients. *Brain and Language, 43,* 107–120.

Schneiderman, E. I., & Saddy, J. D. (1988). A linguistic deficit resulting from right-hemisphere damage. *Brain and Language, 34,* 38–53.

Schuell, H. M. (1965). *The Minnesota Test for Differential Diagnosis of Aphasia.* Minneapolis: University of Minnesota Press.

Schuell, H. M., Jenkins, J. J., & Jimnez-Papn, E. (1964). *Aphasia in adults.* New York: Harper & Row.

Schwartz, A. S., Marchok, P. L., Kreinick, C. J., & Flynn, R. E (1979). The asymmetric lateralization of tactile extinction in patients with unilateral cerebral dysfunction. *Brain, 102,* 669–684.

Schweigert, W. A., & Moates, D. R. (1988). Familiar idiom comprehension. *Journal of Psycholinguistic Research, 17,* 281–296.

Scott, S., Caird, F., & Williams, B. (1984). Evidence for an apparent sensory speech disorders in Parkinson's disease. *Journal of Neurology, Neurosurgery, and Psychiatry, 47,* 840–843.

Semmes, J. (1968). Hemispheric specialization; A possible clue to mechanism. *Neuropsychologia, 6,* 11–26.

Seron, X., Van der Kaa, M. A., Vanderlinden, M., Remits, A., & Feyereisen, P. (1982) Decoding paralinguistic signals: Effect of semantic and prosodic cues on aphasic comprehension. *Journal of Communication Disorders, 15,* 223–231.

Shank, R. C., & Abelson, R. P. (1977). *Scripts, plans, goals, and understanding.* Hillsdale, NJ: Laurence Erlbaum.

Shapiro, B. E., & Danly, M. (1985). The role of the right hemisphere in the control of speech prosody in propositional and affective contexts. *Brain and Language, 25,* 19–36.

Sharpe, M., Hawton, K., Seagroatt, V., Bamford, J., House, A., Molyneux, A., Sandercock, P., & Warlow, C. (1994). Depressive disorders in long-term survivors of stroke: Associations with demographic and social factors, functional status, and brain lesion volume. *British Journal of Psychiatry, 164,* 380–386.

Sherratt, S. M., & Penn, C. (1990). Discourse in a right-hemisphere brain-damaged subject. *Aphasiology, 4,* 539–560.

Shiffrin, R. M., & Schneider, W. (1977). Controlled and automatic human information processing: II. Perceptual learning, automatic attending and a general theory. *Psychological Review, 84,* 127–190.

Shraberg, D., & Weitzel, W. D. (1979). Prosopagnosia and the Capgras syndrome. *Journal of Clinical Psychiatry, 40,* 313–316.

Sidtis, J. J. (1980). On the nature of the cortical function underlying right hemisphere auditory perception. *Neuropsychologia, 18,* 321–330.

Sidtis, J. J., & Feldman, E. (1990). Transient ischemic attacks presenting with a loss of pitch perception. *Cortex, 26,* 469–471.

Sidtis, J. J., & Volpe, B. T. (1988). Selective loss of complex pitch or speech discrimination after unilateral lesion. *Brain and Language, 34,* 235–245.

Siegal, M., Carrington, J., & Radel, M. (1996). Theory of mind and pragmatic understanding following right hemisphere damage. *Brain and Language, 53,* 40–50.

Sieroff, E., Pollatek, A., & Posner, M. I. (1988). Recognition of visual letter strings following injury to the posterior visual spatial attention system. *Cognitive Neuropsychology, 5,* 427–449.

Silberman, E. K., & Weingartner, H. (1986). Hemispheric lateralization of functions related to emotion. *Brain and Cognition, 5,* 322–353.

Sinyor, D., Jacques, P., Kaloupek, D. G., Becker, R., Goldenberg, M., & Coopersmith, H. (1986). Poststroke depression and lesion location: An attempted replication. *Brain, 109,* 537–546.

Sohlberg, M. M., & Mateer, C. A. (1986). *Attention process training* (APT). Puyallup, WA: Association for Neuropsychological Research and Development.

Sohlberg, M. M., & Mateer, C. A. (1987). Effectiveness of an attention-training program. *Journal of Clinical and Exprimental Neuropsychology, 9,* 117–130.

Speedie, L. J., Brake, N., Folstein, S., Bowers, D., & Heilman, K. M. (1990). Comprehension of prosody in Huntington's disease. *Journal of Neurology, Neurosurgery, and Psychiatry, 53,* 607–610.

Sperry, R. W. (1974). Lateral specialization in the surgically-separated hemispheres. In F. O. Schmitt & F. G. Worden (Eds.), *The neurosciences third study program.* Cambridge, MA: MIT Press.

Spinelli, D., Guariglia, C., Massironi, M., Pizzamiglio, L., & Zoccolotti, P. (1990). Contrast sensitivity and low spatial frequency discrimination in hemineglect Patients. *Neuropsychologia, 28,* 727–732.

Spinneli, D., & Zoccolotti, P. (1992). Perception of moving and stationary gratings in brain damaged patients with unilateral spatial neglect. *Neuropsychologia, 30,* 393–401.

Spitzer, H., Desimone, R., & Moran, J. (1988). Increased attention enhances both behavioral and neuronal performance. *Science, 240,* 338–340.

Springer, S. P., & Deutsch, G. (1981). *Left brain, right brain.* San Francisco: W. H. Freeman.

Stachowiack, F., Huber, W., Poeck, K., & Kerschensteiner, M. (1977). Text comprehension in aphasia. *Brain and Language, 7,* 177–195.

Stamenkovic, M., Schindler, S., & Kasper, S. (1996). Poststroke depression and fluoxetine [Letter to the editor]. *American Journal of Psychiatry, 153,* 446–447.

Starkstein, S. E., Federoff, J. P., Price, T. R., Leiguarda, R. C., & Robinson, R. G. (1994). Neuropsychological and neuroradiologic correlates of emotional prosody comprehension. *Neurology, 44,* 516–522.

Stemmer, B., Giroux, F., Joanette, Y. (1994). Production and evaluation of requests by right hemisphere brain-damaged individuals. *Brain and Language, 47,* 1–31.

Sterzi, R., Bottini, G., Celani, M. G., Righetti, E., Lamassa, M., Ricci, S., & Vallar, G. (1993). Hemianopia, hemianaesthesia, and hemiplegia after right and left hemisphere damage. A hemispheric difference. *Journal of Neurology, Neurosurgery, and Psychiatry, 56,* 308–310.

Stone, S. P., Halligan, P. W., Wilson, B., Greenwood, R. J., & Marshall, J. C. (1991). Performance of age-matched controls on a battery of visuo-spatial neglect tests. *Journal of Neurology, Neurosurgery, and Psychiatry, 54,* 341–344.

Strauss, E., & Muscovitch, M. (1981). Perception of facial expression. *Brain and Language, 13,* 308–332.

Stroop, J. R. (1935). Studies of interference in serial verbal reactions. *Journal of Experimental Psychology, 18,* 643–662.

Stuss, D. T., & Benson, D. F. (1986). *The frontal lobes.* New York: Raven Press.

Suberi, M. & McKeever, W. F. (1977). Differntial right hemisphere memory storage of emotional and non-emotional faces. *Neuropsychologia, 15,* 757–768.

Sundet, K., Finset, A., & Reinvang, I. (1988). Neuropsychological predictors in stroke rehabilitation. *Journal of Clinical and Experimental Neuropsychology, 10,* 363–379.

Swinney, D. A., & Cutler, A. (1979). The access and processing of idiomatic expressions. *Journal of Verbal Learning and Verbal Behavior, 18,* 523–534.

Swisher, L. P., & Sarno, M. T. (1969). Token test scores of three matched patient groups; Left brain-damaged with aphasia; right brain-damaged without aphasia; non-brain-damaged. *Cortex, 5,* 264–273.

Tackett, R. L., Webb, J. G., & Privitera, P. J. (1981). Cerebroventricular propranolol elevates cerebrospinal fluid norepinephrine and lowers blood pressure. *Science, 213,* 911–913.

Tartaglione, A., Bino, G., Manzino, M., Spadavecchia, L., & Favale, E. (1986). Simple reaction-time changes in patients with unilateral brain damage. *Neuropsychologia, 24,* 649–658.

Tartaglione, A., Oneto, A., Manzino, M., & Favale, E. (1987). Further evidence for focal effect of right hemisphere damage on simple reaction time. *Cortex, 23,* 285–292.

Tassinari, G., Alioti, S., Chelazzi, L., Marzi, C., & Berlucchi, G. (1987). Distribution in the visual field of the costs of voluntary allocated attention and of the inhibitory after-effects of covert orienting. *Neuropsychologia, 25,* 55–71.

Taylor, J. (1958). *Selected writings of John Hughlings Jackson.* New York: Basic Books.

Terrell, B., & Ripich, D. (1980). Discourse competence as a variable in intervention. *Seminars in Speech and Language: Aphasia and Pragmatics, 10,* 282–297.

Tham, K., & Tegner, R. (1996). The baking tray task: A test of spatial neglect. *Neuropsychological Rehabilitation, 6,* 19–25.

Tompkins, C. A. (1990). Knowledge and strategies for processing lexical metaphor after right or left hemisphere brain damage. *Journal of Speech and Hearing Research, 33,* 307–316.

Tompkins, C. A. (1991). Automatic and effortful processing of emotional intonation after right or left hemisphere brain damage. *Journal of Speech and Hearing Research, 34,* 820–830.

Tompkins, C. A. (1995). *Right hemisphere communication disorders: Theory and Management.* San Diego: Singular Publishing Group.

Tompkins, C. A., & Baumgaertner, A. (1998). Clinical value of online measures for adults with right hemisphere brain damage. *American Journal of Speech-Language Pathology, 7,* 68–74.

Tompkins, C. A., Baumgaertner, A., Lehman, M. T., & Fossett, T. R. D. (1997). Suppression and discourse comprehension in right brain-damaged adults: A preliminary report. *Aphasiology, 11,* 505–520.

Tompkins, C. A., Bloise, C. G. R., Timko, M. L., & Baumgaertner, A. (1994). Working memory and inference revision in brain-damaged and normally aging adults. *Journal of Speech and Hearing Research, 37,* 896–912.

Tompkins, C. A., Boada, R., & McGarry, K. (1992). The access and processing of familiar idioms by brain-damaged and normally aging adults. *Journal of Speech and Hearing Research, 35,* 626–637.

Tompkins, C. A., Boada, R., McGarry, K., Jones, J., Rahn, A. E., & Ranier, S. (1993). Connected speech characteristics of right-hemisphere damaged adults: A re-examination. *Clinical Aphasiology, 21,* 113–122.

Tompkins, C. A., & Flowers, C. (1985). Perception of emotional intonation by brain-damaged adults: The influence of task processing levels. *Journal of Speech and Hearing Research, 28,* 527–538.

Tompkins, C. A., Lehman, M. T., Baumgaertner, A., Fossett, T. R. D., & Vance, J. E. (1996). Suppression and discourse comprehension in right brain-damaged adults: Inferential ambiguity processing. *Brain and Language, 55,* 172–175.

Triesman, A. M. (1988). Features and objects: The fourteenth Bartlett memorial lecture. *Quarterly Journal of Experimental Psychology, 40A,* 201–237.

Treisman, A. M., & Gelade, G. (1980). A feature integration theory of attention. *Cognitive Psychology, 12,* 97–136.

Trupe, E., & Hillis, A. (1985). Paucity vs. verbosity: Another analysis of right hemisphere communication deficits. *Clinical Aphasiology, 15,* 83–92.

Tucker, D. M. (1981). Lateral brain function, emotion, and conceptualization. *Psychological Bulletin, 89,* 19–46.

Tucker, D. M., Watson, R. T., & Heilman, K. M. (1977). Discrimination and evocation of affectively intoned speech in patients with right parietal disease. *Neurology, 27,* 947–950.

Tucker, D. M., & Williamson, P. A. (1984). Asymmetric neural control systems in human self-regulation. *Psychological Review, 91,* 185–215.

Ulatowska, H., Allard, L., & Chapman, S. (1990). Narrative and procedural discourse in Aphasia. In Y. Joanette & H. H. Brownell (Eds.), *Discourse ability and brain damage: Theoretical and empirical perspectives* (pp. 180–198). New York: Springer-Verlag.

Uryase, D., Duffy, R. J., & Liles, B. Z. (1991). Analysis and description of narrative discourse in right-hemisphere-damaged adults: A comparison with neurologically normal and left-hemisphere-damaged aphasic adults. *Clinical Aphasiology, 19,* 125–137.

Vallar, G. (1993). The anatomical basis of spatial hemi-neglect in humans. In I. H. Robertson & J. C. Marshall (Eds.), *Unilateral neglect: Clinical and experimental studies.* Hillsdale, NJ: Lawrence Erlbaum.

Vallar, G., Bottini, G., Rusconi, L., & Sterzi, R. (1993). Exploring somatosensory hemineglect by vestibular stimulation. *Brain, 116,* 71–86.

Vallar, G., Bottini, G., Sterzi, R., Passerini, D., & Rusconi, M. L. (1991). Hemianesthesia, sensory neglect, and defective access to conscious experience. *Neurology, 41,* 650–652.

Vallar, G., Papagno, C., & Cappa, S. (1988). Latent dysphasia after left hemisphere lesions: A lexical-semantic and verbal memory deficit. *Aphasiology, 2,* 463–478.

Vallar, G., & Perani, D. (1986). The anatomy of unilateral neglect after right-hemisphere stroke lesions: A clinical/CT-scan correlation study in man. *Neuropsychologia, 24,* 609–622.

Vallar, G., Sandroni, P., Rusconi, M. L., & Barbieri, S. (1991). Hemianopia, hemianesthesia, and spatial neglect: A study with evoked potentials. *Neurology, 41,* 1918–1922.

Vallar, G., Sterzi, R., Bottini, G., Cappa, S., & Rusconi, M. L. (1990). Temporary remission of left hemianesthesia after vestibular stimulation. A sensory neglect phenomenon. *Cortex, 26,* 123–131.

Van Dijk, T. A., & Kintsch, W. (1983). *Strategies of discourse comprehension.* New York: Academic Press.

Van Lancker, D. R. (1991). Personal relevance and the human right hemisphere. *Brain and Cognition, 17,* 64–92.

Van Lancker, D. R., & Kempler, D. (1987). Comprehension of familiar phrases by left- but

not by right-hemisphere damaged patients. *Brain and Language, 32,* 265–277.

Van Lancker, D. R., & Klein, K. (1990). Preserved recognition of familiar personal names in global aphasia. *Brain and Language, 39,* 511–529.

Van Lancker, D., & Sidtis, J. J. (1992). The identification of affective-prosodic stimuli by left- and right-hemisphere damaged subjects: All errors are not created equal. *Journal of Speech and Hearing Research, 35,* 963–970.

Van Lancker, D., & Sidtis, J. J. (1993). Brain damage and prosodic errors reconsidered: Reply to Heilman [Letter to the Editor]. *Journal of Speech and Hearing Research, 36,* 1191–1192.

Volpe, B. T., Le Doux, J. E., & Gazzaniga, M. S. (1979). Information processing of visual stimuli in an "extinguished" field. *Nature, 282,* 722–724.

Wade, D. T., Legh-Smith, J., & Hewer, R. L. (1987). Depressed mood after stroke: A community study of its frequency. *British Journal of Psychiatry, 151,* 200–205.

Walker, B. B., & Sandman, C. A. (1979). Human visual evoked responses are related to heart rate. *Journal of Comparative and Physiological Psychology, 93,* 717–729.

Wallace, G. L., & Canter, G. J. (1985). Effects of personally relevant language materials on the performance of severely aphasic individuals. *Journal of Speech and Hearing Disorders, 50,* 385–390.

Wapner, W., & Gardner, H. (1979). A note on patterns of comprehension and recovery in global aphasia. *Journal of Speech and Hearing Research, 29,* 765–772.

Wapner, W., Hampy, S., & Gardner, H. (1981). The role of the right hemisphere in the appreciation of complex linguistic materials. *Brain and Language, 14,* 15–33.

Warrington, E. K., & McCarthy, R. A. (1987). Categories of knowledge: Further fractionations and an attempted integration. *Brain, 110,* 1273–1296.

Watabe, K., Nakai, K., & Kasamatsu, T. (1982). Visual afferents to norepinephrine-containing neurons in cat locus coeruleus. *Experimental Brain Research, 48,* 66–80.

Watson, R. T., & Heilman, K. M. (1979). Thalamic neglect. *Neurology, 29,* 690–694.

Watson, R. T., Miller, B. D., & Heilman, K. M. (1978). Nonsensory neglect. *Annals of Neurology, 3,* 505–508.

Watson, R. T., Valenstein, E., Day, A. L., & Heilman, K. M. (1984). The effect of corpus callosum lesions on unilateral neglect in monkeys. *Neurology, 34,* 812–815.

Watson, R. T., Valenstein, E., & Heilman, K. M. (1981). Thalamic neglect. *Archives of Neurology, 38,* 501–506.

Wechsler, A. (1973). The effect of organic brain disease on recall of emotionally charged versus neutral narrative texts. *Neurology, 73,* 130–135.

Weinberg, J., Diller, L., Gerstman, I., & Schulman, P. (1972). Digit span in right and left hemiplegics. *Journal of Clinical Psychology, 28,* 361.

Weinberg, J., Diller, L., Gordon, W. A., Gerstman, L. J., Lieberman, A., Lakin, P., Hodges, G., & Ezarchi, O. (1976). Visual scanning training effect on reading-related tasks in acquired right brain damage. *Archives of Physical Medicine Rehabilitation, 58,* 479–486.

Weinberg, J., Diller, L., Gordon, W. A., Gerstman, L. J., Lieberman, A., Lakin, P., Hodges, G., & Ezrachi, O. (1979). Training sensory awareness and spatial organization in people with right brain damage. *Archives of Physical Medicine and Rehabilitation, 60,* 491–496.

Weinman, E., & Ruskin, P. E. (1994). Anger attacks in poststroke depression: Response to fluoxetine [Letter to the Editor]. *American Journal of Psychiatry, 151,* 1839.

Weintraub, S., & Mesulam, M. -M. (1985). *Verbal and Nonverbal Cancellation Test.* Philadelphia: F. A. Davis.

Weintraub, S., & Mesulam, M. -M. (1987). Right cerebral dominance in spatial attention: Further evidence based on ipsilateral neglect. *Archives of Neurology, 44,* 621–625.

Weintraub, S., & Mesulam, M. -M. (1988). Visual hemispatial inattention: Stimulus parameters and exploratory strategies. *Journal of Neurology, Neurosurgery, and Psychiatry, 51,* 1481–1488.

Weintraub, S., Mesulam, M. -M., & Kramer, L. (1981). Disturbances in prosody: A right hemisphere contribution to language. *Archives of Neurology, 38,* 742–744.

Weisenburg, T. H., & McBride, K. E. (1935). *Aphasia.* New York: Commonwealth Fund.

Werth, R. (1993). Shifts and omissions in spatial reference in unilateral neglect. In I. H. Robertson & J. C. Marshall (Eds.), *Unilateral neglect: Clinical and experimental studies* (pp. 211–231). Hillsdale, NJ: Lawrence Erlbaum.

Weylman, S. T., Brownell, H. H., Roman, M., & Gardner, H. (1989). Appreciation of indirect requests by left- and right-brain damaged patients: The effects of verbal context and conventionality of wording. *Brain and Language, 36,* 580–591.

Whitehead, R. (1991). Right hemisphere processing superiority during sustained visual attention. *Journal of Cognitive Neuroscience, 3,* 329–334.

Whyte, J. (1992). Neurologic disorders of attention and arousal: Assessment and treatment. *Archives of Physical Medicine Rehabilitation, 73,* 1094–1103.

Wilkins, A. J., Shallice, T., & McCarthy, R. (1987). Frontal lesions and sustained Attention. *Neuropsychologia, 25,* 359–365.

Willanger, R., Danielsen, U. T., & Ankerhus, J. (1981). Visual neglect in right-sided apoplectic lesions. *Acta neurologica Scandinavica, 64,* 327–336.

Wilson, B. A., Cockburn, J., & Halligan, P. (1987). *Behavioral Inattention Test.* Suffolk, England: Thames Valley Test Company.

Winner, E., Brownell, H. H., Happe, F., Blum, A., & Pincus, D. (in press). Distinguishing lies from jokes: Theory of mind deficits and discourse interpretation in right hemisphere brain-damaged patients. *Brain and Language.*

Wood, R. L. (1986). Rehabilitation of patients with disorders of attention. *Journal of head trauma rehabilitation, 1,* 43–53.

Winner, E., & Gardner, H. (1977). The comprehension of metaphor in brain-damaged patients. *Brain, 100,* 719–727.

Yokoyama, K., Jennings, R., Ackles, P., Hood, B. S., & Boller, F. (1987). Lack of heart rate changes during an attention-demanding task after right hemisphere lesions. *Neurology, 37,* 624–630.

Yorkston, K., & Buekelman, D. (1977). A system for quantifying verbal output of high-level aphasic patients. *Clinical Aphasiology: Conference Proceedings* (pp. 175–179). Minneapolis: BRK Publishers.

Young, A. W., Newcombe, F., & Ellis, A. W. (1991). Different impairments contribute to neglect dyslexia. *Cognitive Neuropsychology, 8,* 177–191.

Zaidel, E. (1983). A response to Gazzaniga: Language in the right hemisphere, convergent perspectives. *American Psychologist, May,* 542–546.

Zaidel, E. (1985). Language in the right hemisphere. In D. F. Benson & E. Zaidel (Eds.), *The dual brain* (pp. 205–231). New York: Guilford Press.

Zarit, S. H., & Kahn, R. L. (1974). Impairment and adaptation in chronic disabilities: Spatial inattention. *Journal of Nervous and Mental Disease, 159,* 63–72.

Zihl, J. (1989). Cerebral disturbances of elementary visual function. In J. W. Brown (Ed.), *Neuropsychology of visual perception* (pp. 35–58). Hillsdale, NJ: Lawrence Erlbaum.

Zoccolotti, P., Antonucci, G., Judica, A., Montenero, P., Pizzamiglio, L. & Razzano, C. (1989). Incidence and evolution of the hemineglect disorder in chronic patients with unilateral right brain damage. *International Journal of Neuroscience, 47,* 209–216.

Zoccolotti, P., Scabini, D., & Violani, C. (1982). Electrodermal responses in patients with unilateral brain damage. *Journal of Clinical Neuropsychology, 4,* 143–150.

Index